JUST EAT IT

—

How Intuitive Eating
Can Help You Get Your Shit Together Around Food

Laura Thomas, PhD, RNutr is a Registered Nutritionist who isn't afraid to say it like it is. Having had her own strained and weird relationship with food, she now helps her clients build healthy attitudes to food by helping them tune in to their own innate hunger and satiety cues and disconnect from diet tools like meal plans and calorie trackers using a process called Intuitive Eating and other non-diet approaches.

In 2016 Laura launched *Don't Salt My Game* – a podcast that calls out diet trends and myths, and tells what you really need to know to stay on top of your game. Laura was the Nutrition Consultant for the BBC1 documentary *Mind Over Marathon* where she supported people suffering with mental-health problems train for the 2017 London Marathon. She makes regular media appearances and has appeared on *BBC Global News*, BBC News Facebook Live stream and *Channel 5 News*. She has written for *Hip and Healthy*, *Huffington Post*, *New Scientist* and *Spectator Health*, and she provides comment for publications such as *Men's Health*, the *Guardian*, *The Pool*, and *Red Magazine*. She is currently studying for a Master of Science in Eating Disorders and Clinical Nutrition at University College London.

JUST EAT IT

HOW INTUITIVE EATING CAN HELP YOU GET YOUR SHIT TOGETHER AROUND FOOD

———

Laura Thomas, PhD, RNutr

bluebird
books for life

First published 2019 by Bluebird
an imprint of Pan Macmillan
Pan Macmillan, 20 New Wharf Road, London N1 9RR

Associated companies throughout the world
www.panmacmillan.com

ISBN 978-1-5098-9391-1

Visit **www.panmacmillan.com** to read more about all our books
and to buy them. You will also find features, author interviews and
news of any author events, and you can sign up for e-newsletters
so that you're always first to hear about our new releases.

CONTENTS

INTRODUCTION

—

What do you want to eat? Close your eyes for a second and just let that question sit with you. What did you pick out? Is it something that you usually eat? Is it something you have rules around? Is it something on your food shit list? You know that place that all 'bad' foods get relegated to, apart from at Christmas time when you're in full 'fuck-it' mode and they get a free pass but go straight back in the 'Things I Don't Eat' category on 1 January.

When was the last time you even asked yourself what you'd like instead of what you 'can' or 'should' eat?

I work with people like this, every day. People who spend 90% of their day worrying about what to eat. People who have spent an egregious amount of time thinking about if their fruit salad was too high in sugar, or anxious about whether Paleo or plant-based is better. People who conceive elaborate rules about what, when, and how much to eat. People who need a PhD in maths to figure out how much they have to work out in order to 'earn' a cookie based on what they've already eaten that day, and how much carbs and protein are in their other meals. People who have dedicated enormous amounts of time, money, energy and other precious resources to solving the problem of what to eat. People who are fearful and anxious about feeding their bodies. People who don't know how to understand and interpret their hunger and fullness cues and don't trust themselves around food. People who hate their bodies with the fire of a thousand suns. People who punish their bodies with extreme exercise and deploy elaborate systems of hunger avoidance (Diet Coke, anyone?). People who feel guilty for feeding their bodies. An essential and fundamental require-ment for living has become so fraught and stressful that we delegate the responsibility to an app on our phones. WE TRUST OUR PHONES MORE THAN WE TRUST OUR BODIES.

This shit is exhausting.

I know because I have been this person. Despite having a PhD in nutritional sciences, I have experienced being in a weird, strained, and troubled relationship with food: calorie-tracking, juice-cleanses, gluten-free-plant-based-no-oil-whole-foods-'eighty-ten-ten'. Check. Check. And check. I even went through a raw vegan phase (I shit you not). Compulsive exercise, only allowing myself to eat half a plate of food, or chewing gum and downing glasses of water to silence hunger – you name it, I've been there. In fact, I'd go so far as to say, the more I learned about nutrition, the weirder it got.

I have two degrees in nutrition. I've done research at an Ivy League university. I read scientific journals for fun. But I still had a really messed-up relationship with food.

I'm not telling you this for sympathy or pity, or because I've come out the other end and have all the secrets and answers; I'm telling you so that you know I've been there too. I get it. I'm laying all my shit out on the table, because at no point in this book do I ever want anyone to feel shamed or judged; so many of us have problems with food, but rarely do we talk about it.

Having an education in nutritional sciences doesn't immunize you against being weird around food. In fact, often the more you know, the worse you get. Studies have shown than nutritionists and dietitians have the highest incidence of orthorexia and rigid eating. I mean, no shit, right? More on that in a second, let's get back to my sob story first.

Having had a pretty turbulent childhood – divorce and moving and more divorce and new schools – food was a constant in my life. It's no wonder that I became a chubby kid. Food was comfort, food was soothing.

But because kids are dicks I soon got nicknames like Thunder Thighs, and was subject to constant, relentless, teasing at school, especially from boys. This just made me sadder, and hungrier, and I used food to deal with difficult emotions. One summer, when I was around thirteen or fourteen, I went to Summer Camp in America. I loved it. I made friends, got a tan, played, swam, and did fun kid stuff. When I went back to school that fall, it felt like the whole school was talking about my summer at 'fat camp'. It wasn't a fat camp, I was drinking 'real' Coke and eating peanut butter and jelly sandwiches all summer. But I was also more active than usual and actually had fun playing games and dancing, and doing kid shit away from the school bullies. It was also 40°C and we walked for miles a day back and forth to the Fillin' Station (seriously) on the other side of camp. I inevitably lost a few pounds, but, unsurprisingly, put it straight back on when I got home.

Layer on well-meaning but painful comments from parents and family ('can't you just have a piece of fruit or some chewing gum?', 'your skirt is riding up at the back, you're too big for it', 'it's just puppy fat, she'll grow out of it') plus dieting talk all around me, messages that fat was bad, and a tall, athletic brother, and what do you get? A recipe for food fucked-upness.

At around sixteen I started restricting what I ate, and intentionally got very active. I lost a lot of weight. My new thinness was congratulated and reinforced. Boys were suddenly interested (the same ones who had called me Thunder Thighs).

This carried on through university, but my eating got weirder. I started reading books on nutrition; not academic texts, which would have been great, but fear-mongering, spirulina-peddling-type books. I told you I was laying out all my shit. Now, instead of just limiting how much I ate, I started cutting out more and more food groups until I was left with a salad and some tofu. This coincidentally was around the time I decided to go vegan, which was largely due to ethical reasons, but I also got it in my head that milk caused breast cancer (it doesn't), so then there was nothing left to eat.[1] This restriction would almost inevitably lead to me sneaking out to get a Dairy Milk hit like a chocolate junkie. As we'll learn, deprivation often leads to bingeing. Fortunately, I snapped out of that phase pretty quickly; tofu salads don't have anything on cold pizza on a drunken walk home with friends after a night out.

But when shit hit the fan in my final year of uni, I gained a lot of weight. Stress eating was my thing. A few months later I moved to the US to do my PhD and this, combined with not walking anywhere and comfort eating (in Texas, anyone from not-Texas is super foreign and it took a while to make friends), meant I was the biggest I'd ever been and I hated myself deeply.

The binge/restrict cycle went on all through my PhD (remember I was studying nutrition, what the hell was I thinking?). Break-ups? Didn't eat. PhD exam stress? Ate too much. New cities and new jobs meant fluctuations in my weight. I hated my body, I hated tracking everything I was eating only to ultimately faceplant into a jar of peanut butter at night. Remember, this is all confounded by being around nutrition and dietetics students who on the surface of things have it all figured out, but many of whom were also struggling. Calorie-counting, portion control, food rules and a vendetta on bad carbs are not only normal, that's literally what we're taught and many of us dutifully played the part. Underneath it all though, the struggle was so real.

Good thing then that I came across the concepts of Intuitive Eating, and the anti-diet movement. At first I was sceptical but after doing some research I was like 'holy shit, this is genius'. I started reading blogs, books, and published research, and over time I began to chill. I started eating what I wanted, when I was hungry (wow, eating when you're hungry; revolutionary, but you'd be surprised at how many people straight up ignore it), I exercised because it felt good, not because I needed to burn off my food. I stopped seeing food as a problem. My weight stabilized. OK, I wasn't a size 8, but after years of restriction and over-eating, and beating myself up, this felt good. I didn't have to micro-manage what I was eating, and it gave me the time and energy to do more interesting and important things.

Look, I don't want this book to be all about me. It's not about me; it's about helping you feel less weird around food. But I just need you to know that I know what it's like to be in that place where your life revolves around food and weight and being hungry, and eating thirty rice crackers to try and fill yourself up.

And this isn't everyone's experience of studying nutrition, of course. I have a bunch of friends from my nutrition programmes who have a totally uncomplicated relationship with food. But I'd say they're in the minority. I remember going out to lunch with some faculty to a Mexican restaurant while I was working on my PhD; their salsa and guac were next level. But instead of getting down with the house nachos chips, one faculty member was so careful about her eating that she brought along her own rice crackers to dip in the salsa (no guac, duh). At the time I remember thinking, 'huh, that's weird'. I had my own shit going on though, so it didn't really occur to me how messed up that was until way later. When we consider that this was the behaviour of someone influencing and educating cohort after cohort of nutrition and dietetics students, hundreds or even thousands of future dietitians and nutritionists, it's a pretty scary thought, and an indictment on our attitudes towards health and nutrition.

In a sample of 2,500 Registered Dietitians in the US, 12.9% were found to be at risk for an eating disorder, and almost 50% were at risk for orthorexia nervosa, a mental illness that manifests as an unhealthy obsession with healthy eating, to the point where it has serious physical ramifications. Nutrition students have been shown to have a twofold risk of eating disorders compared to students in other disciplines like biology. It's not clear if studying nutrition *causes* disordered eating, or whether people with eating problems are drawn towards these courses to sort out their issues. A third possibility is that people with disordered eating are attracted to nutrition as a way of legitimizing their behaviours; some preliminary research suggests that students are attracted to dietetics because of a pre-existing interest in food and nutrition that may become more restrictive during their degrees. However, research is ongoing to try and get answers to these questions.

It's not just nutrition and dietetics students who are at risk of having problems with food, though; it's estimated that 45.5% of medical professionals exhibited symptoms of orthorexia[2] and in a small study of Ashtanga yoga teachers, 86% were found to have symptoms consistent with orthorexia, particularly in yogis who were vegetarian.[3] Male students enrolled in sports science courses have been shown to have a ten-times greater risk of muscle dysmorphia (a type of body dysmorphia characterized by thinking that one isn't sufficiently muscled, and a compulsion to exercise) than the general student body. And while we don't have much information about the general population, bodybuilders and weightlifters are another group at risk of muscle dysmorphia.[4]

I have provided red flags for eating disorders in the resources section, but for now I want to talk about eating problems more generally. I want to differentiate between clinical eating disorders, which have diagnostic criteria and which, although being incredibly serious, are thankfully relatively rare in the population, in contrast to disordered eating, which is common. *Too* common.

THE CONTINUUM OF EATING

Our eating behaviours lie on a continuum between intuitive eating and clinical eating disorders. We'll talk more specifically about what intuitive eating really means in a second, but for now, let's define it as just regular eating without any hang-ups. We all have a different 'normal', so it looks slightly different on everyone. Having said that, in general it means:

- not having food rules
- not excluding things from your diet (unless you have an allergy/ethical/religious reason)
- not feeling stressed or anxious about food
- not feeling guilty about eating cakes or crisps or other foods you enjoy
- having flexibility in your eating
- enjoying food
- tuning in to your hunger and fullness signals (most of the time)
- eating foods that make you feel energized and well (most of the time)

Intuitive Eating	Disordered Eating	Clinical Eating Disorders

When I started my clinical practice, I noticed that a lot of my clients were eating balanced and nutritious foods, but that their relationship with food was disordered. They had been chronic dieters or had sub-clinical disordered eating. They had arbitrary rules and restrictions and were caught in a pattern of binge/restrict, binge/restrict. When clients first come to see me, they sit towards the middle-right of the chart on the previous page; my goal with them is to get them to have more days towards the left, and fewer days towards the right. Take a moment to think about where you sit. How would it feel to have more days where food feels uncomplicated and you can eat without feeling stressed about food? Sounds pretty good, right?

DISORDERED EATING

—

Let's take a look at what we mean by disordered eating. Here's the academic definition:

> Disordered Eating describes abnormal eating behaviours that may include skipping meals, binge eating, restricting certain food types, or fasting. These eating patterns are deviations from the cultural standard of three meals a day, which is often found in Western cultures. Disordered Eating indicates any deviation from these cultural norms, including food restriction, skipping meals and over-eating. These deviations from cultural norms may be related to later development of an eating disorder but they do not necessarily indicate that an eating disorder is present.[5]

Yeah . . . that's pretty vague, and while this definition is helpful, I also think it's limited because it only talks about *behaviours*. But we know that eating isn't purely a physical experience; it's an emotional one too. Therefore, I propose we add an emotional dimension to this definition that includes:

disordered eating behaviours that may include skipping meals, binge eating, restricting certain food types, or fasting, which represent a deviation from the cultural norm, accompanied by a sense of shame, guilt, or anxiety, or other negative mood state in relation to eating food.

Essentially, what I'm concerned about is whether you feel distressed about eating. So, raise your hand if you currently have, or have ever had disordered eating. *All raise hands*. Yup. Disordered eating is the norm in Western society. Robust estimates of disordered eating are hard to come by, but it's thought to affect between 50% and 75% of women.[6,7] Whichever way you slice it, that's an enormous number of people. Think of your three closest friends. According to these statistics, between two and three of you have a level of disordered eating. In a sample of over 1,600 adolescents, 61% of females and 28% of males reported disordered eating behaviours (e.g., fasting or skipping meals, consuming very little food, smoking cigarettes to lose weight).[8] And in a more recent study of adolescents in the UK from 2018, amongst the fourteen-year-old sample surveyed, 17.9% had significant concerns about their shape and weight, and in the sixteen-year-old sample, 40.7% had some form of disordered eating behaviour (fasting, purging, or binge eating), 11.3% of those were concordant with an eating disorder diagnostic criteria.[9] If over 40% of adolescents have disordered eating behaviours, do we for a second believe that number doesn't gain compound interest as women get older, their bodies change, they join the workforce, have babies, get diseases and injuries, and cycle through diet, after diet, after diet, leaving us even more screwed up about food, exercise, and body image?

Most weight-loss diets are, by definition, disordered eating – whether it's Weight Watchers, intermittent fasting, the alkaline diet, or keto. I don't think that comes as a huge surprise to anyone. And 35% of 'normal' dieters progress to pathological dieting. Of those, 20–25% progress to partial or full-syndrome eating disorders.[10] What's perhaps even more problematic, because it's so insidious and normalized, is the list of arbitrary food rules we build up in our heads, even when we're not on an official diet, that still make us stressed about food. The tips we pick up from women's magazines, the remnants of diets past, weird shit our mums said to us when we were kids, plus the advent of calorie- and movement-tracking apps that take us away from the internal regulation of our eating. Or maybe it's just restricting certain food groups you perceive to be 'bad', either being fully on or spectacularly falling off the bandwagon, or simply going to bed every night promising yourself that 'tomorrow I will be good'. All of these things can make us feel weird about food and can easily manifest as disordered eating or emotional distress around food or body image.

I want to be careful and thoughtful here though. I don't want to suggest that just because you sometimes sleep past breakfast on the weekend, or because you're not a big fan of chicken, that you have disordered eating. Although my clinical experience teaches me that disordered eating is common, I don't want to suggest problems that don't exist. It's important to take individual lived experiences into consideration here too. In other words, what I'm interested in is whether food and eating are causing you problems, or whether you're just kind of fussy. If you are engaging in disordered eating behaviours and they are causing you emotional distress, that's when the real problems begin. If you've ever felt kind of weird or freaky around food, then this book is intended for you.

Not only is disordered eating incredibly common, but it has been so deeply ingrained in us, that we think it's normal. In fact, for some of you reading now, this might be the first time it's occurring to you how much time and energy you've been devoting to this stuff. That realization, in and of itself, can feel pretty intense. But don't worry, I've got you! The framework I use with my clients who have lost their way with food and eating is called intuitive eating. It's a systematic approach to deconstructing food rules, wiping out food worry and anxiety, and gently relearning how to eat, from the ground up, using your own internal signals of hunger, fullness, pleasure, satisfaction, stamina, and a sense of well-being. In these pages I'll share with you my approach to intuitive eating. However, it's not intended to be a rigid or prescriptive plan. These are guidelines for helping you figure out a way of relating to food that feels right for you. In fact, by the end of the book, I actually hope you'll think a lot less about food. Of course, food plays a really important role in our lives, but it shouldn't be all-consuming, and it shouldn't be the least bit distressing.

And even if you've been protected from our society's weird obsession with dieting, and you've never had body-image issues or a funky relationship with food (you lucky thing, you), this book can still help you approach food and nutrition in a way that won't totally mess you up.

HOW IT'S GOING TO GO DOWN

I figured that it's helpful for you to have a sense of where we're going with this; I've structured the book much like I would when working through these concepts with a client. Although the concepts all bleed together and overlap when I'm going through them with clients, I've tried to present them in a way that makes the most sense. We'll begin by unsubscribing from diet culture, then develop some self-compassion; something that will be critical in allowing the process to run its course while allowing you to remain curious instead of beating yourself up for not doing it 'right' – remember that intuitive eating will look slightly different on everyone. We'll then spend some time working on body image before I teach you how to tune in to sensations of hunger; sounds easy, but it's perhaps not as simple as you think. After that, we'll work on developing unconditional permission to eat via the process of food neutrality. We'll explore mindful eating and reconnecting with the pleasure in food. We'll discuss how to find your fullness level and how to build your emotional coping toolkit so that food isn't the only thing in there. Finally, we'll talk about intuitive, joyful movement and gentle nutrition – how to apply nutrition information without turning it into another rigid set of rules. Before we get to the nuts and bolts though, I'll discuss some of the reasons why we become disconnected from our innate ability to feed ourselves in the first place.

I'm conscious of this becoming another 'this worked for me, so it will work for you too' book. I'm not promising you the earth. For a lot of the people I work with, intuitive eating and non-diet approaches aren't miracle cures; they're tools to help you get your shit together around food. Whatever that looks like for you. Whatever that means to you. There are parts of this book that will resonate with you, there are parts that won't. I'm not here to tell you what to do; I'm here to help you figure out what's best for you, your body, and your health. Think of it as a collaboration. You already know so much about your body, and I can help you draw out that knowledge and apply it in a new way, backing up the rationale with nutritional science. If a tool or concept resonates with you, use it. If not, can it. My intention is that it will challenge some of the BS that has been drilled into us for generations about how we should look, eat, and behave, to give us the space and freedom to live fuller lives and be of service to our families, friends, and communities and to accomplish our own goals and dreams. What could we achieve if we weren't obsessing about food and our bodies? Could we be better friends, parents, children, partners, or volunteers? Could we get that project off the ground or take up learning a new language or skill? Intuitive eating isn't a means to an end like a diet, but a set of tools and skills to give you freedom from food and to open up the rest of your life outside of food and body worry.

KEEPING AN
INTUITIVE EATING JOURNAL

—

I know, I know, a journal, just another thing to add to the to-do list. But seriously, if you can, I want you to consider keeping a journal about your experiences with intuitive eating. I get that it's kind of a pain, so if it's easier, just start a note on your phone, but if you can, get yourself a physical notebook. Here's why: keeping a journal can help you reflect back on all the progress and changes you've made, so even when you feel like 'nothing's happening', or you're 'doing it wrong', you have something to go back to and reflect on. It can help put progress and changes into perspective (and we'll discuss what 'progress' looks like through a non-diet lens soon). It's a place to answer the questions and do the exercises and activities dotted throughout the book. It can also act as a place to record your thoughts, attitudes, and beliefs around food and see how they change over time.

You're going to want to split your journal into two parts.

Part 1 – exercises and activities: this is where you'll answer questions, do activities and exercises from each of the chapters in the book, and do the bulk of 'the work'. I'd recommend putting a date and title on each entry, and if it's helpful write out the question you're answering so you know what it was in reference to when you look back over it. Be as creative as you like in your journal – use coloured pens and pencils, cut-outs from magazines, redraw images from the book or write out quotes that resonate with you, add stickers, highlight things. Own it in whatever way you like and make it yours.

Part 2 – food and eating: the second part will follow more of a template that we will build on. We'll start after chapter 4 to begin to chart our hunger levels. The intention here is that you can build up a picture of hunger, fullness, satisfaction, and work on chipping away at judgements about food. It can help you connect the dots as you learn to trust your body (there are some examples below). However, if writing down your food feels a lot like keeping a food diary or tracking . . . don't do it. Just ditch it. An intuitive eating journal can be enormously positive and helpful, or it can trigger diet mentality. Please only do it if you feel like you can approach it from a place of curiosity and non-judgement. Alternatively, you could journal every now and then if that feels like a good compromise for you. Here's what it looks like. If approached with a non-diet mentality, a journal can give you clues as to why things played out the way they did (for instance, if you let yourself get too hungry or didn't eat enough in the morning, did it cause you to eat past the point of comfortable fullness in the evening?).

INTUITIVE EATING
JOURNAL

Journal Entry One

Date:
Meal: brunch
Hunger/fullness level before: 2
What I ate: avocado on sourdough toast with a poached egg
Hunger/fullness level after: 5
Feelings: tired, stressed, anxious
Notes: Really wanted the French toast but freaked out about it not being healthy enough. Left ½ of my toast as it was white sourdough, and felt this was too many carbs. Worried there wasn't enough veg, should have had a side of greens. Ended up eating really fast and feeling bloated and guilty.

Journal Entry Two

Date:
Meal: dinner
Hunger/fullness level before: 3
What I ate: beef burger with cheese on bun, side salad and sweet potato fries
Hunger/fullness level after: 7.5
Feelings: calm, tired, excited to eat
Notes: Satisfying meal; felt good. Enjoyed the food and company. Left a few fries and part of bun. Would definitely eat that again!

ARE YOU AN INTUITIVE EATER?

—

Before we go any further, it might be helpful to do a quick assessment of your own eating behaviours – take this quiz to get a sense of whether or not you're an intuitive eater. Don't worry, this isn't to freak you out, and if you get a high score it doesn't necessarily mean you have an eating disorder. It's just an indication of where you're at right now. My hope is that by working through this book your eating behaviours normalize, becoming progressively less disordered.

The following is an adaption of the Intuitive Eating Scale – 2 (IES-2) developed by Tracy Tylka, a psychologist and researcher, and her team at the Ohio State University to objectively measure intuitive eating.[11] It has been shown to be inversely associated with disordered eating, meaning the more you are an intuitive eater, the less you display symptoms of disordered eating.[12]

In this adapted version, the lower your IES-2 score, the more of an intuitive eater you are.

How many of the following do you agree with?

Unconditional permission to eat

- I try to avoid certain foods high in fat, carbs, sugar, or kcals
- I have forbidden foods that I don't let myself eat
- I get mad at myself for eating something unhealthy
- If I crave a certain food, I don't allow myself to have it
- I follow rules that dictate what/when/how much to eat

Eating for physical rather than emotional reasons

I eat when I'm feeling:

- Emotional (anxious, depressed, sad . . .)
- Lonely
- Bored
- Stressed out . . . even though I'm not physically hungry
- I use food to help me soothe negative emotions

Reliance on hunger and satiety cues

- I don't trust my body to tell me when to eat
- I don't trust my body to tell me what to eat
- I don't trust my body to tell me how much to eat

- I don't trust my body to tell me when to stop eating
- I can't tell when I'm slightly hungry
- I can't tell when I'm slightly full

Body–food choice congruence
- Most of the time, I don't want to eat nutritious foods
- I don't often eat foods that make my body perform well
- I don't often eat foods that give my body energy and stamina

For each statement you agree with, give yourself one point and calculate your total score. If you scored...

15–19 → OK, first of all, don't worry; you may have some problems with disordered eating but this isn't unusual and there are lots of things that can help you develop a healthier relationship to food. If you frequently feel overwhelmed, anxious, or unnecessarily worried about food, or are preoccupied with what you eat and your body image, you might consider seeking professional help – see the resources section at the end of the book. Ask your healthcare professional if this book is appropriate for you to use alongside any other tools or therapies they recommend.

ACTIVITY

In your journal – write out your score. In which sub-sections did you agree with most of the statements? This can help you determine which areas you might need most work in. You can refer back to this quiz periodically to check in and see how you're doing and figure out which area you may need to focus on. One little note though: sometimes your score can go up initially; don't worry about this – it's not unusual for this to happen. It's also important not to get caught up on this number – it can be a nice way to measure progress, but I rarely work with people who get a 'perfect' score, and that's not really the objective here. The point in going through the intuitive eating process is to help you get your shit together.

10–14 → Food rules dictate a large portion of your eating behaviour; you might feel stressed out about what, when, and how much to eat a lot of the time, or be reliant on apps, calorie trackers, rules, and meal or diet plans to guide your eating. This book will give you the tools and confidence to move away from disordered eating towards intuitive eating.

5–9 → You may not be on an official diet, but there may still be some areas that you want to work on to help you become more in tune with your body.

0–4 → You're in a pretty good place with food! You may have a few small areas to work on to make sure you are 100% solid in your relationship to food, but overall, you're doing great.

A FEW TIPS BEFORE WE GET STARTED

Before we get started, I want to share a few tips to help make the process easier. It's worth writing these out in your journal to refer back to as a reminder in case of a wobble.

1 Set nutrition to the side for the short term – I realize this sounds totally bizarre coming from a Registered Nutritionist, but trust me on this. Putting nutrition on the bench in the short term allows you to make food choices based on preference and satisfaction rather than on what you think you know about nutrition. It allows you to explore how different foods make you feel and to be curious about what you eat, rather than feeling guilty for eating less than perfectly. Focusing on nutrition too early undermines the IE process. Setting nutrition aside in the short term won't affect long-term health!

2 Stick a pin in the idea of weight loss – many of you will pick up this book with a sense that it will help you lose weight, and that's OK. There's a lot of pressure on people to lose weight, so I totally understand this. But, I invite you to set that goal aside for the time being, you can always return to diets and weight loss down the line if that's something you still want to pursue. But intuitive eating is not about dieting or weight loss – if you are making food choices based on achieving a goal weight, then it's all too easy to turn IE into 'the hunger and fullness diet'. This comes with an omnipresent threat of restriction and deprivation that can drive the scarcity mindset – a feeling that you can have the rug pulled out from underneath you at any second and be forced back to restrictive dieting. I'll give you specific tools for body acceptance and ditching the diet mentality soon, but for now, just let the idea sit with you. Besides, dieting and the pursuit of weight loss are usually part of the reason we have a screwed-up relationship to food in the first place, so it's unlikely to be the way out! Think about it; the things that break us cannot heal us.

3 Be kind to yourself – we will talk a lot about self-compassion, but it's worth reiterating that this stuff is hard, for many of us we are undoing years and years of conditioning. Beating yourself up when things don't feel like plain sailing will only make it harder. Go easy, be gentle. It will help you cultivate a sense of curiosity instead of perfectionism.

4 Be patient – IE is an iterative process and it's not perfect. In fact, it's really messy, nuanced, and there are loads of caveats. There's no prize for rushing to the end, so take your time. There's a lot of deprogramming and relearning that needs to be done – the more you try and rush through the process without it running its course, the more likely you are to feel bananas. Slow down, take your time, and try and enjoy the process. Just because you have decided you're ready to give up diets and give yourself unconditional permission to eat, doesn't mean you'll automatically become an intuitive eater; if you try and race to the end without putting in the work, it will bite you in the butt!

5 No mistakes – only learning opportunities. In IE there are no mistakes, fuck-ups, or failures, only learning opportunities. Clients always tell me that they've 'screwed up' or that they're failing. You can see how this sounds a lot like being mean to yourself. Instead of berating yourself, ask what you can learn from this experience, what information is it giving me?

And just so you know, although in the long term the goal is to think a lot less about food, exercise, and your body, in the short term you might feel hyper-focused. This is totally normal, and will eventually subside (how long it takes somewhat depends on how long you've had a complicated relationship with food), but if at any point it ever feels like too much, don't be afraid to reach out for help. Talk to a therapist or a Registered Nutritionist or Dietitian who specializes in intuitive eating.

ONE MORE NOTE: WHO IS THIS BOOK FOR?

I am writing from my perspective as a cis-het, straight-sized, able-bodied white woman; that's my experience, and I can't claim to know other experiences. I am aware of, and care deeply about, the experiences of and issues around food, body image, and self-acceptance faced by marginalized groups and communities, and I don't want to imply for a second that these issues do not deserve attention, they absolutely do. But because those are not my experiences, I cannot, and wouldn't want to, speak for those groups. I do, however, want to make it clear that absolutely everyone is welcome here, unconditionally. If there is something here for you, please take it. I want to add too that the concept of intuitive eating and intuitive movement are inherently ableist, directed at those of us who are neurotypical; please adapt concepts where you can, and disregard ones that don't apply or are not useful to you (working with an Intuitive Eating specialist, Registered Nutritionist or Registered Dietitian can help circum-navigate some of these problems). This book is aimed at women with eating problems, as they have historically been at the receiving end of diet culture and patriarchal oppression, but I recognize that they are not the only group who have suffered, and that problem is compounded by intersecting identities. Please know that I'm constantly learning and evolving my approach to be more inclusive. I also acknowledge the privilege tied up in my body, my socio-economic position and my education. My intention here is to leverage it into helping empower people to throw off the constraints of diet culture, so we can focus on the real issues of justice and equality.

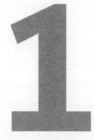

WHY IS OUR RELATIONSHIP WITH FOOD SO MESSED UP IN THE FIRST PLACE?

—

The reasons our relationship with food becomes messy and complicated aren't straightforward. Body dissatisfaction, diet rules that get lodged in our heads, being on the receiving end of body shaming or weight-related teasing, genetic factors, trauma and abuse, and our personality types can all lead to disordered eating, and in extreme cases to eating disorders. But all of these individual variables are compounded by a society that prizes thinness and reinforces a narrow standard of beauty: diet culture.

There has been constant, relentless scrutiny on our bodies since the advent of media and advertising, but in the age of social media, where we are bombarded with images of 'perfect' bodies and adverts for skinny teas and waist-trainers, this pressure has reached a critical mass. Here's the thing though, in a world where 'diet' has become such a dirty word that even Weight Watchers have dropped it, pursuit of weight loss has become passé and people have ditched diets in favour of the more rarefied and esoteric (read: trendy) 'lifestyle' movements like clean eating, wellness and even veganism. In an attempt to distance ourselves from overt dieting, we have developed new, creative ways to engage in disordered eating behaviours. These trends have provided us with a socially acceptable way to micro-manage food intake and manipulate our bodies into conforming to a standard that is unrealistic for most.

On the surface of it, trends like clean eating seem fairly innocuous and many have argued if they're helping inspire people to eat more fruit and vegetables, then what's the harm? But these movements are not harmless, and as we'll see, a lot of people who got caught up in these trends are now trying to piece their relationship with food back together. And while not everyone who got on board with these trends has come out the other end with disordered eating, for so many of my clients 'wellness' has produced anything but. As a result clinicians are reporting an increase in people with orthorexia nervosa, an eating disorder characterized by an unhealthy obsession with healthy eating.[1]

Anecdotally, I see a lot of women (and some men!) who have been misled by irresponsible influencers and pseudo-nutritionists who trade in fear-mongering and peddle their #nutribollocks at the expense of people's relationship to food. We'll talk more about nutrition myths born out of the clean-eating era in chapter 7 but I know many of you will hold concerns about the purity or cleanliness of your food, so I'm sharing some information here about the characteristics of orthorexia. There is more information about other eating disorders in the resources section at the back of the book. As well as orthorexia, we're going to explore some of the socio-cultural structures that perturb our relationship to food; I don't pretend for a second that this is an exhaustive exploration, but I hope it can help you begin to piece together your own history and narrative and begin to allow yourself to heal and repair that relationship.

What is orthorexia?

Orthorexia nervosa (ON) was first described in the 1990s by Steve Bratman, a US physician, and is a type of disordered eating that in some cases can morph into a full-blown eating disorder. It isn't officially recognized as an eating disorder in either the Diagnostic and Statistical Manual of Mental Disorders (DSM) or the International Classification of Diseases (ICD), but it is becoming increasingly recognized amongst nutrition professionals and eating disorder campaigners as a problematic way of eating that's associated with a lower quality of life, nutrient deficiencies and social isolation.[2,3,4,5,6] ON is defined as an unhealthy obsession with eating healthy, 'pure', or 'clean' food.[7] The term is derived from the Greek 'orthos', meaning 'correct'. The proposed diagnostic criteria for ON is listed below in two parts: **1** mental preoccupation and compulsive behaviour leading to **2** clinically significant impairments/outcomes.

There is some overlap between ON, anorexia nervosa (AN) and obsessive-compulsive disorder (OCD). Both AN and ON share traits of perfectionism, cognitive rigidity, and guilt over food transgressions, while OCD and ON share intrusive thoughts and ritualized food preparation. Whereas AN and bulimia nervosa and binge eating disorder are often concerned with quantity of food, people who suffer with ON are generally concerned with the quality of the food they eat.

The proposed criteria for ON include
CRITERION A

Obsessive focus on 'healthy' eating, as defined by a dietary theory or set of beliefs whose specific details may vary; marked by exaggerated emotional distress in relationship to food choices perceived as unhealthy; weight loss may ensue as a result of dietary choices, but this is not the primary goal. As evidenced by the following:

1 Compulsive behaviour and/or mental preoccupation regarding affirmative and restrictive dietary practices* believed by the individual to promote optimum health.**

2 Violation of self-imposed dietary rules causes exaggerated fear of disease, sense of personal impurity and/or negative physical sensations, accompanied by anxiety and shame.

3 Dietary restrictions escalate over time and may come to include elimination of entire food groups and involve progressively more frequent and/or severe 'cleanses' (partial fasts) regarded as purifying or detoxifying. This escalation commonly leads to weight loss, but the desire to lose weight is absent, hidden or subordinated to ideation about healthy eating.

CRITERION B

The compulsive behaviour and mental preoccupation becomes clinically impairing by any of the following:

1 Malnutrition, severe weight loss or other medical complications from restricted diet.

2 Intrapersonal distress or impairment of social, academic or vocational functioning secondary to beliefs or behaviours about healthy diet.

3 Positive body image, self-worth, identity and/or satisfaction excessively dependent on compliance with self-defined 'healthy' eating behaviour.

* Dietary practices may include use of concentrated 'food supplements'.
** Exercise performance and/or fit body image may be regarded as an aspect or indicator of health.

DIET CULTURE

—

Diet culture is probably the biggest culprit in terms of fucking up our relationship to food, our bodies, and ourselves. Defining diet culture is tricky; it's pervasive and ubiquitous, yet really stealthy and sneaky. It demands thinness no matter what the cost on our mental or physical health. A simple way of thinking about it is the culture that upholds the thin ideal as the standard of beauty. Sometimes it's obvious: an advert for a slimming club. Sometimes it's more insidious: an absence of body diversity in the media, a diet masquerading as a healthy 'lifestyle', even the 'war on obesity'.

I think the best way to illustrate it is with some examples of just how normalized diet culture is. I took these examples from the Women's Health UK website in May 2017 from an article about smoothies. The tagline of the piece went like this:

'Up your nutrient intake, aid your **fat loss mission** and taste some delicious blends with these healthy smoothie recipes.'

Diet culture makes it our mission, our life's work, to be thin. It keeps women in the pursuit of the thin ideal, no matter what the cost – our physical and mental health, our relationships, or the drain on our time, money and other resources. Another example:

'Yes, this healthy smoothie recipe is fairly high in calories and fat but sometimes you've earned it!'

OK, two things here: **1** FOOD IS SUPPOSED TO HAVE CALORIES. That's the whole point in food, it gives us energy and keeps us alive. The sentiment that food should have no calories is quintessential diet culture, duping and deluding us into being fearful of the very thing that keeps us alive. And **2** You never, ever, ever have to 'earn' food; it's a fundamental requirement for life. It's not contingent on how much you've worked out, or how 'good' you've been. You always deserve to eat. And finally:

'Your chocolate protein shake just got a clean and lean detox upgrade.'

We'll discuss the concept of 'clean' food later, but this begs the question, why should your smoothie be lean? IT'S A FUCKING

SMOOTHIE, not the recession budget. It's a bunch of fruits and milk blended up, but it's treated as though it will either be the making of your thin self, or your undoing. The connotation, once again, is that you should be fearful of food and of fat; an essential nutrient that serves an important biological role.

The language of diet culture is common parlance; we don't stop to question or critique the subtext, which is essentially: this is a strategy to help you achieve the thin ideal when all your problems will be solved, and you will be thin and life will be perfect. But as we'll see, this couldn't be further from the reality; diets usually fail, make us miserable, and fuck up our relationship to food, our bodies and ourselves.

In her book *Body Positive Power*, Megan Crabbe describes diet culture like this:

> It is so deeply ingrained in us that we barely even notice it's there, it's just the way things are, nothing to be questioned. Diet culture is why we hate our bodies. Not because we're hideously flawed, and not because of some unchanging truth about what it means to be beautiful, but because we have been taught to. We have been taught to hate our bodies by the culture we live in. A culture that has convinced over half of us that shrinking ourselves is a worthwhile and necessary pursuit. How diet culture has been created is simple: people realized that a lot of money can be made from teaching us that our bodies are a problem, and selling us the solution.

The problem is that we become so obsessed with reaching this arbitrary ideal that we put our lives on hold until we get 'there'. How many times have you thought, I'll wear the bikini *once* I lose weight. I'll start dating *once* I lose weight. I'll run around with the kids *once* I lose weight. I'll start living my life *once* I lose weight.

Diet culture keeps women suppressed, both financially and emotionally, by seducing them with claims that that they will be happy once they reach a certain weight. But the reality is that you can change how you feel about yourself without losing weight, whereas dieting may exacerbate body-image issues.

ACTIVITY

Diet culture forces us to compare ourselves with other people. Think back to how many times you have walked into a room, a party or a meeting or whatever, and the first thing you did was size yourself up against the other women in the room? Am I the thinnest? Most attractive? Youngest? We mentally rank ourselves relative to everyone else in the room, and as long as we're doing that, we will never consider ourselves good enough, because there will always be someone thinner, hotter, younger, and prettier. Notice the next time you do this; see if you can check yourself. Can you change the narrative in your head? Perhaps coming up with your own personal mantra might help: 'we are more than bodies' or 'our worth isn't reflected in our bodies'. Come up with two to three phrases you can whip out when you find yourself body-checking other people, and write them down in your journal – feel free to Google some ideas if you're stuck. 'Body-positive quotes' is a good starting place.

Diet culture is omnipresent; it is the predominant culture. It's the air we breathe. It's all around us. And it's not just the blatant juice fasts, detox teas, skinny coffees, and the magic 'fat blasting' pills. It's woven into the fabric of everyday life so seamlessly we barely notice it's there at all; in advertising, TV shows, movies, anti-cellulite products, diet-talk in the office, being 'good', being 'naughty', #fitspo, #cleaneating, and 'health' magazines.

Diet culture normalizes disordered eating, which in and of itself is an issue. But disordered eating can be a slippery slope to a full-blown eating disorder in people who are predisposed or at risk. Of course, not everyone who goes on a diet will develop an eating disorder, but almost everyone who has an eating disorder has been on a diet.[8,9] It's estimated that 35% of people who embark on 'normal' diets will go on to develop pathological dieting, and of those 20–25% will progress to clinical eating disorders.[10] Given the number of people who attempt dieting, this isn't inconsequential. In the same period that 'clean eating' and wellness culture were at their peak in the UK (2010–2016) hospital admissions from eating disorders doubled.[11] And in the same time frame, male hospital admission for eating disorders rose by 70%.[12] Now, we definitely can't claim cause and effect here, and these numbers may reflect growing awareness of eating disorders, but experts also acknowledge the role that unrealistic body standards play in the development of low self-esteem and eating disorders.

BLOGS AND SOCIAL MEDIA
—

We've all heard the advice to 'clean up' our social media feeds. I tell my clients to get rid of things that make them feel like garbage. Usually in one of our first sessions I'll make them whip out their phone and justify why they're following certain people or accounts. This isn't just me being nosy (although that's def part of it) but because I want to understand the type of content they're consuming every day and get real about whether it's helpful or harmful to their body image and self-esteem. When I'm looking through their feeds, I'm thinking about what proportion of the accounts they follow are devoted to health, nutrition, 'healthy' or 'clean' food, and fitness. Are they following pseudo-nutritionists without legitimate credentials who are sprouting nutribollocks that makes people fearful of food? Are there messages of punishing yourself with exercise or around 'earning' foods? Are there people pushing restrictive diets and food rules? For a lot of people, their social media feeds have disproportionate levels of fitspo or healthspo; they're not reflective of our overall interests. If you think about it, we might spend a few hours at the gym or at a yoga class every week, max, and a relatively small proportion of our days actually eating. So why are our social feeds 90% salads and people doing handstands on the beach? Where are the Rupi Kaur quotes? Where are the 'who's a good boy?' memes. Where are the intersectional feminists? Where are your favourite musicians and authors?

Comediennes? Where are the BoPo babes and the 'all bodies are good bodies' inspirational quotes? Where are your actual friends and the people whose lives you're invested in?

Following a narrow range of accounts can give the impression that you should be working out and eating açai bowls all day, every damn day. For instance, fitness trainers are notorious for posting daily workout pictures and aren't always transparent about how often they really work out. They may have taken a whole bunch of pictures and video on the same day to stockpile content that they then drip feed to their followers. This gives a distorted picture of reality and reinforces a level of exercise that is likely to be unhealthy for most. (If you're worried that you might be over exercising, check out the quiz in chapter 11.)

I'm going to get you to take a critical look at your social media feeds in a bit, but first I want to explore not only why social media can make us feel like shit, but how it can fuck up our relationship with food.

It isn't clear whether following certain social media accounts can, in and of itself, *cause* problems with food and body image, if people who are predisposed to troubled eating and poor body image are drawn to these types of accounts, or if social media triggers these behaviours in people who may have a predisposition. Either way, we know that following majority #cleaneating and #fitspo can skew our sense of 'normal'. Whereas in everyday life all kinds of foods exist, and there are a range of diverse body types, if you're following certain types of accounts on social, it's easy to believe the whole world is ripped, and they're all eating perfectly curated smoothie bowls or porridge; we don't see the cornflakes and the fry-ups, we don't see the post-partum bodies or the disabled bodies. All we see are unrealistic standards and consumerism dressed up as unrealistic aspiration.

In 2014, American researchers published one of the first studies specifically looking at the types of messages on 'healthy-living blogs' in the *International Journal of Eating Disorders*; out of blogs which had won health blogging awards in the previous year, they selected the twenty-one blogs with the most page views. They found that 86% of the bloggers were runners, and that 14% were CrossFitters. The majority of bloggers shared pictures of themselves in the 'about me' section of their blogs, and of those 57% used self-objectifying language and 57% posed their pictures in a way that appeared to make themselves look thinner than they actually are (body angled at 45 degrees, hands on hips etc); 76% of bloggers were on a diet or had recently dieted and 52% included some form of negative or guilt-inducing message about food. More than half of the blogs analysed described fat or being in a bigger body in a negative way. The authors concluded that most of the content focused on appearance, especially promoting the thin ideal (which we'll talk about soon), and disordered messages around food and nutrition. There are blogs that are devoted to promoting dysfunctional behaviours and attitudes towards food and exercise. These blogs are called 'pro-ana' (ana being short for anorexia), meaning that they detail strategies for maintaining a very low body weight, or 'thinspo' – messages that are intended to motivate or inspire people to maintain unhealthily low weights. Then there are blogs like the ones described in this study; blogs that are about healthy eating and healthy lifestyles on the surface, but are more closely related to the disordered and dysfunctional pro-ana blogs than they first appear.[13] And although lots of people might find these types of blogs inspiring or a good source of information from a regular person (i.e. not a qualified healthcare professional), they can also, by normalizing disordered eating and extremes of exercise, be potentially damaging for people who are troubled eaters. Healthy-living blogs and their accompanying social media feeds are enormously popular and influential but many of them are promoting unhealthy attitudes to food, body image, and exercise.

Let's talk about another influential trend: fitspo, short for 'fitspiration' – the hashtag was intended to help motivate people to reach their health or fitness goals, usually through exercise and dieting. At the time of writing, there are 54,798,330 photographs on Instagram tagged #fitspo. In 2016, a study published in the journal *Body Image* reviewed text and images from a total of fifty fitspiration websites and again found they promoted messages on 'appearance, eating, and exercise similar to pro-ana sites'. Of the sample of fitspo sites, 92% of websites showed images of women – a vast majority of which (98.34%) met culturally defined standards of beauty ideal (clear, blemish-free skin, straight white teeth, shiny hair) and were thin (98%). In comparison, only 10% of websites showed images of women with a 'curvy' body. Almost 50% of the websites contained pictures of women in bathing suits/bikinis and 50% contained images of women in underwear; 45% of the sample contained images of women posing to appear thinner/smaller. And finally, sexually objectifying images were found on 85% of websites. In terms of the text on websites: 33% of messages were sexually objectifying (i.e. 'one run closer to being sexy as fuck') and 93% of messages connected exercise to appearance (i.e. 'would you rather be covered in sweat at the gym or covered in clothes at the beach'). Almost half of the websites contained negative messages about fat, 20% of messages were promoting restrictive eating, and a further 26% contained guilt-inducing messages about food.

Undoubtedly, viewing these types of websites can make us feel bad about ourselves, but how does viewing #fitspo and healthy-living blogs influence our relationship to food? It's not straightforward to measure these things in a research setting, but a 2017 study set out to get a better understanding of the relationship between social media use and orthorexia symptoms among young women in the UK. They surveyed over 700 women who were active members in 'healthy food communities' on various social media platforms about their food restrictions and social media habits. They found there was a strong relationship between Instagram use and orthorexia symptoms. If the researchers were using conservative estimates of orthorexia rates, they found that 49% of their sample would have been considered as having orthorexia; if they applied the more commonly used but slightly more lenient cut-off for orthorexia, the rate shot up to 90%. However you interpret these results, it's a really troubling statistic. The authors of the paper said: 'Because Instagram is an image-based platform, users may be more likely to follow advice or imitate the diets of Instagram "celebrities" as they feel a more personal connection than they would on a text-based platform. Although often not based on scientific evidence, individuals are encouraged to cut out various food groups from their diets, potentially leading to an unbalanced diet and deficiencies. Moreover, this advice may encourage psychological problems around food.' No other platform showed this association; although Twitter users seemed to be slightly protected from orthorexia, probably because the focus is on text as opposed to images.[14]

Overall, research looking at the relationship between consuming media on the internet and body image shows it is associated with greater internalization of the thin ideal, appearance comparison, weight dissatisfaction, and drive for thinness. Over 3.2 billion new photographs are added to social media networks *every day*. That's 3.2 billion opportunities for us to compare ourselves with the idealized versions of other people. Every. Single. Day. Images where people have found the perfect light, filter, outfit, pose, make-up and hair for their selfie.[15]

I spoke with Dr Amy Slater, a Senior Research Psychologist in the Centre for Appearance Research at the University of West of England and asked her about the role that social media plays in shaping how we feel about our bodies, and how it might influence our relationship with food.

'In my research, I've been trying to look in more detail at what type of feedback young people are giving and getting on social media. We know they're often about appearance: "Oh you look so great, you look so skinny here, you look so beautiful". So even though those comments are positive I would propose that that would still have a negative influence on body image and eating. And we've found this in real life when I've asked girls to report on the types of comments that they get on their appearance; it's not only negative comments but it's also positive comments that are related to poorer outcomes. Social media is putting increased emphasis on our bodies. If people are constantly commenting on how you look, then you have to keep monitoring your body and keep performing appearance-based beauty ideals. And the quantification of the feedback is there, you know if you put something up today and you get a hundred likes and you put something up the next day and you only get twenty likes, what does that mean? Maybe you changed your hair or whatever, and now you're thinking "oh I got fewer likes, fewer comments", and you worry about what that means. To me, the dangerous part is it's constant and it's asking for evaluation on appearance; we're putting ourselves out there, asking to be evaluated, aren't we?'

The corollary of this, of course, is that our self-worth gets tangled up with how we look, and that's a very precarious foundation on which to build a relationship with yourself.

SELF(IE) OBJECTIFICATION

Basing our self-worth on other people's evaluations is one thing, but is the constant body scrutiny on social media contributing to a phenomenon where we begin to view ourselves as an observer? Does it encourage us to value our bodies in terms of how they look instead of what they can do? Abso-fucking-loutely. Self-objectification theory was developed in the nineties and posits that 'in American Culture, girls and women tend to see themselves through a veil of sexism, measuring their self-worth by evaluating their physical appearance against our culture's sexually objectifying and unrealistic standards of beauty'.[16] The male-gaze is the tendency for women to be viewed by society through the eyes of heterosexual men, as objects of male pleasure, primarily there to fulfil men's sexual desires. When we self-objectify, we turn the male-gaze in on ourselves and view ourselves as sexually desirable objects. This may not be conscious behaviour, but when we view our own image, we are thinking 'would I fuck me?' Self-objectification can manifest as body surveillance/checking and constant monitoring of body and appearance, as well as disordered eating.

Amy's research sought to understand whether or not selfies could contribute to the phenomenon of self-objectification. The idea is that selfies encourage self-objectification by encouraging people to scrutinize and evaluate their own images from an outsider's perspective. This scrutiny is then reinforced by others liking and commenting on the pictures after they are posted to social media sites in an effort to seek external validation. Over 1 million selfies are taken every day globally, with Australians reported to take the most on average. Amy and her team surveyed over 250 young female college students between the ages of eighteen and twenty-nine on their behaviours related to taking selfies; they also asked questions to determine if the women engaged in disordered eating, self-objectification, and whether or not they had body-image concerns. They found no relationship between how long the women spent on social media, or how many selfies were posted, and disordered eating or body-image concerns, but they did find that women who were heavily invested in selfie taking/editing had more body-image concerns and disordered eating. They also found that self-objectification explains the link in the relationship between how invested people were in their selfie taking – spending a lot of time picking and editing photos, or staging the photo in the first place – and body-related and eating concerns.[17]

Amy told me: 'Self-objectification has some really serious implications for girls and women, in that even if you're just thinking about the cognitive resources, the financial resources and the time resources thinking and worrying about your body . . . I argue (and it's not just me; many argue), that that is something that is disproportionately experienced by women and girls in our society.' I agree with Amy. Most of the clients I see identify as female; however, we know that males and trans people also suffer as a consequence of increasing pressure to look aesthetically appealing. A recent study showed that men who self-objectify were more likely to edit their photos and posted selfies more frequently than those who didn't self-objectify.[18]

Similar studies have also shown that higher levels of body-related and eating concerns were found in twelve- to thirteen-year-old girls engaging in more social media-related selfie activities, including online photo sharing, and higher frequency of manipulation of photos (editing to cover spots or make themselves appear thinner) but body-image concerns were not related to how long the girls were online. They also found a relationship between higher investment in selfie activities and greater overvaluation of shape and weight, and body dissatisfaction, all of which are core features in disordered eating.[19]

So, what's the big deal? Why should we be concerned with self-objectification? Scientist believe there are four major consequences of self-objectification.[20]

Body shame and negative affect: Negative affect simply refers to negative mood states, like anxiety, depression and sexual dysfunction. Body shame manifests in the intense desire to escape or hide from the gaze of others; often accompanied by feelings of aimlessness, powerlessness and a deep desire to want to manipulate body appearance through fashion, diets, exercise, beauty products and, in extreme cases, surgery or eating disorders.

Appearance anxiety: A culture that objectifies the female body presents women with a continuous stream of anxiety-provoking experiences, requiring them to maintain an almost chronic vigilance both to their physical appearance and to their physical safety (as, for example, women who more closely fit the cultural ideal are assigned greater blame for their own rape as compared to women who less closely fit the ideal).

Reduced or disrupted flow states: 'Flow' is the idea that you are totally in the zone with something; whether it's a conversation, a good book (oh hey!), a piece of work, cooking, a painting or writing. Self-objectification, body-checking and being anxious about how we look can take us away from the moment, however transiently, to think about how our bodies look. This uses up precious cognitive resources, which could be spent on projects that better align with your values and relationships, or on fighting the goddamn patriarchy. Flow is considered to be an optimal state of being, but self-objectification takes us out of our flow.

Lack of interoceptive awareness: Interoceptive awareness is our ability to perceive sensations in our bodies, such as hunger and fullness. According to self-objectification theory, because women, in a culture that objectifies the female body, are vigilantly aware of their outer body appearance, they may be left with fewer perceptual resources available for recognizing, and responding to, internal cues like hunger and satiety, heartbeat, and perceived blood glucose levels. There's also an argument that self-objectification encourages women to go on diets to try and control their weight, and therefore appearance, which also desensitizes them to physiological cues or interoceptive awareness. If you're constantly thinking about your outward appearance you've got less internal awareness of what's going on inside your body.

THE SWIMSUIT BECOMES YOU

—

In a classic experiment from 1998, 'The Swimsuit Becomes You', researchers wanted to induce self-objectification in men and women to see what effect it would have on the two groups. They first asked women to change into either a revealing swimsuit or a modest sweatshirt, and while wearing the clothes, answer questions about body image; the idea being that trying on the swimsuit would induce self-objectification, but not so for the sweatshirt. And they found the swimsuit wearers did self-objectify more than the sweatshirt wearers, leading to increased body shame, which in turn predicted restrained eating (a measure of disordered eating). The researchers wanted to know if they could replicate the experiment in men, so in a second experiment, they repeated the test with both men and women, and while they were trying on either the swimsuit or sweatshirt, they were asked to perform a maths test. Trying on swimwear led women to feel shame and disgust, whereas men felt shy and silly. They found that women self-objectified more than men, supporting the idea that society socializes women to internalize an objectifying observer's position towards their own bodies. The researchers noted that the situation fostered a sense of being on display, despite the fact that both men and women were alone in the changing room. Inducing self-objectification decreased maths performance only for women, providing empirical evidence that self-objectification consumes mental resources. Let me say that again in case it was unclear. Self-objectification turns women into nescient airheads, rendering us incapable of fully participating in the world. The researchers also found that, as in experiment one, self-objectification led to feelings of body shame, which caused women to restrict their food intake.[21] Women who wore the swimsuit felt reduced to feeling 'I am my body' – in effect, the swimsuit becomes you. What this experiment tells us is this: self-objectification leads to negative body image, which leads to disordered eating and uses up our brain power. Seems like a high price to pay for a cute selfie.

THE SWIMSUIT BECOMES US ALL

Since the original experiment in 1998, many researchers have been interested in replicating and expanding on the findings of the original study, which was limited only to white people (a big issue in body-image research). In 2014, researchers from Rice University induced self-objectification in 176 men and 224 women of Caucasian, African American, Hispanic, and Asian American descent who were required to wear a one-piece bathing suit as in the original experiment. And although they found that white women were more susceptible to negative experiences related to body image, men and members of other ethnic groups more typically considered to be resilient to these experiences can be negatively affected by situations that induce a state of self-objectification. All participants in this study (i.e. all ethnicities and all genders) performed worse on the maths test when they were in the swimsuit condition.[22] The point here is that we all collectively suffer as a result of increased body-checking; what else could we accomplish if we weren't constantly checking ourselves out? In yet another riff on the 'Swimsuit Becomes You' study, a study titled 'Those Speedos Become Them' found that gay men were more vulnerable to the effects of self-objectification than heterosexual men, with the gay men experiencing more body shame and dissatisfaction and disordered eating when in their Speedos compared to straight men.[23]

THIN IDEAL INTERNALIZATION

Just about everywhere we look, from TV adverts, to magazine covers, to our favourite movies, we are bombarded with images of thin and attractive people, particularly women. In the West we have a narrow view of what's deemed to be a 'good' body. Thin has become synonymous with attractive and we rarely see images of bodies that stray too far from this narrow standard of beauty. If we do see a fat body, it's usually the 'funny friend' or a caricature of a fat person portrayed as lazy or stupid. Rarely is a fat person the hero or the love interest. Researchers believe that constant exposure to media makes it difficult for people to differentiate between media portrayals of the thin ideal and reality. This means that when there is greater exposure to thin ideals over other body types, an individual may internalize this as the societal definition of attractiveness.[24] Think for a second about your commute to work, or next time you're at the supermarket notice the diversity of body shapes and sizes. Now compare that with what you see in movies, on TV shows, and in magazines. For the most part, we only see one body type represented in the media: thin. Whereas out in the wild there's a huge range of sizes. But because we are exposed to and have internalized thinness as the standard, we are always comparing ourselves against it, creating a disconnect between society's demands on women, and normative female bodies. That is, just the average, non-supermodel, non-celebrity, non-athlete, regular woman. Women portrayed in the media are typically 15% below the average female weight, a thin ideal that is biogenetically difficult, if not impossible, for the majority of women.[25]

Worryingly, the thin 'ideal' has become thinner over time, increasing the discrepancy between media representation and the average woman, making the ideal even more difficult to achieve. The average body mass index (BMI) of Miss America winners has decreased from around 22 in the 1920s to 16.9 in the 2000s.[26] Researchers have argued that this image, combined with our culture's intense focus on dieting, has contributed to the current epidemic of eating disorders.

The weight of female models in the media is often much lower than the criteria for anorexia.[27] A recent study looked at high-street mannequins in UK shops and found that 100% of the female mannequins would be considered underweight and too thin to menstruate, compared to only 8% of the male mannequins considered underweight (although they didn't look specifically at how muscled the mannequins were, which may play into body-image concerns in men).[28] Think about all the times something has looked sensational on the shop mannequin, but didn't look so cute on you. Do you shrug it off as an unrealistically thin mannequin or do you beat yourself up for not fitting into bullshit beauty standards? My guess is it's probably the latter.

The thin ideal is thought to influence eating behaviour in two main ways:

1 Social comparison leading to negative affect, or mood – in other words, you feel bad about yourself because you don't measure up to others.

2 Over internalization of the thin ideal.

Women are socially conditioned to compare their bodies to other women's bodies. We are comparing ourselves to images of 'ideal femininity' (aka thinness) in the media all day, every day, albeit subconsciously most of the time. And now with the advent of social media where we barely have any reprieve from these ideals, our relative 'inadequacies' are constantly, relentlessly reinforced. This isn't exactly a recipe for self-acceptance; social comparison leads to negative affect (or mood states) like depression, anxiety, and insecurity, as well as negative self-appraisals and low self-esteem. Exposure to the thin ideal in the media has been shown to trigger food intake in people who are restrictive or restrained eaters.[29]

The second way that the thin ideal can lead to eating disturbances is through internalization of the ideal; women embody the message that the only way to be cooler/more popular/more successful/more lovable is by becoming thinner. Research has shown that women who internalize the thin ideal engage in disordered behaviours related to food and exercise, have heightened body dissatisfaction and set unrealistic body 'goals'. Internalization of the thin ideal is a risk factor for the development of disordered eating and body dissatisfaction.[30]

A 2004 experiment studied how looking at photographs from three major women's magazines (*Glamour*, *Vogue* and *Cosmo*) influenced the way women felt about their bodies, and how it affected their mood. Women were given either copies of adverts from the magazines that portrayed the thin ideal or control adverts – neutral images of cars, make-up and jewellery without any people in them. Just thirty minutes of looking at the thin-ideal images increased body dissatisfaction, negative mood states (anger, anxiety, depression, and confusion) and eating disorder symptoms and decreased self-esteem.[31] If thirty minutes of this stuff can make us feel like that, imagine the cumulative effect over a lifetime.

But it's not just psychological health that suffers from internalizing the thin ideal and body dissatisfaction: evidence suggests it can lead to physiological problems like a weakened immune system and poor sleep quality too.[32]

––––

Pay attention next time you flip through a magazine or are watching TV. How many people fall outside the narrow range of socially 'acceptable' body types? More importantly, how do you feel after spending half an hour flicking through these magazines? If the research is anything to go by, I'm guessing you don't feel too hot.

ACTIVITY

While you're scrolling through social media or flipping through a mag, take a moment to notice all the examples of diet culture, the thin ideal and self-objectification. Notice how often people in the office engage in diet chat or body talk. Keep a note of some of these in your journal and reflect on how ubiquitous they are. How does it make you feel now you're paying more attention?

FAT PHOBIA

—

Through its propagation of the thin ideal, diet culture perpetuates the status quo of stigma and prejudice against fat people. Just like prejudice based on the colour of someone's skin, their sexual orientation, their age, gender, physical ability or their religion, it's *never* OK to hate on someone because they have a bigger body than what we typically see in the media. You wouldn't be mad at a dalmatian for being bigger than a pug. No way – you'd be up for snuggles with either.

Yet in diet culture fat bodies are demonized and 'othered'; pushed to the margins and oppressed. We'll talk more specifically about the health consequences of fat phobia and weight stigma in chapter 5 but for now let's focus on some of the sociopolitical consequences. Weight stigma has been linked to:

- lower educational attainment in children[33]
- increased weight-related bullying and teasing in children (which may lead to disordered eating and eating disorders)[34,35]
- being penalized in the workplace in terms of salary, employment opportunities and promotion decisions[36]
- negative stereotypes such as lazy, undisciplined and gluttonous[37]

I try and distance myself from the word 'obesity' as I recognize that it can be painful for some people to be attached to this label (even if it's used with 'person first' language, i.e. person with X). This is because it's a medicalized label that reduces a person down to a number, flattens the experience of living as a fat person, and pathologizes body fatness. It breeds shame and stigma, and while I don't claim to know the breadth of experience of living as a fat person, I did grow up as a fat child and teenager and know the pain caused by weight-based bullying and stigma. Now, as a nutrition professional, I've seen how weight stigma plays out in a health context with my clients; we'll discuss that in more detail later, but suffice to say, it's not pretty.[38] Part of my intention with this book is to leverage my professional privilege to help raise awareness of weight stigma in nutrition and medicine and provide a non-shaming, non-stigmatizing resource for fat people who want to improve their relationship with food or learn more about nutrition without the assumption that they need to or should lose weight.

And a note on the word fat: I use fat here in the reappropriated sense, as an ally to the fat activist/fat positive movement; fatness is inherently political and I am fully aware that to most in my line of work, fat activism is professional heresy. I think about this a lot and I've decided I'm OK with that, because to me it's the most ethical way to practise and prevents me from causing harm to my clients. I understand that for many people this word might be uncomfortable and I invite you to use whichever word is more fitting for you: 'plus-size', 'curvy' etc. However, I want to make it clear that when I say fat, I am using it as a neutral descriptor, just like 'thin' or 'tall', 'blue', 'brunette'. If the word fat feels uncomfortable, try sitting with it until it sounds less scary.

In Western society we have a dichotomy whereby thinness is reinforced and rewarded, thereby conferring power and status to those who achieve the thin or beauty ideal. Fat is feared, belittled, discriminated against. Fatness is penalized and punished. This is an injustice: injustice leads to inequality and I am not here for that.

Interview with Michelle Elman (@scarrednotscared), fat-identifying body-positive author of *Am I Ugly?*

Why are people reappropriating the word fat? And why is this important?

Much like how the LGBTQ+ community embrace queer and the black community often use the N word, it's about taking your power back from a word that was used to hurt and disempower marginalized communities. The word fat at its core is a descriptor. It is a fact and it is its connotations in society which have led to the immediate interpretation that it's an insult. The associations are what need to change, not the word itself. The word itself is no different to words such as tall. The way the word fat is censored, either shushing people who use it or calling it the F word or following it up with 'you aren't fat', even though you are, embeds shame and implies it is something that shouldn't be spoken of freely but something that you should be embarrassed about. It also adds to the fear of fat. If the word itself is so scary that parents shush people when it's being used around their kids, their kids quickly learn it is a bad word and therefore fat is a bad thing.

What should people do if the word fat makes them uncomfortable?

They should challenge their perceptions and associations around the word. If you are a fat person, it often will be associated with unpleasant memories when it was used to hurt and shame. Remember that it's the association that is the problem and not the word. No word should hold that much power over an individual. Changing the meaning to it simply being a descriptor will really help. Ask yourself what you hear when you hear fat? What does the word fat say about you? Because if your answer is anything other than 'I wear a higher dress size and I hold more fat on my body', then that perception needs to be updated to be more accurate.

> ### Is it OK to use other labels
> ### like 'plus-size', 'curvy'?
> The plus-size community are still divided on other euphemisms, especially because at this stage it is not acceptable to call other people fat, even if you mean it as a descriptor. Body-positive advocates using fat to describe themselves is part of the way to changing the narrative around fat, but until we have normalized it in the general population, there will always be a need for other euphemisms due to other people's discomfort and fear of offending people.

HEALTHISM

—

Another consequence of diet culture is healthism; a term coined by Robert Crawford and defined as a 'preoccupation with personal health as a primary – often the primary – focus for the definition and achievement of well-being. A goal which is to be achieved primarily through the modification of life styles.' In English, this idea that your sole purpose in life is to be chasing after 'perfect' health. Of course the subtext being **1** that there is such a thing as perfect health, and **2** health is a personal obligation. The latter of these completely ignores things like social connections, and the health of our communities. This is further complicated by the fact that we think weight equals health, albeit subconsciously in the context of healthism. On the surface, sure, we're told it's about preventing disease, but have you ever seen any fat wellness gurus? Exactly.

In her book *Fat Activism*, Charlotte Cooper expands on Crawford's definition and explains healthism as follows: 'Healthism refers to the idea that health is a moral project that is the responsibility of the individual. Here, health is not merely the absence of illness, it's about presenting yourself to the world as glowingly well, athletic, able-bodied, and full of vitality.'

I think what Charlotte has described here sums up pretty much every wellness guru on the planet! In diet culture a premium is placed on 'health' and the pursuit of health. This is inherently ableist, classist, and fatphobic. Healthy people are considered more valuable, worthier. 'Unhealthy' people are moral failures. And because health, within the healthism paradigm, is conceptualized as a personal choice, or simply something that is a personal responsibility which can be achieved through the 'right' behaviours, it fails to consider the multiplicity of factors that influence health. We have known for a long time that the majority of health outcomes are determined by social factors known as the social determinants of health.[39,40] In the context of healthism and diet culture, nutrition is king: according to every wellness wanker I've ever met, if you just eat 'right' you'll achieve health, as though it was a level on Mario and nutrition was the boss you had to destroy. If you just align your chakras with a turmeric latte, you won't get cancer. Ever. Look, nutrition is important, I'm not saying it isn't, but relative to social determinants of health, it's small-time in terms of its influence over health at a population level. Current estimates suggest that only 38% of health is determined by individual behaviours, including individual psychological assets (self-efficacy, optimism, and conscientiousness), negative mood and affects (stress, anxiety, depression), drug use (alcohol, tobacco, and other substances), sleep pattern, physical activity, sexual health and, wait for it . . . nutrition. The other 62% is attributed to social circumstances, genetics, medical care, and the physical environment (pollution, air quality).[41] And let's be real, Sweaty Betty leggings do sweet FA to reduce the socio-economic disparities that lead to health inequalities and may even increase socio-economic disparities.

The way we construct health as a society determines our under-standing of how we access health. If health is constructed as a set of practices that include: collagen supplements, excoriatingly expensive superfood blends, clean eating, coconut water, alkalizing unicorn tears, more coconut water, and dehydrated, activated dragon shit, then it's easy to see how people feel alienated from it.[42]

A kind of reductionism or one-dimensionalization seems to occur among healthists: more and more experiences are collapsed into health experience, more and more values into health values. Health, or its supreme 'super health', subsumes a panoply of values: 'a sense of happiness and purpose', 'a high level of self-esteem', 'work satisfaction', 'ability to engage in creative expression', 'capacity to function effectively under stress', 'having confidence in the future', 'a commitment to living in the world', the ability 'to celebrate one's life', or even 'cosmic affirmation'. 'Health is more than the absence of disease ...' writes one of the new pulpiteers, 'it includes a fully productive, self-realized, expanded life of joy, happiness, and love in and for whatever one is doing.' In the 'high level wellness' ethic, 'health is freedom in the truest sense – freedom from aimlessness, being able to express a range of emotions freely, a zest for living'. In short, health has become not only a preoccupation; it has also become a pan-value or standard by which an expanding number of behaviours and social phenomena are judged. Less a means toward the achievement of other fundamental values, health takes on the quality of an end in itself. Good living is reduced to a health problem, just as health is expanded to include all that is good in life.

Healthism is a system for quantifying and judging bodies; for creating another standard that is unrealistic, if not impossible. It's no longer enough to be 'thin'; we also have to perform 'health' too. Health isn't merely the absence of illness; it's conquering and mastering our bodies. It's the social signalling that we are 'well' because we have a green juice in one hand and a yoga mat slung over the shoulder. It's about glowy skin, bright eyes, youthful abounding energy, and evading the inevitable. It's about being in control.

In the twenty-first century, healthism has replaced overt diet culture as a means of achieving the thin ideal via what you and I know of as 'wellness'. 'It's for my health' is the new way of legitimizing semi-starvation in a society where 'diet' has become a dirty word. From my perspective and clinical experience, I think it also flattens and commodifies the concept of health; making it into something that you have to buy into to make it count. I'm reminded of a particular client who'd spend her whole lunch break rushing to the hottest new juice bar that was on the other side of town from her office. Or she'd spend her weekends trekking all over London to go to one particular gym class – that actually left her feeling more drained than energized – just because it was Instagram-chic. Was that green juice more nourishing than soup and a sandwich from Pret? Did that class do more for her physical and mental well-being than a walk in the park? Nope!

REDUCTIONIST NUTRITION
—

Related to the concept of healthism is that of reductionist nutrition, sometimes known as nutritionism.[43] In the context of the reductionist nutrition paradigm, foods and diets are understood in terms of their most basic units, that is to say, their nutrient and biochemical composition. From a scientific perspective, it's important for us to be able to identify and isolate specific compounds, as well as understand the biochemical mechanism by which they prevent disease. This can lead to new drug discoveries and a better understanding of human biology. However, when we are communicating messages about nutrition, a reductionist, single-nutrient focus can be misleading and confusing to people, particularly if they have a troubled or disordered relationship to food.

In the context of reductionist nutrition, food is reduced to nutrients: grams of protein, fat, and carbohydrate. Bloggers tell us we need to 'remineralize' (WHAT DOES THAT EVEN MEAN?) and take super-potent vitamin supplements.

We are taught to think of food in terms of its constituent parts, rather than in terms of taste, satisfaction, satiation (or ability to quash hunger), tradition and culture, or simply how it makes us feel. In the reductionist nutrition paradigm, specific foods are judged in isolation from other foods, the wider diets, and broader frames of reference. This approach to evaluating foods often leads to certain foods being either vilified or fetishized, as in the case of 'super-foods', on the basis of their nutrient composition. For instance, the denigration of eggs, on the basis of high cholesterol levels, is an example of decon-textualization of a single food from the diet as a whole. We now know that dietary cholesterol from foods like eggs and prawns has little impact on our blood cholesterol, and both are great sources of other nutrients.[44] Yet the cholesterol myth still persists today, just one consequence of the reductionist approach. We also know that food is more than the sum of its parts, with some nutrients working synergistically, and so discussing nutrients outside of the context of foods is unhelpful at best.[45]

The media are especially culpable over vilifying individual foods or nutrients; they're currently going batshit over sugar. And if sugar is the super-villain, protein is the hero, with his side-kick 'good fat'. The sensationalization and fear-mongering brought about by reductionist headlines communicating the findings of individual studies can make it seem like a single bite of a cookie or a burger is going to send you to the hospital.

————

The main issue I take with this approach to relating to food is what I see in my clinical practice almost daily: food fear and anxiety. In my office I have food emojis that I've printed out and laminated and Blu-tacked onto the wall. I'll ask my clients to pick out the foods that represent their favourite dishes. A memorable example was a client who said she was experiencing some guilt around her once- or twice-a-month Chinese takeaway. So I asked her to pick out the emojis that comprised the meal, a sweet 'n' sour pork dish with rice. She grabbed the pineapple, a chilli pepper, the pork, and a bowl of rice. And then I asked her to write down words to describe the meal on Post-it notes and stick them next to the emojis. Here's what she said: saturated fat, white carbs, cholesterol, and sugar. She did muster up a 'tasty' too, but it was clear that the vigilance on 'bad' nutrients under-mined the experience of eating the food in the first place. So I helped her reframe these thoughts with a focus not just on nutrition but on the experience of eating food. Here's what my Post-its said: BALANCED!, protein, energy, vitamins & minerals, fibre, satisfying AND tasty.

I don't think it's wrong to discuss nutrients *per se*, and gentle nutrition is something we'll talk about later on in the book. My concern is that a hyper-focus on 'good' and 'bad' nutrients results in dichotomous, all-or-nothing, absolutist thinking; it's reductionist. What I find with people who have eating problems is that they know too much about food and nutrients, and this becomes a source of anxiety for them. Remember that nutrition isn't all or nothing. Unless we're knocking back a bottle of olive oil, we're rarely eating individual nutrients. And the presence of sugar or saturated fat doesn't negate other beneficial nutrients. Dairy is a great example: sure there's some saturated fat up in there, but there's also protein, calcium, vitamin D, B12 and iodine and other important nutrients.[46] In fact, dairy is considered to be beneficial for heart health.

We've already discovered that nutrition isn't the be-all and end-all of health, as well as the fact that health isn't a moral obligation. Food and eating are as much about pleasure, memories, and community.

DIETS
—

And here's what it's all been building towards. The thing that, arguably, has the biggest influence on our relationship to food. Diets.

According to Mintel, in the period 2015–2016, 48% of people in the UK tried to lose weight. When only women were considered, the number increased to 57%. Among those who have tried to lose weight, two-thirds say they are trying to lose weight all or most of the time.[47] It's been reported that 40% of parents encourage their children to diet, and that parents engage in weight talk with children as young as two years old. TWO![48]

Nearly a third of children aged five to six chose an ideal body size that was thinner than their current perceived size. By age six, children are aware of dieting and may have tried it, and there is a preference and desire for thinness seen amongst six-year-old girls, but not six-year-old boys.[49] In addition, 25% of five-year-olds recommend dieting behaviours (not eating 'junk' food, eating less) as a solution for a person who has gained weight, and by the time they're seven years old, one in four children has engaged in some kind of dieting behaviour.

Young kids can join diet programmes – at a time when young girls are developing and laying down fat for growth spurts and puberty. It's totally normal for young girls' weight to increase, many need to go out before they can go up; it's what bodies do. Yet we are pathologizing this phenomenon and putting young people on diets. As though puberty isn't hard enough without being on a motherfucking diet.

Just so we're clear here. If you're a parent and you've put your kid on a diet or made comments about their body shape I don't want you to freak out, you haven't permanently, irreparably damaged your kid, and this is in no way a judgement. I'm not a parent, so I'm not sure what I would have done in your situation, but I do know this, you were doing what you thought was best for your kid. That's what parents do. Ditto, if you've ever been on a diet, are currently on a diet, or thinking about going on a diet, I don't want you to feel badly about that either. Diets are the norm, women are socially conditioned to think that diets are an inevitable part of the female experience (and more and more dudes feel this pressure too). Diets teach us that there's a 'right' and a 'wrong' way to eat, and by extension our choices are either 'good' or 'bad'. That then dictates how we feel about ourselves. They fill our heads with a bunch of external rules, many of which are conflicting, arbitrary, or based on extremely questionable science. Think about it like this – diets and pseudo-diets consist of a bunch of draconian rules that even when followed meticulously are destined to fail. Diets have a spectacularly high failure rate, even when you stick to them like glue. Not because you've done anything wrong, but because, biologically, our bodies have evolved not to shrink away. However, because the pressure to lose weight is so high, and the 'right' and 'wrong' ways of eating have become lodged in our brains, we end up with a lot of noise in our heads about what, when and how much to eat. It might be guilt associated with eating a 'bad' food. It might be bargaining and negotiating with yourself: 'if I eat this cookie, I will run an extra X miles on my run tomorrow'. It might be weird rules about not eating gluten or sugar. Whatever it is, it prevents us from being in our bodies, and eating in accordance with hunger, fullness, pleasure, and sustenance. These food rules become an external barometer by which we determine our self-worth. The number on the scales dictates our ability to accept who we are inside. Self-compassion becomes contingent on hitting a calorie or macro goal. And all of this is upheld by a system that preys on our vulnerabilities and insecurities. This of course all plays out through feeling batshit-crazy around food. But by figuring this stuff out in the microcosm of food, we learn skills that can be applied to other areas of our lives: self-acceptance and compassion, mindfulness, and emotional resilience.

———

My hope is that by teaching you about the sociocultural structures that have us spellbound into thinking that dieting is not only normal but the only way of existing, we can begin to challenge some of these norms, become the experts of our own bodies, and take our power back. It's only by educating ourselves that we can begin to liberate ourselves from the hold that dieting has over us. I don't expect this to happen overnight or all at once. For some women this is an ongoing process; just take it at a pace that's comfortable for you. My sense, though, is that once you start to recognize how pervasive diet culture is in everyday life, you can't unsee that shit. Once you've come far enough down the road, there's no turning back.

OK, so we know that dieting and disordered eating is the default way of eating and being for many women, but what's the harm? Sure, it feels vaguely uncomfortable that our kids are dieting, but if they've got some extra pounds lying around, surely they could stand to go on a diet?

We're going to talk a lot more specifically about why diets don't work in chapter 2, but let's consider what the scientific literature has to say about the effects of diets. Studies have shown that dieting leads to:

- body and food preoccupation (basically obsessing about food and body)
- body dissatisfaction
- increased stress

- disordered eating
- eating disorders (in those who are predisposed)
- lowered self-esteem
- depression[50]

Guys! What part of that is HEALTHY? Exactly; sweet fuck all. When we talk about health, we can't compartmentalize physical and mental health.

So, what if you're not on an 'official' diet? Maybe you turned in your Slimming World membership years ago. Oh, or maybe you're not dieting but you just don't 'do' gluten. And you have no sugar in your house? A lot of the women I work with are no longer on a *diet* diet. But they still have a bunch of lingering (usually conflicting) rules, 'bad' foods, and guilt associated with eating said bad foods. Eating is still associated with some sort of compensatory behaviour or negative emotions. So, despite the fact that you're no longer on an official diet, you may inadvertently have dieting characteristics. Sure, there may be more flexibility and less rigidity than an official diet, but are they all that different in reality?

Let's define what we mean by rigid and flexible dietary control, and then take a look at whether flexible control is closer to intuitive eating or rigid dietary control.

Rigid dietary control is an all-or-nothing, black-and-white approach to eating – you're either eating *no cookies* or *all of the cookies*. You might be avoiding or straight up refusing desired higher-calorie foods or foods high in fat/carbs/sugar. And if you do eat those foods, you probably feel a strong sense of guilt and probably end up overeating or bingeing. You might be following a strict calorie limit (or macros if that's your bag) in order to control your weight. You're probably also eating 'diet foods' to prevent weight gain. Do you remember the banana ice cream trend, where we were all encouraged to freeze bananas, blend them up and call it ice cream? Yikes! You might also be skipping meals altogether.

Flexible dietary control is generally considered a 'balanced' approach to eating – it's essentially what most nutritionists or dietitians would recommend: things like taking smaller than desired servings of food to control weight (portion control), being conscious of foods eaten, taking weight into account when making food choices, and compensating for the foods you do eat (i.e. intentionally eating less and/or 'healthier' alternatives at the next meal) if you perceive that you've eaten too much or an 'unhealthy' option at the previous meal. Sounds fairly sensible, right?

Not so fast; research has shown that, although these two concepts *appear* to be distinct and separate from one another on the surface, they conceptually overlap too much to be considered discrete entities. In other words, it's impossible to teach someone strategies to increase flexible control without inadvertently increasing rigid control. So, if I teach you 'appropriate' portion sizes, you couldn't learn them without applying a degree of rigid dietary control. Portion control is an *external* regulation of food.

On the other hand, if I were to tell you a portion of food was however much was needed to satisfy your hunger, that's an *internal* regulation of food, aka intuitive eating. Intuitive eating has been suggested as a viable alternative to both flexible and rigid dietary control.

Conceptually, intuitive eating and flexible dietary control should be distinct. Intuitive eating relies on internal hunger and satiety cues, and compensation occurs naturally (e.g. not being hungry after a large meal), whereas flexible control relies on external cues for eating (e.g. portion control, weight, and nutritional information), and compensation is conscious and effortful. EFFORTFUL. Making decisions about feeding your body shouldn't be a goddamn chore.

Intuitive eating entails eating mainly in response to physiological hunger and satiety cues – those who eat intuitively are attuned to and trust their hunger and satiety signals to guide their eating. If intuitive eaters eat more at one meal they will naturally eat less at the next meal because they are less hungry (as opposed to conscious restriction); therefore IE has been described as a flexible and adaptive eating behaviour. People who eat intuitively are less likely to be preoccupied with food or dichotomize food as good or bad – instead they often choose food for the purposes of satisfaction (i.e. taste), health, energy, stamina, and performance.[51]

Intuitive eating and flexible dietary control are not the same construct. Flexible control is more closely related to rigid control than to intuitive eating.

Studies have shown that rigid/flexible dietary control is associated with restrictive eating behaviours, food group exclusions, disordered eating and compensatory behaviours that lead to feelings of restriction and deprivation (even subconsciously). They're also related to negative body image.[52,53]

People often worry that if they're not applying some form of control over their eating they will just eat and eat and eat until they burst. But research shows that not only is intuitive eating associated with less eating restraint (restrictions) but also less disinhibited eating (bingeing or eating past the point of comfortable fullness).[54,55] I love seeing this play out with clients; people who at the start of our work together are convinced they can't have delicious foods in the house because they'll decimate them in thirty seconds flat, to then having foods in the house that they had more or less forgotten about because they were no longer such a big deal.

IF NOT DISORDERED EATING, THEN WHAT?

As we've established, eating behaviours sit on a spectrum from intuitive eating, to disordered eating, to eating disorders. If you've been towards the right-hand side of that spectrum, then it can feel totally overwhelming and scary to let go of those disordered behaviours and food rules, and begin to get back to a place where you feel comfortable and safe around food; intuitive eating and other related non-diet approaches are tools that we can use to get our shit together and help rebuild a healthy relationship to food.

Intuitive eating has had a renaissance lately in the UK, which is exciting. But as with every trend that gets popular and goes mainstream, nuances and subtleties are lost and confusion follows. People have a tendency to make snap judgements, rather than actually doing the research to find out what it is. Side note: if I hear a fitness blogger say that intuitive eating is 'just eating whatever you want' ONE MORE TIME, I am going to gouge my eyes out with a spoon.

So, let's take a second to talk about what intuitive eating *really* is. The intuitive eating model was developed in 1995 by two Registered Dietitians based in the US, Evelyn Tribole and Elyse Resch. These two pioneers proposed an intervention to help their patients get off the dieting merry-go-round once and for all. This was the nineties, so we're talking peak Atkins, the era of the Grapefruit Diet, and a time when dangerous diet pills like Fen-Phen (fenfluramine/phentermine) were available on prescription. Tribole and Resch had been in the business of what was considered sensible weight loss at the time, producing meticulous calorie-controlled and nutritionally flawless meal plans for their clients that were *textbook* in terms of macronutrients, vitamins and minerals. Their clients followed these plans to the letter, and predictably lost weight. But a few years out, despite sticking to their meal plans, clients began regaining weight. The clients naturally blamed themselves, internalizing that blame and guilt for failing their diets. But Tribole and Resch were smart, they turned to the available scientific evidence at the time and developed an intervention that was designed to help people move away from external regulation of food intake (diet plans and food rules), and towards internal regulation based on physical hunger, satisfaction, and satiety (fullness) cues.

They developed ten principles to build their intervention around:

1 Reject the Diet Mentality
2 Honour Your Hunger
3 Challenge the Food Police
4 Make Peace with Food
5 Discover the Satisfaction Factor
6 Respect Your Fullness
7 Honour Your Feelings Without Using Food
8 Respect Your Body
9 Exercise – Feel the Difference
10 Honour Your Health with Gentle Nutrition

They found that the intervention helped people reach the weight that was healthiest for them, but also helped heal their relationship with food and body image. They published this method as a book in 1995; it has subsequently had two further editions, and a boat load of academic research has been done using the principles as a basis for the interventions, now considered to be an evidence-based practice that helps people build a healthier relationship with food and their bodies.[56,57] It's now widely used in clinical practice alongside in-patient eating disorder treatment, and in the outpatient setting with sub-clinical eating disorders or disordered eating.

And while the research is in its relative infancy, lots of promising findings have been made supporting the benefits of this approach.[58, 59,60,61] I've summarized these in the table over the page.

Increased	Decreased
blood glucose control	binge eating/disinhibited eating
mental health	disordered eating
psychological flexibility	dieting
body appreciation and satisfaction	thin-ideal internalization
interoceptive awareness and responsiveness	blood pressure
proactive coping	LDL 'bad' cholesterol
positive emotional functioning	
life satisfaction	
unconditional self-regard and optimism	
greater motivation to exercise for enjoyment rather than guilt or appearance	
dietary variety	
HDL 'good' cholesterol	

Intuitive eating is a specific intervention, with ten principles that guide the process. I'm going to say this a lot, but THEY ARE NOT RULES. IE is about deconstructing rules and learning to eat in accordance with physical cues, as well as recognizing and understanding emotional cues. Recognizing, understanding, and acting on internal cues is fundamental to the IE process:

Biological eating cues: Hunger and fullness (or satiety cues) have a physical sensation.

Emotional feelings: Every emotion has a physical sensation.[62,63]

States: Physical states like sleepiness or needing to pee have a physical sensation.[64]

Dieting, food rules and restrictions move us away from the internal experience of our bodies and disconnect us from these physical sensations. You might not have a clue what these mean at this point, but that's OK. Throughout the book I'll teach you tools that help you become more aware of, and responsive to, these physical cues and sensations. I know it sounds kind of new-agey, but there's some solid science behind it, so stick with me!

This is how I like to explain intuitive eating to my clients and maybe it will help you conceptualize IE better too: imagine a baby who has just been weaned, eating at their high chair. They have a variety of foods in front of them – some blueberries, some chopped-up avocado, black beans, potato and sweetcorn. The kid doesn't think 'oooh, this is too many carbs' or 'does this fit my macros?' Nah, most kids will pick and choose what they need to satisfy their hunger; a little bit of everything until they feel full, at which point they start throwing shit on the floor or feeding the dog. They instinctively, intuitively pick a balance of foods that will help them meet their nutritional requirements for energy and growth. The theory is that we're all born with the innate ability to regulate our own feeding. When we're young we're highly attuned to our innate sense of hunger and fullness. Babies will tear the house down when they're hungry, demanding to be fed. They'll also turn their head away or clamp their mouth shut when they're done. Not surprisingly, they manage just fine without a calorie tracker.

We're pretty willing to accept that babies and children can regulate their own feeding, but less willing to trust that our own bodies can do the same. It's true that for many of us, the innate abilities to feed ourselves become . . . complicated; let's take a look at why that is.

'You can only go out to play once you clean your plate.'

'You can only have ice cream once you've finished your dinner.'

'You shouldn't have that.'

'Eat up, you need energy to grow big and strong.'

'Don't eat that, it's bad for you.'

Over the years, well-intentioned comments from parents, teachers, grandparents, and other caretakers can cause us to override our innate hunger and fullness cues, causing them to weaken and atrophy. Child feeding practices can also influence how and what we eat; research has shown that when parents apply excessive overt restriction on foods that are allowed, it can inhibit the child's ability to self-regulate their appetite. When parents use food as an emotional coping tool, it may teach children to use food to alleviate or distract from negative emotions. And pressuring kids to eat has been shown to result in more emotional eating.[65,66,67] The reasons why we dissociate from an internal regulation of foods is enormously complex and we'll explore some more reasons soon. It's unlikely that your issues with food are just because your mum was weird about food and your aunt was always on a diet, but this might all be part of the puzzle.

Through the process of IE, people can learn to get back in touch with the signals their body is sending. They can become more aware of and responsive to these cues. Most people eat according to rules, restrictions, some external app, plan or tracker, or maybe even just the clock, instead of their internal GPS. This can cause a disconnect between body and mind. Most people don't value or trust the signals their body sends to them and don't believe that they could ever learn to eat without rules or systems to guide them. So, the process isn't as straightforward as: just eat when you're hungry and stop when you're full. It can take time, and it can be a bumpy road in places, but this book will give you the tools to help you along the way. I hope you can begin to piece together your own history and narrative about your relationship to food and begin to allow yourself to heal and repair that relationship.

BECOME A DIET CULTURE DROPOUT

—

Diet culture teaches us we're not good enough as we are. It teaches us we need to control our bodies through rigid dieting (like clean eating) and over exercising; how many times have you seen something gross like 'sweat is just fat crying' or 'no excuses'. It teaches us that we'll be cooler/funnier/more successful if we force our bodies to look a certain way. But that comes at a huge cost in terms of our mental health and our relationship to food.

Diet culture teaches us to conform. Follow the diet rules. Obey the food police. Check yourself. Stay in line. Monitor and micromanage your body. It keeps us busy with the work of perfecting, refining, 'gains', 'body goals', and whatever other bullshit. It teaches us disordered eating is the norm. And that chasing the thin ideal is part and parcel of the 'work' of being a woman; it's what we're socialized to do. Do we even know that there's another way to live? A way in which we're liberated from food and body preoccupation? A way of living in which our precious resources aren't squandered on chasing a narrow and exclusionary idea of what you should be.

The biggest lie of diet culture is that you will be happy when you reach this elusive body standard.

How much time, energy, effort, and money do you spend chasing the lies of diet culture? What would it be like if you were to disobey? Disrupt the status quo? Rebel? Break the rules? Riot? Rise up?

What would we achieve if we were to cast off the expectations of diet culture? The ones we never signed up for in the first place but have somehow been trying to live up to our whole lives? What if we decided to be brave, bold, ambitious, and say 'FUCK YOU' to diet culture? Who would we be if we didn't define ourselves by our workouts or how 'clean' we ate? What is our identity outside of 'the healthy one'? The dieter? Start that project, develop your politics, make noise, get angry, stand for something, be what they said you couldn't be, be fucking brilliant. Not at boring squats and meal prep, but at living your whole life to the fullest. Do you want to be remembered for your visible abs? Or do you want to be remembered for your fire and passion? You already have everything you need, RIGHT NOW, to achieve your dreams. Not two dress sizes from now. Not a juice cleanse or Paleo diet from now. Stop hiding behind diet culture and LIVE! Because at the end of the day, how many cookies you ate or how heavy you lifted is trivial and it's time for the REAL work to begin. Through these pages I invite you to join me in becoming a diet culture dropout, a dissident, a rebel. Let this book be your guide to unsubscribing from diet culture once and for all.

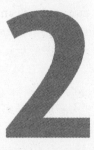

DITCH THE DIETS

'm not gonna insult you by bringing up the whole 'diets don't work' trope. You know they don't work, otherwise you wouldn't be here reading this. What you might not know though, is that diets have something like an 80% plus failure rate but at the same time we have a diet and weight-loss industry estimated to be worth $176 billion worldwide, and projected to be worth $245 billion by 2022.[1] The diet industry is profiting from our insecurities, our desperation, our failure. Yeah, sure, a diet might work in the short term to help you lose some pounds, but sooner or later, despite you fully leaning in, you start gaining weight again.[2,3] It's easy for us to blame ourselves at this point: 'I must be doing something wrong', 'I can't stick to the diet'. But what the diet industry don't want you to know (I'm guessing, they haven't actually told me this) is that it's not you, it's them.

There's no standardized definition of a diet, and there are SO MANY different types, it sometimes makes it hard to know what a diet is, especially now that diets have shape-shifted into 'wellness' and 'lifestyles'. For the purposes of this book, a diet is anything that restricts what, how much, or when you eat food.

For example: the Paleo diet restricts what you eat as it has a whole bunch of food rules (and contributes to food fear, but we'll get to that). Calorie-counting apps like MyFitnessPal restrict how much you eat (and encourage you to 'earn' food through exercise). Intermittent fasting determines when you eat (and ignores the fact that it is your God-given right to have breakfast).

Like I said before, in my practice, I see a lot of people who may not be on a formal diet, but have developed all sorts of weird rules about what, when, and how much to eat. There's all this negotiation and bargaining that goes on. 'If I eat this cookie then I have to run an extra two miles tomorrow', 'I've already had bread today so I can't eat sweet potatoes'. Basically, they pick up little nuggets from different diets and apply the ones that seem most reasonable to them (or the parts they think they can stick to, like Paleo people eating bacon). I remember one client who thought dairy was like drinking bleach, but would then eat coconut ice cream and yoghurt to the point of making herself feel sick (restriction often leads to bingeing). These self-imposed food rules, plus the subtle diets that masquerade as 'lifestyles' that slip in under the guise of healthism, are almost more insidious than the obvious Slim Fast-type diets. I call them pseudo-diets.

PSEUDO-DIETS

You might be thinking, 'uhhhh, I'm not on a diet'. And sure, you might not be going to Weight Watchers or Slimming World, but let's talk about all the subtle ways we can be on a diet or attempting to control our eating. Maybe your plan was to 'eat clean', maybe challenge yourself to the Whole 30; just do what the bloggers do. It's a *lifestyle*. It's about *balance*. It's a fucking diet. Sure, it's subtle, not easy to spot. But once you know the signs of a diet, you cannot unsee them.

All the signs are there: rules about what, how much, or when to eat. But here are some other things to look out for.

- Can you break rules? Diet.
- Can you 'mess up'? Diet.
- Can you have 'cheat days'? Diet.
- Does it have off-limits foods? Diet.
- Do you count points? Diet.
- Does it promote 'guilt-free' foods? Diet.
- Is someone trying to sell you something? Diet.
- Are you being told what, how much, or when to eat? Diet.
- Is it a case of eat like me, look like me? Diet.
- Do you have to count calories, macros or track activity? Diet.
- Do you have to follow a meal plan?* Diet.

All of these things take decisions about food and eating away from you and place them under external control: a diet or lifestyle guru, an app, a meal plan, an activity tracker. They reinforce the idea that you're not to be trusted, 'You don't know how much is the appropriate amount of food to eat, so let me tell you'. 'You're an incompetent jerk

---

* Unless you are in recovery from an eating disorder in which case a meal plan might be part of your treatment.

who doesn't know how to feed yourself' is the message they send. And although rationally we understand that the best person to make food choices for you is you, we internalize this idea that we have no clue what we're doing. This heightened attention to food intake creates a cognitive boundary that interferes with a more intuitive regulation of food intake. This overly cognitive focus moves people away from sensitivity to their own hunger and fullness cues and instead creates a preoccupation with psychological, cultural, or social signs to eat. We feel consumed about 'right' and 'wrong' food choices, which leads to anxiety, stress, and guilt. It also removes any sense of pleasure or enjoyment from our food.

How to spot diet buzzwords

If you see any of these words associated with food and nutrition then they should set off alarm bells that they're trying to restrict your eating in some way. DO NOT RECOMMEND.

PSEUDO-DIET BUZZWORDS

IIFYM	Restrict
Cheat Meal	Syns
Quit Sugar/ Sugar-free Diet	Calorie Counting
	80/20 Rule
Clean Eating	Whole 30
Meal Plan	Health Kick
Gluten-free Diet (when not coeliac)	Unrefined Sugar-free
Intermittent Fasting	Plant-based (when not for ethical reasons)
Low Fat	
Low Carb	Juice Cleanses
Paleo/Grain-free	Rest Plans
Cleanse	Detox
Grain-free	Dairy-free (without allergy)
Unprocessed	

THE BIOLOGY OF DIETS

OK, now you know how to recognize a diet in all its subtle forms, you might still be like 'what's wrong with diets, aren't they supposed to make us healthier?' After all, there's an 'obesity' epidemic and OMG! Argh! (Cue brain short-circuiting.) Let me break it down for you.

The psychological, physiological, and social stress of diets and the pursuit of weight loss outweigh (not sorry) the benefits.[5,6] This is counter-intuitive to the messages we receive every single day in the media and from doctors that say we have to do everything we can to control our weight. We'll discuss the link between weight and health later on (chapter 5), but for now let's talk about what happens to our bodies when we try and force them below their genetically and environmentally determined weight (known as your 'set point weight').

HERE'S WHAT HAPPENS WHEN YOU GO ON A DIET OR PSEUDO-DIET

In the early stages of a diet you're all like 'I got this, this is no big deal', you're pumped and excited and you go to the shop and buy all the chia seeds and coconut oil and drop the GDP of a small country. You might even lose some weight in the first few days – you'll have heard of the term 'water weight'. What this means is that you're depleting your glycogen stores. Glycogen is made of long chains of the sugar glucose joined up together and stored in the muscles and liver so that when your blood sugar levels get low, you have a quick, readily accessible source of glucose good to go. Glycogen is a bulky molecule and it attracts a lot of water, so along with the glycogen stores, you're storing a bunch of water. When you're dieting, exercising intensely, or not eating for long periods of time (like overnight), glycogen is burned to help keep your blood sugar levels from falling too low. So, in diet mode, you can end up using up some of your glycogen reserves, and all the water that was associated with it. This makes it seem like you're doing great on your diet and you keep feeling jazzed; it gives you the bump of encouragement you need to keep going.

Next you're in a negative calorie balance (burning more than you eat) and you start to break down protein (from muscles) and fat to make sure you can carry out critical biological functions (remember your calorie *needs* haven't really changed, just how much you're feeding your body). You'll lose a bit more weight.

Then, your body gets the memo that food is in short supply; food is scarce. Evolutionary mechanisms to get you off your butt and go forage for food kick in. Your appetite changes; a wider variety of foods start to sound good.[7] Four-day-old stale bread? Sure, sounds *delicious*. A complicated cascade of neurotransmitters and hormones get triggered, sending signals to your brain telling you to eat. That can manifest as cravings for really specific foods or just a really general hunger. I remem-ber doing a stupid juice cleanse once and so desperately wanting to chew food; that ended up with me diving head-first into chocolate cake.

This is where things can start to fall apart. If you manage to ride out the hunger and the cravings for long enough, you might start to notice that your weight loss plateaus. This is because your body is making adjustments to compensate for the new lower energy intake. It can't differentiate a diet from genuine food shortage or scarcity, so it makes adaptions. Metabolic processes slow down.[8,9] It becomes more efficient at extracting every calorie out of food. You end up needing to eat even less to maintain the new weight loss.[10] Your body will do whatever it needs to do in order to defend your weight because that's what evolution favours – not people who rot away after a few days of no food. You are a product of hundreds of thousands of years of natural selection and evolution, which is a pretty cool bragging point, but I digress.

Back to the diet. You've plateaued, you are frustrated, and then you say 'fuck it'. You have a bad day, an argument with your boyfriend or your mum, your boss is a dick, or maybe you start your period. Dieting, after all, is stressful: research has shown that if you're just restricting energy intake, in and of itself, and eating whatever you want (à la macro counting), you may have a raised cortisol level. While straight up restricting food groups is associated with a higher stress load,[11,12] add on your usual life stress, and your ability to keep your shit together will be totally compromised. You end up having a huge blow-out. What might feel subjectively like a binge leaves you feeling guilty and anxious. Like a failure. So you start the restriction and exercise again the next morning and the cycle continues.[13,14,15]

Here's the thing, though. YOU are not a failure. Your body's just doing what it needs to do. The diet failed you, *you did not fail the diet.*

THE DIET CYCLE
—

This is how we get stuck in the diet cycle, a constant battle with your body. Maybe it's a slim-down for summer, a wedding, a class reunion, your TV debut, or just because you feel unhappy with something else in your life. The effects are the same: a vicious cycle; rinse and repeat. Dieting then becomes yo-yo dieting, or weight cycling if you wanna be fancy.

Over twenty years ago researchers reviewed the 'adverse medical, metabolic, and psychological health outcomes linked to weight cycling'. They found that weight cycling is associated with higher mortality (death rate), higher risk of osteoporotic fractures and gallstone attacks, loss of muscle tissue, hypertension (high blood pressure), and chronic inflammation.[16] Not to mention disordered eating, lower self-esteem and self-worth, and more emotional distress and emotional eating. Dieting is also a risk factor for weight gain in the long term. Not that there's anything wrong with gaining weight, it's a normal part of life, which we'll discuss in more detail in chapter 5, but it underscores the futility of dieting. Dieting and weight cycling may also be associated with more visceral adipose tissue – the type of fat that accumulates in your abdomen and is thought to be associated with type-2 diabetes, heart disease, breast cancer, colorectal cancer and Alzheimer's disease.[17] This is in contrast to subcutaneous adipose tissue, which is spread more evenly around our bodies (hips, thighs,

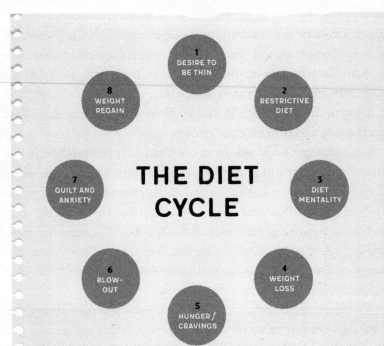

THE DIET CYCLE

1 DESIRE TO BE THIN
2 RESTRICTIVE DIET
3 DIET MENTALITY
4 WEIGHT LOSS
5 HUNGER/ CRAVINGS
6 BLOW-OUT
7 GUILT AND ANXIETY
8 WEIGHT REGAIN

1 A new diet or 'lifestyle' is usually pretty exciting, you're pumped about becoming the version of you you always wanted to be. And if you're being totally honest, that's probably something to do with changing the shape/size of your body.

2 So you follow all the rules: HIIT four times a week plus a couple of yoga classes to keep you chill. You ditch gluten, dairy, sugar and anything 'processed'.

3 You become hyper-vigilant of food choices, carefully pick which restaurant to eat at, compulsively check labels, track activity/calories/macros/whatever.

4 You start to see some changes in your body and feel encouraged.

5 But the cravings start to kick in and you can't keep up with the exercise.

6 You end up saying 'fuck it' and eat all the food.

7 You feel shitty about all the food.

8 You might gain back a little weight. So, you're back at the start – the restrict/blow-out cycle continues. Maybe next time you try Whole 30 or Paleo. You convince yourself that THIS is the one that will stick, but the cycle goes around and around until you decide to break it.

Adapted from Lucy Aphramor.[18]

arms etc) in what is considered to be a much healthier distribution.[19] Visceral adipose tissue, in both fat and thin people, is considered to be the main determinant of health risk (compared to the relatively benign sub-cutaneous adipose tissue).[20]

But with the physiological and psychological risks associated with dieting, there's GOT to be a better way!

To summarize: body weight is defended by a powerful biological system that reacts to a negative energy balance by lowering metabolism and increasing hunger signals, so that you become a little bit obsessed with food and a wider range of foods taste good. So on one hand, your metabolism is slowing down and on the other, food is more and more appealing. And you have a complex cascade of hormones and neurotransmitters driving this phenomenon. It's not greed or lack of willpower. It's biology!

A meta-analysis (one of the best-quality studies we have) of 29 weight-loss studies revealed that on average, participants regained 77% of the weight they initially lost after five years.[21] But we have to bear in mind that's a *best*-case scenario. In science we generally only publish studies that have the most promising findings and those interventions are usually very structured with lots of support from a nutritionist, dietitian, nurse, or personal trainer.[22] The average person attempting weight loss at home might not have the same level of support. In other words we don't publish weight-loss studies where people don't lose weight, so the finding that participants regain 77% of their initial weight is likely to be higher! In fact, a more recent meta-analysis study from 2017 wanted to see how 'successful' dieting was in the wild, so they looked at the data from 11 randomized controlled trials and 14 observational studies of commercial meal-replacement, calorie-counting, or pre-packaged meal programmes.[23] They found that almost 60% of people who started a commercial weight loss programme (CWLP) such as Weight Watchers, Jenny Craig and Slimming World, were unable to meet their target weight-loss goal of 5%. Side note: these programmes are actually available on the NHS. WTAF? The authors of the study concluded that 'our research demonstrates that, although CWLP may help individuals to lose weight in the short term, the amount of weight lost is often not enough to be clinically meaningful'. If you were thinking of signing up to one of those programmes, you should know that the average cost per kilogram of weight lost at Weight Watchers was US$155, and US$424 for Jenny Craig. And bear in mind that you're paying top dollar just to gain the weight back in the long run, and probably feel shitty about it too.[24] So, only around 40% of people lose 5% of weight in the first place, and of those, almost 80% fail. Those aren't great stats.

THE BIGGEST LOSER
—

Do you remember that US TV show *The Biggest Loser*? The one where Gillian Michaels screams at everyone as a motivational tool for weight loss? Each year fifteen or so contestants are split into teams and they battle it out to lose the most weight over a thirty-week period. One by one they get knocked off and the last one standing (i.e. the one who lost the most weight) wins a butt load of cash. Invariably everyone loses a ton of weight; they have a team of trainers pushing their bodies to extremes with punishing exercise and strict nutrition plans. It would be hard not to lose weight under those conditions. Interestingly though, one team of scientists decided to see what happened *after* the show. You know, after the after. Did the participants' weight go back up? What about body fat? And how did it affect metabolism? Were there any long-term consequences or did the participants just live happily ever after?

As suspected, six years after initial weight loss, both weight and body fat rebounded back up to around the same level as before they started. However, their metabolism never recovered! The average metabolism for participants before they started the show was approximately 2,600kcal per day. That's the average energy they spent on general metabolic processes like breathing, digestion, fuelling their brains and keeping their hearts beating, and maintaining their current weight. Six years later, they were only spending approximately 1,900kcal to do the same thing, even though their weight had gone back up (contrary to what people assume, larger people burn more calories than smaller people). Scientists estimated that their metabolism was 500kcal LESS than would be expected (they assumed metabolism would have increased as weight was regained, but that wasn't the case).[25]

Obviously this is a pretty extreme example, and a very small sample size (there were only sixteen participants tested and they acted as their own control, rather than having a separate control branch). That said, it does seem to suggest that dieting can irreversibly lower your metabolism. One of the study's authors, Kevin Hall, had this to say: 'Metabolism appears to act like a spring, the more effort you exert to lose weight, the more it stretches out, and the harder it will spring back, regaining and holding onto the fat that was lost.'[26]

Michael Rosenbaum, Professor of Paediatrics and Medicine at Columbia University Medical Center in New York puts it this way:

> Your body is working to defend your energy stores – really your fat mass. When that fat mass is diminished (either by eating less or exercising more) most of us respond by changes in brain circuitry that increase our tendency to eat and changes in neural and endocrine systems, and especially muscle, that make us more metabolically efficient – it costs fewer calories to do the same amount of work.[27]

This is why diets don't work. But this isn't news. We've known this for over seventy years.

THE MINNESOTA STARVATION EXPERIMENT
—

During WWII, an early nutrition researcher named Ancel Keys wanted to understand the implications of food rationing and semi-starvation. He got together a group of thirty-six healthy men who were conscientious objectors but who wanted to help with the war effort. They were started out on a 3,200kcal diet – pretty typical for young, active men – for twelve weeks.

Then their calories were slashed in half and food was restricted until they were essentially in a semi-starved state for six months. The men were receiving 1,600kcals' worth of food a day (which is more generous than most diets, tbf) and the researchers found that:

- Their metabolic rate decreased by 40%
- The men were obsessed with food – one dude wrote an entire cookbook during the time of the study
- Several men failed to adhere to their diet and reported episodes of bulimia
- Some men stole food and binged
- Some men exercised deliberately to obtain more food rations
- The men's behaviour changed and there was an onset of apathy, irritability, moodiness, and depression – sound familiar?

Anyone who has experienced any level of disordered eating has an idea of what those guys were going through. We also have to remember that these men weren't being bombarded with the same pressures to lose weight and diet culture that we are today, and we can speculate that would only add to their frustrations and obsessions with food.[28]

THE SIDE EFFECTS OF

DIETING

THAT NO ONE EVER TALKS ABOUT

- BINGEING
- SLOWED METABOLISM
- LOSS OF MUSCLE MASS
- REBOUND WEIGHT GAIN
- FOOD OBSESSION
- DISORDERED EATING
- LOSS OF YOUR INNATE HUNGER AND FULLNESS CUES
- SHAME, GUILT, AND ANXIETY WHEN THEY INEVITABLY FAIL

Side effects of diets include:

● **Slower metabolism:** Your body can't tell dieting apart from actual food scarcity and starvation, so to compensate for the shortage of calories your metabolism slows to try and conserve energy. You become more efficient at doing more with less. In other words, your body becomes really good at storing fat.[29,30,31]

● **Overeating and bingeing:** Dieting leads to bingeing. It's science. Say you skip breakfast to try and be 'good'. Your brain is pissed. It sends out neurotransmitters and hormones like ghrelin and neuropeptide Y – both of which are super-potent orexigenics, meaning that they stimulate appetite. So as the day goes on, these guys build up, you give in (to your normal biological urge to eat) and once you pop you can't stop. Sound familiar? Yup.[32,33,34,35,36]

● **They undermine your own innate ability to recognize hunger and fullness:** Think about it; if you're following a diet plan down to the letter, you're relying on someone else to tell you what, when, and how much to eat. THEY DON'T KNOW YOUR LIFE. I never give clients diet plans.* Who am I to say when they're hungry and what they're hungry for? We'll explore how to tune in to your body's cues in chapter 4.

● **Relying on someone else to tell you what to do can so easily result in eating too much or too little:** Let's say you're doing one of the points systems. You've used up all your points for the day, but you're still hungry. You either go hungry or you beat yourself up for going over. Neither of them sound like good options to me. Likewise, if you have some points left over, you're probably not going to let them go to waste, even though you're not hungry.

* A big caveat to the 'no meal plans' is for people recovering from severe restrictive eating disorders, in which case a meal plan is essential for nutritional rehabilitation until weight is restored.

- **Rebound weight gain:** Your weight can go up higher than your original weight – I mean, doy! How many people do you know who've sustained weight loss over long periods of time? Now how many of those people are content and not furiously counting calories or going 'beast mode' at the gym? Right, so everyone else is probably heavier than their original weight and feeling pretty shitty about that (because that's what society has decided they should feel), and now they're trying to figure out the next diet they're going to attempt.
- **Food obsession:** You can't stop thinking about your next meal, when you're allowed to eat again, you spend hours picking out recipes on Pinterest and trawling Instagram for #foodporn, figuring out how you can make 'healthy' gluten-free, sugar-free, low-cal substitutions. You have no mental bandwidth left for living your life.
- **Deprivation backfires:** You know when you were a kid and your mum told you not to do the thing, so you did the thing? Yeah. I see this all the time with my clients. They say certain foods are off limits, foods they enjoy eating but deem 'bad'. They do without it instead of satisfying their craving for it. Next thing they know, they're shoulder deep into a bucket of Phish Food, feeling sick and guilty. And the next morning you're skipping breakfast to 'make up' for it. Rinse and repeat.

BUT IT'S NOT A DIET, IT'S A LIFESTYLE!

—

As we've already seen, over the past five or so years, the focus has shifted away from overt dieting towards 'wellness' and 'health'. Clean eating, gluten-free, sugar-free, dairy-free, whole food plant-based, and the rest, all claim to be lifestyles not diets. But when we compare them with the diet checklist, they're still giving us rules about what, when, or how much to eat and the subtext is usually about weight loss. Almost all the clients I see have bought into one of these lifestyles at some point after they realized traditional diets didn't work for them anymore. But if we are totally honest with ourselves, these lifestyles have more to do with control (of food, of body) than with health and are predicated on food restrictions and fears.

'IT'S ABOUT ABUNDANCE, NOT RESTRICTION'

—

This is classic wellness garbage. Bloggers and Instagram gurus claim their lifestyle is about all the things you *can* have, and by focusing on all the whole, 'unprocessed' foods and abundance of organic grass-fed nutribollocks you can have, you won't feel restricted or deprived. And somehow, miraculously, you will stop thinking about food and live your best life.

There are no words to describe this level of absurdity; any time you cut out a food group, you are restricting yourself. It creates a **scarcity mindset** and a sense of deprivation. You are placing that food on a pedestal and saying 'I can't have that' or 'that is a bad food', even if it's subconsciously or just on an emotional level. Restriction and deprivation almost always backfire in one or more of the following ways:

- in the form of food obsessions and food preoccupation
- eating past the point of comfortable fullness
- eating 'bad' foods with a sense of urgency and intensity
- binge eating

- trying to compensate for eating 'bad' foods through exercise or further restrictions
- feeling a sense of guilt, shame, or anxiety about eating 'bad' foods, or even just not eating as 'well' or as 'optimally' as you could
- perpetuating the binge/restrict cycle
- generally feeling weird around food
- having no mental bandwidth left to think about and focus on more important life stuff

Eating shouldn't come with rules; it's not a game, it's not something to be mastered and conquered. It's a tool for helping us lead happy, fulfilling lives. But when our eating is wrapped up in food rules, restrictions, deprivation, and good and bad foods, it feels the exact opposite of living a happy fulfilling life.

THERE IS NO SUCH THING AS A PERFECT DIET

—

All the nutrition gurus will make you think that there's a perfect way of eating: 'Just follow my rules and you'll look and feel great; the happiest, healthiest, hottest version of you.' But these claims are pretty much entirely fabricated, or at least based on a sample of one; they're anecdotes at best. We're going to take a closer look at specific food myths in chapter 7 but for now, what you need to know is that there's no such thing as a perfect diet, and people can thrive on a variety of foods and eating patterns. Through intuitive eating, you get to figure out what works for you, and that might look totally different from anyone else around you. You could have the 'healthiest' diet ever, but if you don't have a healthy relationship to food, then it's not really that healthy, is it? A recent meta-analysis (the highest level of evidence that we have available) suggests that anxiety can increase the risk of type-2 diabetes.[37] If you have food rules that make you feel stressed out, anxious, or guilty around food then it's probably not great for you. Likewise, if you have to engage in restriction and disordered eating to maintain your weight, then it's not the weight your body is naturally comfortable at.

Dieting or pseudo-dieting is bad for you and there's solid science to back that up. But when you've pretty much spent your whole life on a diet or pseudo-diet, it's tough to break the habit. Learning how to recognize and reject diet culture (in all its subtle guises) will help you break the diet cycle.

THE PROBLEM WITH DIET MENTALITY

—

Diet mentality is the tether between diet culture and our eating habits. When we receive messages about health or thinness through the lens of diet mentality, the outcome is disordered eating and exercise patterns. The diet mentality is antithetical to intuitive eating. It's impossible to eat according to your biological hunger and fullness signals if you're also monitoring carbs and calories or invested in the outcome of weight loss. But changing the mindset of a lifetime can be slow and arduous; I don't want you to freak out if you are having a lot of diet mentality thoughts, that's totally normal in the beginning of the IE process. Acknowledge that they are there and gently let them go. In the diet mentality we often measure our progress in terms of concrete numbers, points, calories, and pounds. How we feel about ourselves is dictated by how well we've stuck to 'the plan'.

Instead of measuring progress in terms of weight lost or calories burned, or even how you look, put weight concerns to the side and begin to trust that biology will work itself out. Start to think of progress in terms of moving away from the diet mentality, learning to trust yourself with food, letting go of the idea of messing up around food, and beginning to recognize your hunger and fullness cues. Sounds easy but it will take time, there's a lot of shit to undo. Be gentle on yourself; this isn't yet another thing to beat yourself up about. Try to recognize when you're using diet mentality thinking; are you acting on those thoughts or can you check yourself and see if you can reframe it as non diet mentality thinking? This is a subtle mindset shift that can have a big impact on how we feel about ourselves.

Diet mentality	Intuitive eating
MOVEMENT + EXERCISE	
I go hard at the gym to make up for food I've eaten.	I exercise and move my body because it feels good, makes me feel energized, and helps me cope with stress, helps me sleep well, makes me feel stronger, helps me move more easily in my body.
I feel guilty if I skip a workout.	I exercise because it makes me feel like a badass.
I work out mostly to burn calories.	I exercise because it helps my mental health.
FOOD + EATING	
I deserve this.	Am I hungry?
I've earned this.	Do I want this?
It's my cheat day.	Will this taste good?
Diet starts tomorrow!	Will I enjoy it?
I need to eat clean/real.	I deserve to enjoy eating without guilt!
I'll work this off at the gym.	I need to eat to survive regardless of whether I've been to the gym.
This is unhealthy	There's no such thing as a perfect diet

HOW TO BREAK DIET MENTALITY

—

I'm going to level with you; this will be really hard for you to lock down because we are all living in diet culture. That means that breaking diet mentality is that bit more difficult; it's kind of an ongoing process where you constantly have to recognize and protect yourself from the diet culture BS. It can be especially hard to recognize when it's dressed up under the guise of health too, so be careful and ask yourself: is this really about health or is it about looking a certain way?

Step 1: Recognize that diets do more harm than good

If you ever feel yourself being tempted by a diet, go back and read the section on the side effects of dieting (see page 81) to remind yourself of the psychological and physiological aspects of dieting that are so damaging. I want you to think back to your own relationship with food and any attempts to control your weight or restrict your food.

Step 2: Get MAD AS HELL about the lies diet culture sells you

How much time do you think you've wasted worrying about your weight, your appearance, the food you eat, the food you don't eat, the exercise you 'should' be doing, tracking calories in MyFitnessPal, or on your Fitbit, or calculating macros? Now think about all of the money you've spent on chia, coconut sugar and spirulina, on the clean-eating cookbook franchises, for spin classes that make you want to pass out, and that spiralizer that's growing cobwebs? How much of that stuff actually made you happy versus how much was making you anxious and obsessive about every calorie that passed your lips?

Take a minute to GET MAD AS HELL at diet culture and the pursuit of 'wellness'. Eventually you'll be able to laugh it up as you become more resilient to the messages, but it's OK to feel pissed off too!

ACTIVITY

Draw or write out a timeline of your relationship with food.

In your journal write (or draw) a timeline of your relationship with food, dieting, over exercise and under exercise, restricting, bingeing, purging behaviour or laxative abuse, or other disordered behaviours. Think about how these things may or may not have coincided with life events (for example: puberty, parents' divorce, getting married, having a baby, a death in the family, going to university, a new job or moving house, job or financial worries). Think about your parents' attitudes towards food, dieting, and exercise. Did you have off-limits or bad foods? Was food used as a reward? Did family or relatives comment on your eating habits or physical appearance? Was food always available or did you live with the threat of not having enough to eat?

This is usually a very complicated story but reflecting on it can help us draw parallels between these early experiences and our current behaviours. Reflect on your timeline and answer the following questions in your journal. This can be an emotionally challenging activity, so only do it if it feels comfortable and have some self-care practices lined up for afterwards, such as checking in with your support system.

- Do you think these early habits and experiences led to feeling weird around food as an adult?
- To what extent do our parents help shape our relationship to food?
- What are your memories of dieting or trying to control your weight as a child/teen?
- Did your parents place restrictions on what/how much you could eat?
- Was food freely available when you wanted it?
- Was there always enough food to go round?
- Do you remember your parents dieting or having body issues?
- Did they, or other people in your family, comment on your body shape or size?
- Did any of your siblings or relatives suffer from an eating disorder?

Step 3: Ditch the diet tools

Diet tools can keep us tethered to the diet mentality so we'll work at slowly phasing them out. This can feel like a big scary step, but trust me, it's so, SO liberating. If you feel ready to go for it, then go ahead and delete MyFitnessPal, take off the Fitbit/calorie tracker, ditch the scales. Throw out diet books and meal plans (or just donate to charity). Try and catch yourself if you're compulsively checking the calorie information on labels. Ditch your Weight Watchers membership.

If that feels like too much for now, take it slow. Write down a list of your diet tools in your journal in order from most scary to give up to least scary. Tackle them one at a time when you feel ready or have more confidence, starting with the least scary and working your way up. These tools can feel like a comfort blanket, so if ditching them one at a time feels more comfortable for you, then do it that way instead.

Side note: a lot of people tell me that they have a calorie/activity tracker like a Jawbone or whatever, but they don't actually use it. Like it's just there but they never *actually* check it. This is usually given as a weird justification for why they should keep it. My response is this: great! Then you shouldn't have any problem getting rid. Trust me, if it's there, you're using it. Plus, if it makes you feel a bit weird about not having it, that's a pretty good sign that you need to back off for a while. Here's the thing: if you take it off for a bit while you're trying to break the diet mentality, it will always be there if you want to go back to it. From experience though, activity trackers usually trigger the diet mentality, even if it's in a subtle way. Try it for a while and see how it goes.

Step 4: Throw yourself an unfollow party

In other words, take control of your digital environment and unfollow people who are pushing diet culture or diet mentality. I have Instagram in mind here, but really it applies to all social channels as well as media you consume IRL. I've made a quick list of things to look out for that are pseudo body positive or just straight up replacing the word 'clean' with 'real'. I see a lot of talk on social media about balance

ACTIVITY

Get yourself a copy of a glossy/fashion/health mag and start to literally tear or cut out anything that could be conceived as diet culture. This will help you learn to spot it, push back and resist, rather than internalize it as something you should actually care about. This could be:

- 'healthy alternatives' – we'll discuss why these are problematic later, but think sweet potato brownies or raw cheesecake instead of the real deal
- diet foods – rice cakes, zero-calorie noodles, 0% fat yoghurt
- 'swap this for that' calorie reductions. I remember once seeing the suggestion that you swap tablespoons of almond butter for some apple sauce and slivered almonds – IN WHAT WORLD ARE THOSE THE SAME THING?
- meal plans
- diet and weight-loss ads
- surgical and beauty ads
- body-shaming
- lack of diversity in bodies
- anything with an unrealistic aesthetic goal that involves engaging in extreme or disordered behaviours
- headlines that shame or vilify certain foods

How much of the magazine was left once you removed all the diet culture?

but when I look at these meals they're 90% protein with a side of broccoli. What else would you add to this list?

- Promote balance – but don't eat any damn carbs
- Shame certain foods or vilify food groups
- Push unrealistic body standards or unhealthy levels of exercise (for fitness models/regular models, remember it's their job to look a certain way, not yours)
- Use any of the diet or pseudo-diet buzzwords
- Say you have to earn food by working out or you deserve to eat because you've been 'good'. Spoiler – you never, ever have to earn the right to eat, ever
- Post pseudo body-positive pictures that maybe don't acknowledge their own thin privilege or genetic advantages
- Send out confusing or conflicting messages
- Include anything that makes you feel badly about yourself
- Post transformation pictures suggesting that one body type is better than another (when people usually look pretty good in both!)
- Anyone promoting the 'perfect' diet or one diet over another
- Post about number of calories or macros in food

Here's a quick test: if you cover up the caption and it still looks like a #fitspo or #cleaneating pic, ditch it.

Conversely, I want you to start filling up your feed with accounts that are truly body and fat positive. Be careful of things that say 'real women have curves' or 'strong not skinny' because that's still trying to promote one body type over another – the point is there's no right or wrong way to have a body. Tall, short, fat, thin, curvy, muscular, soft, with scars and stripes – it's all good. In the Resources section at the back of the book I have included some accounts I think are great, go check them out; which ones would you add to this list?

A little warning though; people have a tendency to gravitate towards 'barely' plus-size models, and while this might be a good stepping stone, it's easy to forget that these people are still models, and so what they share may still be unrealistic standards. If you find yourself comparing your body to theirs, then it's gotta go. Try following accounts that push you outside of your comfort zone and make sure your feed is truly diverse and representative; this can help challenge any internalized fat phobia. Or just take a break from looking at bodies altogether and follow some dogs or memes or something. Remember that body positivity doesn't just mean loving your own body (although that's part of it). It means accepting and being positive towards ALL bodies.

Step 5: Call out the diet culture BS

Have a little code word you use with your friends or your partner or even just with yourself. When you see something that promotes diets or diet culture, call it 'DCBS', or say 'diets are for dicks', anything that reinforces that diets are trouble. I usually see a lot of diet-culture ads on the Tube, especially around January and as summer gets closer. If I see a Kardashian promoting protein powder or anything claiming there's a good way to lose weight, I snap a pic on Instagram stories and vent to my followers that it's DCBS. It's good to remind yourself, and others, that these things are rarely the solution.

Step 6: Give yourself a break

Seriously, this shit is hard to let go of, most of us have twenty-plus years of diet-culture programming to undo, so go easy on yourself. It will take time, and it's hard! Check out the self-compassion exercises in the next chapter to help you learn how.

How to deal with office diet chat

A lot of clients tell me how they're loving this whole intuitive eating approach, they've cleaned up their social media, they've ditched the dieting tools, but they can't get away from the diet chat. I've set up a free Facebook group for people who are learning to be cool around food to come and vent and share resources. It's a super-helpful escape and a supportive community. But how do you handle people IRL who won't shut up about their new diet? Here are my favourite tips.

1 Flat out ignore it, pretend like you didn't hear it and carry on the conversation with something relevant/interesting.

They say: 'I'm not having that, I'm trying to be good.'

You say: 'I have exciting plans* for my life this weekend.'

(*insert cool exciting plan that doesn't revolve around dieting)

2 Tell them all the reasons why diets don't work – that dieting slows down their metabolism so they have to eat even less to maintain their new lower weight. Or remind them that all the weight will pile back on – kind of a dick move, I don't actually recommend this, but it's a fun thought experiment you can do in your head while you remind yourself that you're glad you're not in that headspace anymore.

3 Stop them in their tracks. Hit them with a comment about how you're loving this new intuitive eating and non-diet book that you're reading. It helps you tune in to your body's natural hunger and satiety cues and allows you to have a healthier relationship with food. A good phrase to memorize is: 'I don't worry about what I eat anymore, I just eat in accordance with my body's natural appetite and I really like how freeing it is.'

4 Tell them to STFU: this takes a bit of cojones, but essentially you politely (or not) ask them to keep their diet chat to themselves as it's derailing your own efforts to move away from diets and towards intuitive eating.

Personally I like number 3. If you can be excited and enthusiastic about this new approach that is free from diets, talk about how you're learning to tell how full you are, and you're looking forward to eating what you want when you want and bust out of diet prison. And remember that it's OK to prioritize your mental health: if people are all up in your shit with their diet talk, you can walk away for some breathing space, excuse yourself and go to the bathroom, take a quick walk, or go get a coffee. If they are close friends or family, you can try and have an honest conversation about how you find their diet talk derailing and would they mind not talking about it in front of you? This is especially helpful if it's someone who you're particularly close to and need them to understand how you're feeling. If they are a good friend, they should be understanding and supportive, and, hey, maybe it's something they want to get involved with too. I've found that dieting is often a distraction for something deeper going on. Perhaps your friend is really signalling that they could use your friendship and are using diet chat as a way to connect. You can also show them the chart of the side effects of diets.

It's tough, and this is exactly why I wanted to write this book and build the community around my podcast (*Don't Salt My Game*) and the Facebook group, because sometimes people out there just don't get it and you need somewhere to escape to. Search 'Just Eat It' on Facebook to join the free community and get help on your IE journey.

DIETING EXPECTATION VS REALITY

———

As you go through the process of intuitive eating, it's pretty normal to second-guess whether or not you should try one last diet. As you learn to make peace with food, and that all foods are equal, you might feel like you're overeating or out of control, and maybe even gaining weight. It becomes tempting to think that a diet will be the solution: maybe if you just lose Xlb you'll be happy with your body and THEN you can give this intuitive eating thing a go. But here's the thing.

Dieting doesn't fix poor body image. It doesn't heal your relationship with food.

A lot of clients tell me that they were really good at dieting, it was 'successful', and they lost a lot of weight. I ask them, at what price? Were they engaging in disordered behaviours? Did it make them happy? Did their relationships improve? Usually the answer is: yes, no, no.

ACTIVITY

It's helpful to take a second to reflect on where dieting has got you in the past and to make a list of the reality of dieting in your intuitive eating journal. Does it cause you to get obsessive about food and body image? Do you cut out on seeing your friends for dinner or drinks? Do you put your life on hold waiting for the day you reach that elusive dress size. Does it make you cranky and miserable?

Expectation	vs	Reality
e.g. Will be very good and follow diet to a T		e.g. Felt restricted and deprived and over-ate 'bad' foods

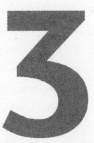

SELF-COMPASSION AND SELF-ACCEPTANCE

—

Something that's critical to the intuitive eating process is developing self-compassion. In intuitive eating, you can't 'mess up'. There's no bandwagon to fall off. There's nothing to fuck up. Unless you try and make IE into a weight-loss diet, you can't do it 'wrong'. It's all just a learning experience, right? But clients tell me a lot that they feel like they've screwed up or they're not doing it right; particularly if they're a bit of a perfectionist or have a tendency to want to control things.

People often come into clinic wanting to totally nail this intuitive eating thing. They want to get an A, get the blue ribbon. But guess what? You're not going to get a certificate at the end of reading this book. You may even get to the end, let it percolate for a while, and then come back to some of the principles. It's not a race and it's important not to blow through the concepts without letting them fully sink in. If you try and rush to the end, you can end up undermining the whole process. I can pretty much guarantee that you'll want to bookmark this page now, because the whole IE process kind of hinges on self-compassion. Being able to give yourself a break when things feel challenging will make the whole thing that bit easier.

Remember, intuitive eating is a process of discovery, a set of tools to help you figure out what works best for your body. Hitting hurdles along the way, although super-annoying, is all part of the process. The difference is how we react and respond to the little bumps and detours; do we berate, blame, and self-criticize ourselves? Or do we meet it with a little self-compassion and understanding? Because chances are you will inevitably faceplant into a tub of Ben & Jerry's at some point, so how do you react to that? Do you beat yourself up or treat yourself with the warmth and compassion of a good mate? Because let's face it, ice cream is delicious and it's normal to want to eat lots of it! Learning simple self-compassion techniques can help us mindfully and non-judgementally examine the situation, without the critical voice that might just exacerbate the problem.

Do you know the Disney-Pixar movie *Inside Out*? It's for kids, but there are definitely some lessons in there for adults too. The premise is that there are a handful of emotions, each represented by a colourful character, at the control centre of a child's mind. These personified emotions (Joy, Sadness, Anger, Disgust, and Fear) are responsible for helping their human, a little girl named Riley, navigate her way through the turbulence of moving cities and schools. The movie portrays what happens when one emotion overrides all the others; in this case Joy tries to bully Sadness into submission, deeming the emotion of sadness to be too painful to be part of a 'core' memory. It then describes the catastrophe of letting one emotion dominate and prevent the other emotions from being expressed and doing their jobs; by the end of the movie the characters learn that *all* emotions are valuable and have an important role to play in helping people navigate life.

I like to use this analogy when I talk to my clients about self-judgement. Obviously, our emotions are much more complicated than just a core few, but the result is the same. For many of my clients, their control centre is dominated by a judgey, critical, tyrannical brute who leaves no space for self-acceptance or self-compassion; it's like a relentless Twitter troll who lives in your brain. This results in a downward spiral of self-flagellation, which can lead to excessive self-criticism, self-hatred, and even depression and anxiety.

One antidote to this is self-compassion, which at first may sound self-indulgent, but is in fact an important facet of living a fulfilling life. I know it sounds woo-woo, but just stick with me, OK? There's some solid science behind it.

Self-compassion is simply compassion directed inwards. Just as we can feel compassion for the suffering of other people or animals, we can extend compassion towards ourselves when we experience suffering, regardless of whether the suffering resulted from external circumstances or from our own mistakes, failures, and personal fuck-ups. First up, self-compassion means being in touch with our own suffering, not dodging it, hiding or disconnecting from it. It also means offering ourselves kindness to help reduce the experience of suffering. Self-compassion also involves offering non-judgemental understanding of your pain, and perceived inadequacies and failures, so that your experience is seen as part of the larger human experience.

According to researcher and Professor of Psychology at UT Austin, Kristin Neff, there are three domains of self-compassion:

Self-kindness: This refers to our ability to treat ourselves gently and kindly, as we might with a friend. For many of us, when shit hits the fan, we have a tendency to internalize the blame and talk crap about ourselves. Dieting is a perfect example of this: think back to a time when you've been on a diet or pseudo-diet and then 'fallen off the wagon'; how have you responded? Did you ruminate on all the things you *could* or *should* have done better; like I *should* have meal-prepped better or I *could* have said no to dessert at dinner last night. This can lead to feelings of stress and frustration. Or do you treat yourself more like a friend would and cut yourself some slack: 'Diets are fucking miserable, and don't work, and you're great just the way you are.' In other words, do you build yourself up, comfort and soothe yourself, or tear yourself down and trash-talk yourself? The latter undermines our ability to self-soothe and comfort ourselves when we're in pain and in need of care.

Common humanity: The second tenant of self-compassion has to do with our shared experience with other people. To put it into terms relevant to this book, *everyone has weird shit going on with food*. OK, maybe not *everyone*, but it's certainly a lot of people. However, because we don't really talk about our weird shit, we rarely consider that other people are also struggling with their relationship to food, exercise, or body image. As Neff puts it: 'All humans are flawed works-in-progress; everyone fails, makes mistakes, and engages in dysfunctional behavior. All of us reach for things we cannot have, and have to remain in the presence of difficult experiences that we desperately want to avoid.' [1]

When we take a myopic view, we get it in our heads that everyone else is *nailing it*: diets, exercise, relationships, parenting, career, spirituality, creativity, life in general. But literally no one has all their shit together, at least not all of the time. Remind yourself that everyone has ups and downs, and that the intuitive eating process is no different. I don't mean to freak you out by saying that, but to reassure you that you're not fucking it up. Self-compassion can help us feel less isolated when we are in pain, by recognizing our common humanity and shared experiences. We're all in this together.

Mindful awareness: Mindfulness speaks to our ability to witness emotions, thoughts, and sensations without judgement, avoidance, or repression. Why is this important in the context of self-compassion? Well, you need to be able to first of all recognize that you are suffering or in pain in order to give yourself compassion. An example I see of this is people who use food to 'numb out'. They use food to push down uncomfortable emotions. Sometimes this is an important coping mechanism (as we'll discuss in chapter 10) but if viewed without mindful self-compassion, we might miss the fact that emotional eating may be a symptom that something else is going on for us. Bringing a gentle awareness allows us to bear witness to our experience, even when it's uncomfortable. Mindfulness also prevents us from over identifying with a particular feeling or emotion to the point that we can no longer differentiate ourselves from our thoughts. 'That kinda sucks' becomes 'I suck'; 'that was disappointing' becomes 'I'm a disappointment'. Mindfulness allows us to examine our thoughts as simply that, thoughts. Not facts. That in turn can put a little distance between you and your thoughts so you don't over-identify with them.

Mindfulness: Informal mindfulness is available to us in any moment of any day; it means bringing our attention to thoughts, emotional experiences, and sensations in the body, non-judgementally.

Meditation: The formal practice of mindfulness that can help train our minds to help us cultivate mindfulness in our daily lives.

WHAT ARE THE BENEFITS OF SELF-COMPASSION?

OK, I get it, self-compassion sounds fairly spiritual and borderline new-age; I was pretty sceptical about the concept when I first came across it too. But the research around it is really interesting and pretty compelling; from an intuitive eating perspective, like I said, it can help us shut down that judgey, hyper-critical voice in our heads that tries to sabotage the IE process. If you ever feel like you're fucking things up with IE, then come back to this section. Do some self-compassion practice and see if that changes your outlook a little (don't worry, I'll teach you how!).

But what's also really exciting about self-compassion is that research is showing that it may also play a role in developing positive body image. For instance, women who are high in self-compassion experience less body shame and body surveillance, engage in less body comparison, and place less emphasis on appearance as an indicator of self-worth.[2,3] Self-compassion has also been shown to be a buffer between the thinness-related pressures from the media, and both thin ideal internalization and disordered eating. A recent systematic review found that self-compassion was consistently linked to lower levels of disordered eating and more positive body image.[4]

A cool study from Amy Slater's group (remember she is the appearance researcher we met in chapter 1) wanted to know if self-compassion messages could help attenuate some of the negative impact #fitspo images on Instagram might have on body image. They randomly assigned women to view fifteen images showing #fitspo, self-compassion, a #fitspo/self-compassion mash-up, or neutral images. The #fitspo images were what you'd expect: images of toned, fit bodies, wearing workout clothes; the self-compassion images were a self-love or body-positive quote on a patterned background. The neutral images were pictures of a beach and things like that. Viewing just the #fitspo images resulted in lower levels of self-compassion, but the women who viewed the self-compassion images showed increased levels of body satisfaction, body appreciation, self-compassion, and better mood, compared to the #fitspo group. Even the group who viewed #fitspo and self-compassion quotes together had better outcomes than just #fitspo alone.[5] Another study showed that just three weeks of self-compassion meditations led to greater reductions in body dissatisfaction, body shame, and self-worth based on appearance, as well as greater gains in self-compassion and body appreciation compared to a control group who didn't receive the intervention. In as little as three weeks you can begin to undo a lifetime's worth of diet-culture bullshit, and that's pretty cool.[6] Self-compassion may also help relieve guilt associated with eating, and help prevent disinhibited eating, or bingeing.[7,8]

Before we talk about how to put self-compassion into practice, let's first take a closer look at a component of self-compassion that's critical, not just to self-compassion but to the whole IE process: mindfulness.

WHY MINDFULNESS?

Look, I'm going to be straight up with you guys; I'm not some super-chill Zen master. Sometimes I meditate, sometimes I don't. Sometimes I'm mindful, other times my husband yells at me for paying too much attention to my phone and not listening to whatever it is he's saying. I know people have this icky stereotype of what a meditator is, like you have to light some incense and chant and sit cross-legged on a floor cushion. That's not really what it's about at all; for me it just means deliberately, but gently, focusing my awareness in the present moment, not ruminating on things that have happened in the past, or what may or may not happen in the future. It's about being in your flow (remember we talked about how self-objectification can disrupt your flow in chapter 1?). To me, it means being able to focus on what my friend is saying when she's having a tough time, and not drifting off thinking about what I'm doing that weekend. It means taking my headphones off and walking down the street, paying attention to the people, the trees, the buildings, the sky; don't get me wrong, I love listening to podcasts and music, but sometimes your brain just needs a little time out, to just be.

Like I said, I'm not some mindfulness guru, so I called in for back-up on this. Fiona Sutherland is an Accredited Practising Dietitian based in Melbourne, Australia, also known as @TheMindfulDietitian. Fiona is a lecturer at Deakin University, a yoga teacher, and a mindfulness and mindful-eating expert. I asked her what mindfulness is and she told me that Jon Kabat-Zinn, the founder of Mindfulness Based Stress Reduction (MBSR), the guy in mindfulness, describes mindfulness as: 'The awareness that arises through paying attention, on purpose, non-judgementally, in the service of understanding and wisdom.' She explained that it means being with our experience, just as it is, without criticizing it. Our experiences may be pleasant, unpleasant, or neutral, but they're usually somewhere in between all of those. Mindfulness allows us to be with our changing experiences with a sense of presence, acceptance, and openness.

People often think of mindfulness and meditation as a means to an end: to reduce stress or anxiety, or to be able to better cope with difficult emotions or situations. However, it's worth reminding yourself that mindfulness is, in and of itself, its own reward. Try and enjoy the practice of meditation in its own right, as opposed to a portal to transform you into some enlightened shaman. If you struggle with wanting to just get to the end so you can get the prize, then you can reframe it as simply ten minutes you're taking out of the day for yourself.

Mindfulness has been shown to increase self-acceptance; self-acceptance is defined as 'holding a positive regard for or attitude towards oneself as a whole, including one's past life experiences. Self-acceptance does not rely on the approval of others or personal achievements.' You're not going to be everyone's cup of tea, but self-acceptance can help you learn to be cool with who you are, without having to live up to anyone else's standards.[9] This can massively help with the IE process, so don't just brush it off, k?

According to the Oxford Mindfulness Centre, part of Oxford University, regular mindfulness practice can help manage depression (alongside other strategies, like medication, as recommended by your doctor), chronic physical conditions, including chronic pain and stress, and overall well-being.

THE SECOND ARROW OF SUFFERING
—

Building on the concept of self-compassion, let's further explore the idea of suffering. There is a Buddhist parable that goes like this:

'If you get struck by an arrow, do you then shoot another arrow into yourself?'

This refers to the fact that shit happens in life: the first arrow. It's inevitable that stuff will happen to us as we navigate our lives; sometimes it's annoying shit, sometimes it's painful shit, other times it's pleasant or happy shit. Pain is inevitable, but suffering is optional. Suffering is the second arrow that we inflict upon ourselves.

When shit goes down, we generally have two options: react or respond. When you get a notification on your phone, chances are you automatically reach for your phone, without thinking. It's like an impulse. Same as when you see a cute dog on the street, you don't hesitate to stop and pet that good boy. Reactivity is like a knee-jerk reaction, whereas responding to a stimulus means taking a beat, pausing, and considering how we want to respond. It's a more flexible way of perceiving, understanding, and behaving; it allows us to have options instead of reacting like a robot. This brief pause opens up space between the stimulus and the response, a moment to consider how or if we want to respond to that stimulus, rather than being on autopilot.

This space allows us to choose how we respond, instead of mindlessly reacting. Take the phone example. If we are reacting every time our phone pops off, it disrupts our flow, it challenges our concentration. By having a mindful pause, instead of compulsively checking our phone, we can decide if we want to engage with the phone or stay with our work, our friend or whatever else it is we're doing. This is where we can summon a little self-compassion if it's a 'shit hitting the fan' scenario. Otherwise, if it's just our phone, we can decide whether we pick it up and let ourselves be distracted from whatever it is we're doing, or if we actually want to pick up our phone and call a friend for a catch-up and some connection.

Let's see how this applies to intuitive eating. Picture the situation. You're super-busy at work, stressed about a deadline, and you've been in meetings all day. All you've managed to eat were a few biscuits set out on the conference table. You're going to get home late, way past dinner time. You're exhausted, and you know there's nothing in the house, so you order a pizza and it arrives just as you've changed out of your work clothes into your sweat pants. By this time you're so beyond hungry that you practically inhale the entire pizza, you're also engrossed in Netflix, and without even realizing you're rapidly heading towards the bottom of a pint of double-fudge-brownie ice cream. When you stop to catch a breath you notice that you now feel uncomfortably full and a bit sick. This is the first arrow. In this moment, you have two options: react or respond.

Reaction goes a bit like this: 'OMG, I'm such a disgusting sloth, I can't believe I hammered an entire pizza and half a tub of ice cream, I'm so gross and I feel so guilty. Tomorrow I'm going to do X, Y and Z to make up for it' and so on. The scenario may play on your mind for days afterwards.

Responding compassionately might go more like this: 'Wow, I was really hungry and have eaten past my point of comfortable fullness [mindful awareness]. I'm going through a lot right now, and don't have the time or energy to take care of myself the way I'd like to, but I'm doing the best I can right now [self-kindness], maybe tomorrow I can take a snack with me to make sure I don't let myself get too hungry at work. I know other people who comfort eat when they're really stressed out [common humanity].'

That momentary pause after the first arrow allows you enough space to intercept the second arrow with a moment of self-compassion. You get to unsubscribe from the suffering, guilt, angst, shame, and other negative emotions associated with eating more than is comfortable. Instead of percolating on what you might perceive as a slip-up, you can use this as an opportunity to show yourself some kindness, and be curious as to what else might be going on. We'll talk more about the 'what else' when we discuss emotional eating in chapter 10, but for now let's think about how we can put this stuff into action.

HOW DO YOU DO IT?

———

Let's start with mindfulness. We'll be applying mindfulness to other aspects of the IE process, so it's worth getting to grips with it now. The website Mindfulness.org is a cool resource, and they have kindly let me reproduce their 'getting started' guide here:

'Mindfulness is a natural quality that we all have. It's available to us in every moment if we take the time to appreciate it. When we practise mindfulness, we're practising the art of creating space for ourselves – space to think, space to breathe, space between ourselves and our reactions.'

Some things to consider before practising mindfulness:

1 **You don't need to buy anything.** You can practise anywhere, there's no need to go out and buy a special cushion or bench – all you need is to devote a little time and space to accessing your mindfulness skills every day.

2 **There's no way to quiet your mind.** That's not the goal here. There's no bliss state or otherworldly communion. All you're trying to do is pay attention to the present moment, without judgement. Sounds easy, right?

3 **Your mind will wander.** As you practise paying attention to what's going on in your body and mind at the present moment, you'll find that many thoughts arise. Your mind might drift to something that happened yesterday, meander to your to-do list – your mind will try to be anywhere but where you are. But the wandering mind isn't something to fear, it's part of human nature and it provides the magic moment for the essential piece of mindfulness practice – the piece that researchers believe leads

to healthier, more agile brains: the moment when you recognize that your mind has wandered. Because if you can notice that your mind has wandered, then you can consciously bring it back to the present moment. The more you do this, the more likely you are to be able to do it again and again. And that beats walking around on autopilot any day (i.e. getting to your destination without remembering the drive, finding yourself with your hand in the bottom of a chip bag you only meant to snack a little from, etc).

4 Your judgey brain will try to take over. The second part of the puzzle is the 'without judgement' part. We're all guilty of listening to the critic in our heads a little more than we should. (That critic has saved us from disaster quite a few times.) But when we practise investigating our judgements and diffusing them, we can learn to choose how we look at things and react to them. When you practise mindfulness, try not to judge yourself for whatever thoughts pop up. Notice judgements arise, make a mental note of them (some people label them 'thinking'), and let them pass, recognizing the sensations they might leave in your body, and letting those pass as well.

5 It's all about returning your attention again and again to the present moment. It seems like our minds are wired to get carried away in thought. That's why mindfulness is the practice of returning, again and again, to the breath. We use the sensation of the breath as an anchor to the present moment. And every time we return to the breath, we reinforce our ability to do it again. Call it a bicep curl for your brain.

While mindfulness might seem simple, it's not necessarily all that easy. The real work is to make time every day to just keep doing it. Here's a short practice to get you started:

How to practise mindfulness

1 Take a seat. Find a place to sit that feels calm and quiet to you. Set a time limit. If you're just beginning, it can help to choose a short time, such as five or ten minutes.

2 Notice your body. You can sit in a chair with your feet on the floor, you can sit loosely cross-legged, in lotus posture, you can kneel – all are fine. Just make sure you are stable and in a position you can stay in for a while.

3 Feel your breath. Follow the sensation of your breath as it goes out and as it goes in.

4 Notice when your mind has wandered. Inevitably, your attention will leave the sensations of the breath and wander to other places. When you get around to noticing this – in a few seconds, a minute, five minutes – simply return your attention to the breath.

5 Be kind to your wandering mind. Don't judge yourself or obsess over the content of the thoughts you find yourself lost in. Just come back.

That's it! That's the practice. You go away, you come back, and you try to do it as kindly as possible.

If you want to take things a little deeper, Fiona recommends that the best way to learn about meditation and mindfulness really depends on how you like to learn. I've summarized some suggestions in the table over the page but feel free to keep searching until you find something that's the right fit for you.

If you are a . . . type of learner	Try . . .	Like . . .
visual	YouTube channels	The School of Life
auditory	apps	Smiley Mind, Stop Breath Think, Headspace, Calm
	podcasts	Mindful 10% Happier
reading	websites	Mindful.org
	books	*Introducing Mindfulness: A Practical Guide* by Tessa Watt *Mindfulness: A Practical Guide to Finding Peace in a Frantic World* by Mark Williams and Danny Penman
hands-on	courses	Mindfulness Based Stress Reduction BeMindfulOnline.com

OK, now you've got the mindfulness thing locked down, let's talk about some ways to cultivate self-compassion. I'd recommend giving these activities some time to sink in before moving on to the next chapter. Starting a mindfulness practice from here on out can help you develop self-compassion and better body image, and help with IE. If you can, try to get into the habit of regular meditation, even 5 minutes a day will help. BUT, if it's not your bag, can it. No rules, remember; do what works for you. Try it, see how you like it, and go from there.

THE SELF-COMPASSION BREAK

(adapted from Kristin Neff)

The self-compassion break is a quick tool to pull out when you're in the midst of a difficult or challenging situation.* You can use it any time you need a little self-compassion. Think of a difficult situation or challenge you're facing; notice how placing your awareness on the situation feels in your body. It could be something stressful. You might feel anxious about letting go of food rules, for instance. Or it could be something unrelated to intuitive eating, like work or relationship worries. Visualize the situation until you notice discomfort in your body. Consider what happened, or what might happen, bring the situation to focus in your mind.

Now say to yourself:

- 'This is a moment of suffering' (mindful awareness of the fact that suffering is happening).
- 'This is really hard right now', or 'I'm really struggling' (we are acknowledging our suffering).
- 'Suffering is a normal part of life, and everyone suffers at some point in their lives' (common humanity).
- 'It's not abnormal to feel this way, many people are going through similar situations' (common humanity).

---

* If the situation is too painful or challenging for you to tackle alone, consider finding a therapist who can guide you through it and help you unpack difficult emotions.

Put your hands, one on top of the other, over your heart. Feel the warmth and gentle pressure of your hands on your chest, and notice it moving up and down with the breath. If you're not comfortable with putting your hands on your heart then place them somewhere comfortable on your body.

Now say something kind and compassionate to yourself:

- 'May I be kind to myself' (self-kindness).
- 'May I accept myself just as I am.'

For the last part, you can switch it up and use a phrase that resonates with you.

- May I forgive myself
- I'm here for you
- It's going to be OK
- I care about you
- May I be free from suffering
- May I safely endure this pain
- You've got this
- You're doing great

GIVE YOURSELF A PEP TALK

—

We are so great at lifting other people up when they are down. When our friends are in a rut, have been through a tough break-up, lost their job, or are just generally in a bad place, we remind them of how super fuckingcool they are. We list all of their amazing characteristics, skills, unique talents, accomplishments and remind them of why they are such a badass. We cannot seem to do the same thing for ourselves, however. Let's change that.

1 First of all, I want you to imagine a situation where your friend was having a really shit time. Imagine a specific friend and a specific scenario. In your journal, write out how you respond. List all the things you'd tell your friend to cheer her up. Imagine you are bringing your A-game. What do you say? How do you say it?

2 Now on the flip side, think of what you would typically say to

yourself in a similar situation. How do you talk to yourself? What's the tone? What type of language do you use?

3 Are there any differences between how you treat yourself and how you treat a friend? If so, why do you think that might be?

4 How do you think things might be different if you were to respond to yourself the way you do to a close friend who is suffering?

5 Now write yourself a pep talk in your journal. Write what you'd say to yourself if you were treating yourself the way you would someone who you love, care about, and admire. It might sound contrived, but just go with it.

GET YOU SOME INSPIRATIONAL QUOTES
—

A lot of my clients really like to use cute little mantras or inspirational quotes to whip out when they need to develop a little compassion for themselves. If this feels icky to you, can it. If mantras and quotes are your bag, then go for it. Even if they're not your bag, but the meditations and journal exercises aren't clicking for you – then just give this a shot, and see if it helps things shift. What I want you to do is go online and have a quick Google for some self-compassion/self-acceptance quotes that resonate with you. I don't care what they say, as long as they are in the vein of being kind and gentle and accepting of yourself. Once you've found a few that resonate with you, you have a few options:
- Write or draw them in your journal
- Use an app like Canva or WordSwag to create an image you can use as a background on your phone or post to your social media (see over page)[11]
- Create a Pinterest board
- Make it the screensaver or background on your computer

Self-compassion or acceptance doesn't just happen overnight, you have to keep working on it and revisiting it. Having these reminders around you will help reinforce the messages and get them into your head. Come back to them as often as you need to.

'Looking outside
of yourself for love
and acceptance
leaves your happiness
in the hands
of others'
Debra Beck

Self-esteem and self-acceptance

**Kimberley Wilson, Chartered Psychologist,
@foodandpsych:**

The psychologist Abraham Maslow developed a framework for understanding human motivation and personality development. Initially proposed in the 1940s and '50s, his 'Hierarchy of Needs' remains a clear and useful description of human psychology. The hierarchy is usually depicted as a pyramid. Moving from the bottom to the top, he proposed that individuals have certain needs that must be fulfilled before they can move on to the next level. So, starting at the bottom we all have basic physical and safety needs for air, food, water, sleep, health, and a roof over our heads etc. Without these things our basic survival is insecure and it is impossible to move on to the further levels of development.

The next two levels describe our psychological needs. First, we need to belong. We all need to know that we are loved, valued, and cared for. We need to know that there is someone thinking about us and to whom we can turn in times of need. The need for Love & Belonging is the psychological equivalent of having a roof over your head. It creates a sense of emotional safety that means you are not always looking over your shoulder or fighting to protect yourself. It frees us up to pursue higher psychological and social goals that help to enrich our lives.

Esteem is the level where many people get stuck and it is the main level that diet culture taps in to. Esteem is the knowledge that we are respected and valuable to others. Self-esteem is the

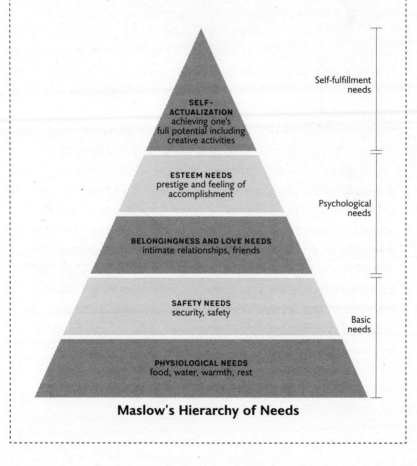

Maslow's Hierarchy of Needs

attitude that we have towards ourselves. Healthy, secure self-esteem develops from having a balanced view of our internal traits and characteristics. Are we kind, hardworking, thoughtful? Having good self-esteem is a predictor of future happiness, relationship success, achievement, and body satisfaction. It goes from the inside out.

Having good self-esteem means we are more likely to have a balanced and positive view of our own bodies. However, the messages of diet culture try to convince us that it is the other way around, trying to suggest that changing our appearance will make us feel better about ourselves. Diets and workout programmes are promoted as being able to create 'body confidence' and helping you to 'love yourself'.

But self-esteem doesn't work like that. It is a psychological not a physical need. Worth that is based only on what we look like is the most fragile foundation for self-esteem, and it cannot last. If we don't have a basic sense of our own worthiness as a person we will always find a fault with an aspect of our physicality. You'll try to twist and change yourself, certain that any moment now, maybe after the next few pounds, something will click and you will suddenly feel good about yourself. But it doesn't happen. It's not enough. It can't possibly be enough because self-esteem is internal.

Healthy self-esteem says 'I'm not perfect, but who is? I am a good person, and that is an important thing. I am loved for who I am. I have skills, talents, or interests that make me unique and the opportunity to use them.' Healthy self-esteem says that, irrespective of what your body looks like, you have something to offer and deserve to be respected.

How to get started (re)building self-esteem

1 First of all, if you have spent a long time being told by the world that your body, face, skin colour etc are not acceptable then it may take a little while to undo that damage and come to a place of self-acceptance. So try to be patient with yourself.

2 Often, poor self-esteem is linked to wishing the real self away. Wishing that we had inherited a different bone structure or metabolism. Wishing we were more outgoing. Wishing our faces met the current fashion for what is considered attractive. This wishing to be the things that we are not takes us away from accepting and appreciating the things that we are. We need to start there. This is my body. This is my body. This is who I am. This is me.

3 Similarly, it is important to allow other people to have their own bodies. What I mean is to stop telling yourself that someone else's body is in any way a reflection or comment on your own. If you see someone out or at the gym with a body you admire, try to catch yourself from thinking 'I wish I looked like that.' That is their body. They are allowed to look different to you. They are allowed to be who they are. It's not a competition.

The tools of IE are complementary to fostering healthy self-esteem (and vice versa). Hopefully, as you go along, you will find you are increasingly accepting of more and more aspects of yourself and your life. If you find you really struggle with your self-esteem it may be important to seek professional support to help you get through any psychological roadblocks.

DO YOUR GOALS ALIGN WITH YOUR VALUES?

—

Our values represent what's important and meaningful for us; clarifying our values can give us direction as to the qualities we want to embody, and how we want people to remember us. Our values can give us clues as to what we want our lives to stand for and how we show up for ourselves and others; the type of person we want to be. Values are what guide our behaviour on an ongoing basis. Values are directions we keep moving in, whereas goals are what we achieve along the way. We live in a society that rates achieving goals more than embodying qualities that align with our values. Getting the degree/job/house/car/partner/kids, hitting the milestones, checking the boxes. Sure, these things come with a temporary sense of accomplishment and happiness, but then it's on to the next goal and the next goal. This can lead to a sense of frustration and exhaustion from always striving for the next thing and the thing after that. Now, there's nothing inherently wrong with goals, and we all have things we want to accomplish, but can we do it in a way that aligns with our values? Might this make the actual process of attaining the goal more fulfilling and satisfying, rather than hinging on the outcome of a goal that you may or may not achieve? Let's use two examples: a goal that aligns with your values, versus one that doesn't.

ACTIVITY

In your journal, I want you to spend a few minutes writing or drawing out your values and what's important to you. These can be pretty much anything you want – there's no right or wrong answer. You can make the values bigger or smaller depending on how strongly you hold them, and give them shapes or colours. You can have as many as you like, but it might be helpful to focus on five or six core values. You can use the list opposite to help you, or do some research into different values if you're struggling to identify what they are for you.

Values: respect for myself and others, compassion, adventure, acceptance, humour, gratitude, acceptance, mindfulness

Unaligned goal: get shredded for summer – getting 'ripped' usually involves engaging in some sort of disordered behaviour, whether that's food or exercise – that's not kind or compassionate. It's also not particularly accepting of your current body. Also, what adventures might you be missing out on in order to pursue this goal?

Let's compare that with the goal of becoming an intuitive eater.

Aligned goal: becoming an intuitive eater is a compassionate and kind approach to honouring your health. It requires self-acceptance of where you are in your process, and allows you to be flexible in your eating so you can have adventures and not worry about what you will eat or if there will be a gym you can go to. It's also conducive to having a sense of humour, because you need to be able to not take yourself too seriously.

WHAT ARE YOUR

VALUES?

LOVE	CHALLENGE	PLEASURE
RESPECT	GRATITUDE	PERSISTANCE
KINDNESS	COOPERATION	HONESTY
COMPASSION	ACCEPTANCE	SELF-AWARENESS
HUMOUR	AUTHENTICITY	MINDFULNESS
FORGIVENESS	CURIOSITY	OPEN-MINDEDNESS
FUN	SERVICE	INDEPENDENCE
ADVENTURE	POISE	JUSTICE
PLAY	FAIRNESS	EQUALITY
CREATIVITY	SELF-CARE	COURAGE

Now write out some of your goals in the major areas of life (again these may be different for you, these are just some suggestions): **love** (close relationships, not just romantic ones), **career** (work/education), **play** (rest/relaxation/hobbies/creativity), **health** (mental, physical, spiritual).

Do your goals align with your values?

Can you adjust your goals to more closely align with your values?

Do your thoughts and behaviours align with your values?

Clarifying your values can help you understand if your current goals, behaviours, and thought patterns are authentic to you and reflect how you want to move through the world.

Side note: when I'm working with clients towards intuitive eating (their goal), they have a tendency to want to skip the process and jump straight to the end. Something that's helpful might be setting intuitive eating as your *long-term* goal; that way there's less temptation to get frustrated or try and force it. You can relax into the process more. If it's helpful, you might want to break your goals down into short-, mid- and long-term goals. Here's a suggestion, but you can make it whatever feels right to you. Just make sure you write it in your journal, and refer back to it when you need to.

Short-term goal: practise food neutrality

Medium-term goal: give myself unconditional permission to eat all foods

Long-term goal: work towards becoming an intuitive eater and supporting my health with gentle nutrition

HUNGER

Everyone on Instagram: 'Listen to your body.'
Me: 'Uhhhhh, how?'

All right, here we go, time to talk about food. Feeding ourselves should, in theory, be pretty simple. You get hungry, you eat something, and you get on with your life. But in our diet-obsessed culture, we think it's kinda OK to just ... not eat and pretend like we're 'not that hungry'. We are made to feel guilty and ashamed for giving our bodies nutrients and energy, either by other people or by ourselves.

Be real, how many times have you felt hungry but just ignored it? Or maybe you've choked back a can of Diet Coke or tried to pacify hunger with a coffee or a cup of tea? Maybe you've even taken up smoking? In my dieting days I'd be so hungry that I'd compulsively chew an entire pack of gum because eating food was basically a criminal offence. Some people have even told me they go to bed early to avoid hunger pangs.

But there's only one way to satisfy physical hunger: by eating food.

The thing that is as fundamental to our entire existence as breathing, sleeping, and going for a pee has become something we're afraid to let ourselves experience, for fear that if we start eating, we won't stop. Our bodies aren't to be trusted, right? Advice given to us in magazines usually comprises strategies to avoid hunger.

Hunger has become pathologized and eating stigmatized. We are told that insatiable appetites are the cause of the 'obesity epidemic', and women in particular are shamed for eating anything other than a salad. Only dudes can eat burgers and steak because they have big appetites that need feeding. The subtext here is that women should eat like little birds; if you control your appetite, you control your weight.

Well, I say fuck the patriarchy.

You don't need to 'earn' food, you don't need to watch your appetite, you need to eat. Period.

Hunger is normal. Hunger is healthy. Hunger tells us that our physiology is working, and regular hunger may be a signal that our hormones are working as they should. The problem is actually when we habitually override our hunger signals they become eroded, as our body learns we're not responding to them. These hunger signals atrophy over time and our ability to respond to them is compromised. If you've been on the dieting merry-go-round or had a degree of disordered eating, you might find that you're out of touch with your hunger and fullness signals.

What's not normal is to voluntarily starve ourselves. Yes, I said starve. Sounds harsh, but it's the reality of most diets. Here's why: our bodies are pretty smart in a lot of ways, but really dumb in others. Bodies can't tell the difference between self-imposed restriction and legitimate starvation states. Think back to the Minnesota Starvation study in chapter 1 for more on this.

HUNGER HORMONES
—

We typically think of hormones in relation to our menstrual cycle, but actually hormones are involved in hunger and appetite and can give us a clue to what's going on with our bodies. Having regular hunger signals can be a sign of good overall metabolic health. In people who have been chronic dieters, who have a history of eating disorders, or who have very low body weight, these signals may have atrophied over time; if you don't respond to hunger signals, your body sees them as being superfluous and ditches them. What's the point in sending them out if you're just going to ignore them?

Hunger is controlled by a complicated cascade of hormones and neurotransmitters, signalling molecules that circulate the body and send messages between organs and tissues and the brain. These mechanisms are not totally understood by nutritional scientists; a lot of the evidence we have comes from animal studies and, although the mechanisms are probably pretty similar to humans, we can't make assumptions.[1] There are a few things we know for sure.

A (VERY) BRIEF INTRODUCTION TO HORMONES AND NEUROTRANSMITTERS

Just a few quick definitions before we get into it: both hormones and neurotransmitters are chemical messengers that communicate information through the body. They help keep your body in homeostasis (a fancy way of saying balance). Hormones are produced by endocrine and exocrine glands in the endocrine system, whereas neurotransmitters are produced by neurons (nerve cells) in the nervous system. The effects of hormones are long term, meaning they can last a few days. Neurotransmitters are fast-acting – I'm talking milliseconds (real fast!). Neurotransmitters usually act locally on nearby cells, whereas hormones can travel longer distances and act on tissues or organs a little further away from the glands they're made in. For example, insulin, a hormone that helps us metabolize energy from foods, is produced by beta cells in the pancreas, and travels in the blood to muscle and other tissue. Serotonin is a neurotransmitter (mainly) produced in the gut and has a direct effect on the nerves that control how quickly food passes through the gut (cool, huh?).

Hunger is controlled by both hormones and neurotransmitters.

Ghrelin

Ghrelin is *the* hunger hormone – I remember it because **g**hrelin makes your tummy **g**rumble. It's a general hunger hormone, meaning that it increases overall hunger (as opposed to specific cravings – we'll get to that). Ghrelin is secreted mainly by the stomach and in smaller amounts in the small intestine, pancreas, and brain, and goes up in response to food deprivation (*cough, diets, cough*). Ghrelin receptors are located in the hypothalamus – a region of the brain that's responsible for appetite control. The more you ignore hunger, the more ghrelin gets produced. This means that the harder you restrict food intake, the harder your body fights back; this is part of why diets fail. Rather than being a lack of willpower or you succumbing to the power of food, your biology is driving you to eat![2] Typically, ghrelin gets suppressed in response to eating a meal, but for chronic dieters, postprandial (after a meal) ghrelin may stay elevated as a result of being in negative energy balance – aka being on a diet.[3,4,5] People who have lost a lot of weight seem to have a higher circulating concentration of ghrelin in their blood to compensate for the weight lost.[6] Ghrelin can be elevated for up to a year after dieting![7,8] It doesn't take Einstein to figure out why people who have lost weight on a diet gain a lot of weight back – they're super-hungry! It's thought that ghrelin is most active in the evening, peaking around 7pm; this can help explain why you're super-'hangry' when you get home from work, *especially* if you skipped lunch or your afternoon snack.[9] The only way to switch off ghrelin is by making sure you eat enough; this 'trips' the fullness hormone leptin (which we'll get to in a bit), kind of like a see-saw. But it's important to understand that if you don't eat enough, your body will keep pumping out ghrelin and you'll keep feeling hungry.

Neuropeptide Y

Whereas ghrelin is a general hunger hormone – neuropeptide Y (NPY) is a neurotransmitter that specifically increases your appetite for, wait for it . . . CARBS. Yup. You have a carb-specific signalling molecule that drives cravings for carbohydrates.[10] That explains A LOT, right? NPY is a neurotransmitter and powerful orexigenic – meaning it stimulates appetite. NPY activity is stimulated by ghrelin, so the two are linked. In cases of food deprivation (looking at you, diets) the hypothalamus pumps out NPY, increasing appetite and, specifically, driving up cravings for carbs. Like ghrelin, the longer you try and ignore it, the bigger the craving gets until you inevitably demolish a whole loaf of bread. This is why, if you don't eat enough during the day, later on you get crazy carb cravings and you need to eat like *right* now, and an apple isn't gonna cut it.[11,12,13,14] You need to get your blood sugar levels up, STAT. The easiest, most efficient way is with something sweet and carby, which is why you crave bread, crisps, and chips.

So, we have these two mechanisms which, when they get ignored, get louder and louder and louder. Until you can't ignore them anymore. When you finally do decide to give into your (totally normal) hunger cues, it isn't a civilized affair with a fork and knife and napkins. Nope, it's usually a standing-up, at-the-fridge, using-your-hands kinda affair. And because you were over-hungry, you inhale your food without chewing properly and gulping down large amounts of air. You go from ravenous to feeling bloated and gross in what seems like thirty seconds flat. And then layer on the guilt and shame. You feel like a total garbage human.

Let's look at this a bit differently for a hot sec, try something a little novel. What if, when you first feel that gentle rumbling in your belly, and you start thinking about what sounds good for lunch, instead of flat ignoring it, you eat? Pretty radical, right? Eating in response to hunger? Just to see what happens. To see if maybe you can break the cycle of going from 'I'm so hungry I could eat a horse' to total food coma.

EATING WHEN YOU'RE HUNGRY IS GOOD FOR YOU!

If you're not yet totally convinced that responding to hunger is a good idea – maybe you still think there's something to the whole 5:2 diet – then check this out. Recent research from Italy suggests that responding to initial signs of hunger supports the self-regulation of food intake, as opposed to relying on external controls that don't work so well.[15] Translated, that means that using internal cues like hunger to help us eat in concert with our needs works better than something like dieting, which we know doesn't work for a lot of people.

And here's what the study showed about the benefits of self-regulation: people who were trained to use feelings of initial hunger to determine when to eat, and began to eat that way, experienced significant improvements in insulin sensitivity, blood sugar control, and HbA1C (a measure of blood glucose control).

The researchers concluded: 'These findings, together with those of an associated study on weight, suggest that the current epidemic of insulin resistance . . . may have its origin in noncognizance of hunger.' They also say: 'By restoring and validating hunger, the IHMP [initial hunger meal pattern — their term for eating when hungry] could help in the prevention and treatment of diabetes . . . This could lessen the high economic burden of health services in industrialized societies.' How neat is that? By responding to early signs of hunger you could actually be lowering your risk of chronic disease like type-2 diabetes![16,17,18] Responding to initial signs of hunger is the first step in relearning how to eat. Sounds obvious and easy, but it's actually kinda difficult to nail. Let's take a look at how to put it into practice.[19]

LISTEN TO YOUR DAMN BODY

—

The idea of listening to our bodies sounds fairly nebulous, but it's actually a concept from physiology, which is the branch of biology that deals with the normal functioning of our body, and that concept is called interoceptive awareness – basically, how well an individual can perceive and interpret the signals their body is sending to them. And this is really cool: the first studies done on interoceptive awareness were conceptualized as people who could accurately perceive their own heart rate without taking their pulse; they just sit quietly and they can feel their hearts beating. Try it: sit in a quiet room. If you have a heart rate monitor watch, compare the value it measured to the number you count in your head over a minute. Pretty neat, right? How close did you guess?

This concept can also be applied to our own hunger and fullness. Interoceptive awareness involves awareness of, and sensitivity to, internal physiological sensations. And people who have higher interoceptive awareness are typically more intuitive eaters too.[20] So how do you begin to develop interoceptive awareness?[21]

The first step is to disconnect from the diet mentality. Like I've said already, this is an iterative process, and something you'll have to work on, but eventually you'll start laughing at messages of diet culture. But, if you're in the diet mentality of having to track everything, calories, activity, macros, or you're following a meal plan, then you're letting apps and meal plans make choices about your food for you. That's the *opposite* of tuning in to what your body is saying, ya know? We've already been over this, but I'll say it again. The first step is to ditch the Fitbit, calorie-counting apps and meal plans. External influences draw you away from recognizing your own hunger and satiety cues. If you haven't already ditched these, now's the time.

The next thing is to begin to understand what the sensation of hunger feels like for you. I've noticed that a lot of times people bounce from one extreme to the other. They go from being wayyyyyyy too hungry and eating ALL the food, to going into a food coma/food baby-type situation. And people aren't familiar with that sensation of *gentle* hunger, that sort of mild rumbling sensation in your belly – the middle ground before you get HANGRY. That's where you need to be eating, not when you're about to gnaw your own arm off.

So I want you to imagine a fuel gauge like in your car that goes from zero to ten. Zero is totally empty; you've hit a wall, you might feel woozy and like you have low blood sugar, you're over-hungry. Ten is stuffed, so full you feel like you're going to burst. Ten is like Christmas Day after turkey and pudding and half a box of Quality Street. Ten is unbuckling your belt full. Then imagine five, right in the middle. A bit like this:

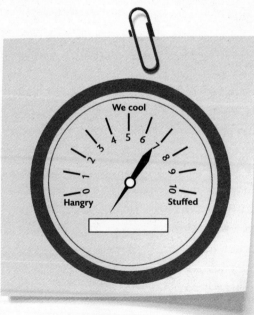

Five is neutral, neither hungry nor full; there's no sensation in your stomach, you're not really aware of it, you're just going about your life. I see most people wait until they're around a 1 or a 2 before they start to eat, and that's a sign you've gone too long without food. Think about a time you've got to that level of hungry, what happens? Do you calmly cook yourself a meal from scratch? Or do you faceplant into a box of Crunchy Nut Cornflakes? Don't worry, me too.

What typically happens when we let ourselves get over-hungry is that we rebound eat. It can feel chaotic and out of control. It might make us feel like we can't be trusted around food, or that we're super-greedy. But the reality is, your body is just doing its thing, tryna get nourishment and energy. This is what Tribole and Resch call primal hunger. You may also end up feeling bloated and uncomfortable.

If we think about the fuel gauge, in general, you need to eat at around a 3, this is what we call *gentle hunger*, and stop when you're satisfied, but not too full – around a 7 (remember you can eat again if you get hungry later). This is entirely subjective and may take a little while to figure out for you. It's also full of nuance and caveats, **this is not a hard and fast rule**; remember we're done with them, so make sure you keep reading for explanations of specific scenarios where this may not apply.

To give you an idea of how to use the chart, I've tried to illustrate what it might look like for the average person (whatever that is, right?), based on my experience working with clients, as well as my own experiences and similar tools used in clinical practice. But this is totally subjective, so it might look different for you, and it can vary from day to day (for example, activity can suppress appetite for a few hours afterwards, so you might need to eat, but not feel physical hunger, which shows you how important it is to refuel!). Use this as a guide if you're not sure where to start. I've roughly grouped them into five categories: over-hungry, gentle hunger, neutral, content, and stuffed. The difference between these numbers can be pretty nuanced and if you've been out of tune with these sensations for a long time, then that more granular detail can be hard to figure out. I don't want you to get too hung up on that and stress about whether you're a 3 or a 4, because the point is, you're hungry, and you need to eat. Simple, right? **Don't over-think it**, instead use the broader categories and go from there. Over time you'll get better at perceiving exactly where you are on the scale. My husband doesn't describe hunger with words anymore, he just gives me a number! So, your challenge from now on is simply to eat when you're hungry. That's it. Whenever you feel physical sensations of hunger, that's your cue to eat; it might be a meal, it might be a snack, but the first step on this journey is just to feed your body when it's hungry. Got it?

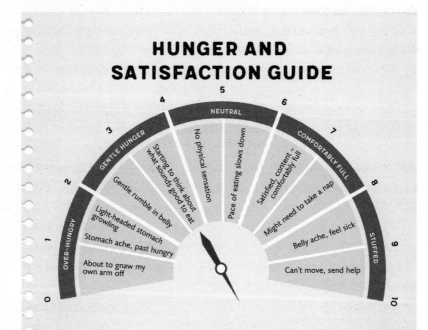

HUNGER AND SATISFACTION GUIDE

That said, I need to be clear about something. You don't need to change WHAT you eat at this point. OK? Let me say that again. YOU DO NOT NEED TO CHANGE WHAT YOU EAT AT THIS POINT. Here's why. I see this happen all the time in my clinic: 'I'm doing this intuitive eating thing now, I'm just going to eat whatever the fuck I like.' And yes, we are going to be breaking down food rules and legalizing foods. BUT. If you go too much, too fast, there's a risk that it will all feel a bit out of control and overwhelming and I don't want that to happen. So take it easy. Focus on allowing yourself to eat when you're hungry, and then we'll start to systematically introduce more variety. You might also notice that focusing on hunger results in changes to your pattern of eating too. That's OK, go with it. Just don't feel as though you have to start going wild with off-limits foods quite yet.

EXERCISES

—

Hunger and satisfaction wheel

Use the blank template below to find the sensations of hunger for you. It's designed to help you understand what the subjective feelings of hunger are like in your body; dizziness, tiredness, hanger, sore stomach, lightheadedness, headache, crankiness – these can all be signs that you're TOO hungry. Try and find the sensations of gentle hunger – a light rumbling in the belly, thoughts about food are more frequent. Eating at this point means you're less likely to get over-hungry; being over-hungry can lead to eating too much and being uncomfortably full – fine every now and then, but if it's every time you eat it doesn't feel so great. I recommend doing this on a day where you don't have a whole lot going on so you can pay attention and tune in. If you're distracted by work or family stuff it can be pretty tough to pay attention. Use the word bank or come up with your own words to help describe the sensations. Don't stress if you don't really feel the subtle sensations of hunger; it will take time to get used to these feelings if you've been regularly overriding them. More on that later. If you're finding it hard to differentiate between two numbers (i.e. the spokes of the wheel), don't sweat it; use the space around the outside (the 'tyre' of the wheel) to help roughly group the sensations into categories (see the example I gave earlier for help). I'd recommend doing it in pencil too (or making a few copies – there's a printout on my website) because you'll probably refine the chart over time.

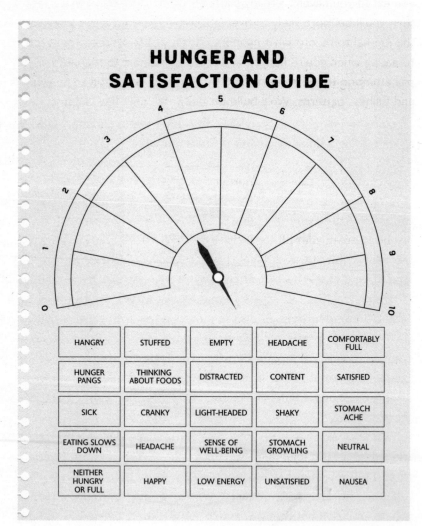

HUNGER AND SATISFACTION GUIDE

HANGRY	STUFFED	EMPTY	HEADACHE	COMFORTABLY FULL
HUNGER PANGS	THINKING ABOUT FOODS	DISTRACTED	CONTENT	SATISFIED
SICK	CRANKY	LIGHT-HEADED	SHAKY	STOMACH ACHE
EATING SLOWS DOWN	HEADACHE	SENSE OF WELL-BEING	STOMACH GROWLING	NEUTRAL
NEITHER HUNGRY OR FULL	HAPPY	LOW ENERGY	UNSATISFIED	NAUSEA

ACTIVITY

Intuitive eating journal

For the next week, practise using the hunger and satiety gauge by keeping an intuitive eating journal to record your hunger level when you eat (if you haven't already started). Try not to dip below a 2, as then you'll be more likely to overeat. And if you do dip too low, use the journal to record what happens. This is just to help you get used to eating when you're hungry, and to help you start to recognize and pay attention to these signals and to bring your attention to hunger and fullness patterns. We'll build on this in the next few chapters.

Remember – this isn't another tool to beat yourself up with. Use it to check in with yourself over the next week. I know it's a pain in the ass to write everything down, so make it easy on yourself, it can just be a note in your phone if that's easier. If you've been tracking and recording things for your whole life then this can feel like just another food diary; if that's the case, ditch it and just notice what those feelings of hunger feel like. Otherwise keeping an intuitive eating journal can be helpful to identify patterns.

Try and be gentle with yourself when you write foods down – don't be too critical, especially when you eat according to hunger. It can feel unnatural and uncomfortable – just remember that eating in response to hunger is NORMAL and HEALTHY. Overriding hunger is the problem.

Some of you may have fears that you won't be able to stop eating, and this is a valid fear, but remember that's not the reality. Typically when I tell my clients to eat more, it manifests as them having more balanced meals and reduced cravings and binges. Sounds counterintuitive but trust me – I've got you on this one! Like I said, this journal is purely to help you bring awareness to eating in response to physical hunger; we'll build on it in time, but for now, honour your hunger and notice what happens!

Hunger body scan

We usually only think about hunger in terms of our stomach growling or feeling really hollow. Or maybe we only know we're hungry when we get to that hangry stage, by which point it's usually a bit too late and you're ready to figuratively and literally bite your colleague's head off.

Using this hunger scan meditation can help you recognize the more subtle and nuanced symptoms of hunger. Record the following script on a voice memo on your phone, and then play it back to yourself. Listen to the meditation once, when you know you're hungry, then go have something to eat, and rescan your body. Sometimes it can be difficult to perceive some of these sensations, but comparing them immediately before and after eating can help make the shift more noticeable. Give yourself about ten minutes after eating before rescanning.

Hunger body scan script
(adapted from Tribole and Resch, intuitiveeating.org)

Record the following on your phone, making sure to pause between each sentence to let yourself assess the sensations. Play it back as many times as you need to feel comfortable recognizing the signs of hunger.

Get yourself nice and comfortable.

Take a few deep breaths, in through your nose and out through your mouth … In through your nose, and out through your mouth. And once more, in through your nose, and out through your mouth . . . And then gently close your eyes…

Let's start by getting in touch with your physical body…

In your head, scan your body starting from your head, and moving down towards to your toes…

How would you describe the physical sensations in your body in this moment? … Pleasant? … Unpleasant…? Or neutral? … There's no right or wrong answer, you're just checking in with yourself.

Just notice the description that best describes how you physically feel, right now… Pleasant? … Unpleasant? … Or neutral? …

Now we're going to look at some key areas that hunger can show up in the body, starting with the more subtle and nuanced signs of hunger...

I'd like you to begin by bringing your attention to your mood...

Sometimes biological hunger is experienced with a shift in mood. You may feel irritable or cranky... Notice your mood right now in this moment... Do you feel a little snappy or curt?... Do you feel a little low?...

If so, these may be signs that you're beginning to experience hunger. Just take notice, without judgement...

Now I'd like you to shift your attention to your overall energy level . . . Sometimes biological hunger is experienced by a dip in energy, characterized by fatigue, or even sleepiness... Do you feel sluggish and tired and it has nothing to do with a bad night's sleep?... Or maybe you feel unusually blah or a bit listless?...

Again, just notice if you experience these initial signs of hunger by a shift in your energy...

Now I'd like you to shift your attention to the more easily detectable hunger signals, starting with your head, so just bring your awareness to your head...

Sometimes biological hunger is experienced as a physical sensation in your head, so just notice any physical sensations in your head right now... How would you describe the way it feels to you?...

Is there a slight ache?... Are you light-headed, or does it feel like you're zoning out?... Maybe you feel a little dizzy, or even a bit faint?... Are you having any difficulty concentrating?... Whatever the sensation, just notice...

If you're experiencing any of these sensations, it's possible that you're experiencing a degree of hunger ...

Just notice it without judgement...

Now, move your attention to your stomach...

What would best describe the physical sensation in your stomach right now?...

Would you describe it as a gentle rumbling or gurgling? Or maybe it feels empty?...Or maybe there's an uncomfortable pain; a stomach ache...

Are there any hunger pangs or a gnawing feeling in your belly?...Or does your stomach feel comfortable or neutral?...

What is the physical sensation in your stomach — be aware that any of these sensations may be signalling hunger...

Perhaps you're experiencing other physical sensations that might be indicating you're hungry . . . Maybe you find yourself salivating at the thought of food and of eating . . . Or maybe you feel kinda shaky and like you have low blood sugar, another physical symptom of hunger indicating you need to eat . . .

Now I'd like you to take a brief scan of all of these elements, starting from your mood . . .

Now your energy level . . .

Now your physical sensations, in your head and your stomach and anywhere else you might be experiencing them . . .

Now I'd like you to consider all of these elements together, and with that overall consideration, I'd like you to rate your hunger level on a hunger/fullness scale from 0 to 10 . . . 10 is so full you feel sick, it's painful . . .

0 is painfully empty, and 5 is completely neutral; neither empty nor full. So how would you rate your hunger right now? . . .

Keep in mind whatever number you rate, it's not right or wrong. It's just a process to help you get in touch and the more you get familiar with the sensations, the easier it will become to tell when you're hungry.

Good. Now I'd like you to take a few deep breaths in through your nose, and out through your mouth. In through your nose, and out through your mouth. And once more, in through your nose, and out through your mouth. Open your eyes, and take your attention back to the room . . .

Awesome, you've just learned how to sense your hunger using a full hunger scan. Use this practice as often as you need until you become comfortable using it on your own on the spot throughout the day, or use the quick body-scan checklist below to check in with yourself throughout the day.

Quick hunger body scan

Snap a picture of the checklist opposite or draw it out in your journal to whip out and refer to throughout the day. Of course, these sensations aren't all unique to hunger, but they may help you narrow down and focus. It may take some experimenting to find out which sensations signal hunger for you, so don't be afraid to eat something in response to these signs and see if it helps!

Now it's your time to put this into practice; over the next week or so try simply responding to those early signs of hunger using the hunger wheel and body scan. You can also use your intuitive eating journal to keep a note of how hungry you are when you begin eating (see the template for keeping your journal on page 20). What happens if you eat when you're super-hungry vs gently hungry? Does food taste as good when you're not that hungry compared to when you have a light rumble in your belly? Remember to bring a level of non-judgemental awareness to this process; you're just gathering information at this stage and eventually you'll get better at responding to these signals without overthinking it.

Mood	Energy	Head	Stomach	Body
hangry	fatigue	achey	gurgling	shaky
irritable	sleepy	light-headed	gentle rumble	quivering
cranky	sluggish	dizzy	emptiness	low blood sugar*
snappy	blah	poor concentration	stomach ache	salivating
moody	meh	distracted	hunger pangs	
low	listless		gnawing	

* Low blood sugar here refers to what subjectively feels like your blood sugar levels are getting lower and it feels like time to eat, but is different from hypoglycaemia, which is a medical condition.

137

Journal questions

How have you been getting on responding to your hunger signals? It can be harder to implement than you'd think! Sounds totally logical and rational to eat in response to hunger, but we don't always do it, for a variety of reasons. It can be all too easy to fall into the hunger/fullness trap, which is just another way of dieting (remember how I said it was so important to ditch the diet mentality?). Have you beat yourself up this week at all for eating while you're not hungry? Has that type of thinking been helpful or constructive, or just made you feel THE WORST?

WHAT ABOUT FULLNESS?

—

I don't want you to focus on the fullness side of the scale for now. Not that it isn't important, but until we've nailed this hunger thing and done a few of the other steps, you may have a hard time stopping when you feel full. That's OK. Especially if you've been depriving yourself of things – remember I said ghrelin can be elevated for up to a year after stopping a diet? It can be hard to stop and your body needs to have the opportunity to fully experience this before it will get the memo that you're allowed to eat these foods whenever you damn well please. Something I've noticed is that people get hung up on the fullness side of things too early, and start beating themselves up for not 'getting it'. So remind yourself that you're not there yet and that's cool too. We'll get to fullness later; set it to the side for now, otherwise it will undermine the whole process. OK?

Can I only eat when I'm hungry?

Nope, not even. This whole approach is about ditching the rules, so whatever you do, don't interpret this as the 'Hunger & Fullness Diet'. That's not what this is about. In order to be cool with food, you're going to have to learn to be flexible and break the rules. That means sometimes eating when you're not hungry to help prevent you getting TOO hungry later.

Let's go through an example: if you're at, say 5 (neutral) but you're going to be heading to a movie later and know you'll get over-hungry if you don't eat dinner, it's OK to be prepared and eat something to bump you up to a 7 until the movie's done and then you can have something else to eat later. In other words, it's OK to eat when you're not hungry! These are guidelines, everything in intuitive eating is a guideline not a hard and fast rule.

The same goes if you're at a birthday party and you've had some nibbles and snacks and you're at a 7 and then someone rolls out a birthday cake; it's cool to have that too. In other words, sometimes we eat past that point of comfortable fullness, we make that conscious choice, which is where mindful eating comes in and we'll get to that in chapter 8. But the key here is to give yourself permission, and eat the cake mindfully and without guilt (and we'll talk about how to do that too). You can always choose to leave a bit of the cake if you decide you don't have room for it (or take a slice home for later!). So the point is that sometimes we do overeat, and that's OK – that's life and it's normal to want to eat a lot of something that tastes good. The key is to let yourself off the hook and develop some self-compassion; you're not bad or naughty for eating cake. But at the same time, feeling over full and eating too much is also not that enjoyable an eating experience either, and when we bring mindfulness into the equation, we're less likely to overeat at every meal. Occasional overeating is totally normal, it's when it becomes an unconscious habit that it's more of an issue. Like I said, we'll deal with fullness later, but for now, let's get back to hunger.

'I just ate, I can't be hungry again, can I?'

DOY! That's not how it works. You can eat something and be hungry again pretty soon afterwards. Have you ever eaten an apple and then been hungrier than when you started? Exactly. A common mistake I see is that when people get to a 3 on the gauge, they eat, say, a banana or a croissant and call it a day. They then wonder why they're hungry again a little while later and berate themselves by saying 'you can't be hungry, you just ate!' If you think about it though, those foods aren't especially filling – they have no staying power! They maybe bump you up to a 3.5 or a 4. So it's no freaking wonder you get hungry again an hour later!

Imagine that was breakfast, and you were starting at a 3 then you might want to have the croissant, the banana AND a yoghurt or a smoothie. That will leave you feeling satisfied and comfortably full, and it's balanced, which means it will have more staying power; that 'stick to your ribs' kind of feeling that gives you energy and makes you feel all cosy inside.

What can happen when you start checking in with your hunger level is that you rely less on the clock to tell you when to eat and less on your plate to tell you when to stop eating. That's what it means to be attuned to your body.

How hungry you get again after a meal or a snack will depend on a number of things, for instance what you ate, how much you ate, how hungry you were to begin with, how active you have been, if you're tired or ill, and so on. In general, foods that are higher in protein and fat might keep you fuller for longer, as do foods that are higher in fibre. Research has found that boiled potatoes are some of the most hunger-satisfying foods you can eat, but a croissant is one of the least satisfying, in terms of sating your hunger.[22] But what if you were super-hungry and really fancied a croissant? Well, you could add some ham, cheese and tomato and make it into a sandwich. Or you could have it with a fruit and yoghurt smoothie to get an extra hit of fibre, fat, and protein. The point is, that meals that are balanced in terms of macronutrients (protein, carbs, fat) are generally more filling and satisfying. That's easy to get intellectually, but how does that feel in your body? You don't have to worry about counting exact ratios of anything; just notice how it feels in your body when you eat a variety of different foods, remembering to be curious and non-judgemental. You are gathering information.

Comfort eating or just hungry?

What I see clients do a lot is backload their meals. What I mean by this is they skip breakfast, they eat a tiny lunch, and come dinner time they feel totally out of control around food. It's what I call the 'fuck-it' effect, where you basically eat the entire contents of the fridge in five minutes flat.

'Fuck it, I'm going to eat whatever I want because I'm so tired/annoyed/stressed/had a shitty day.'

Along with that you might feel guilty, stressed, anxious and scared that someone's going to catch you in the act (which only makes you eat it even faster). But here's the thing. What if you were actually just hungry?

It might just be that you haven't eaten enough throughout the day to adequately nourish yourself so your hunger hormones and neuro-transmitters are poppin' off, screaming out for you to eat. It's biology.

Try this instead: eat 3 balanced meals plus 2–4 snacks/dessert throughout the day. Come dinner time, you might not be so desperate to eat your weight in Pringles (no judgement, been there).

I see this happen with my clients all the time and when I give them permission to eat according to their hunger instead of ignoring it or overriding it, they tend to lessen the amount of emotional eating they're doing. I remember one client in particular realizing that actually she wasn't feeding herself enough food in the morning, she wasn't filling herself up enough to that point of being around a 7 or so, and she ended up snacking more later in the day. And then when she started paying attention she realized that she needed to eat more in the mornings to give herself enough energy for the day and as a result wasn't sniffing around for stuff later in the day or that night. And this is a really common thing I see with clients: that what they perceive as emotional or comfort eating is actually just because they're hungry!

Try not to judge your hunger

Our appetites naturally ebb and flow, this is normal and healthy. I've noticed especially a few days before I get my period I am RAVENOUS; it often takes a a lot more food than normal to feed my appetite. When I first noticed this it kinda freaked me out, but instead of judging it as bad or wrong, or straight up ignoring it, I went with it, to see what happened. Turns out after a few days of eating more, my appetite is slightly less on the days after, and without having to exert control or count anything, it all sort of levels out. Some days you are hungrier than others. Can you go with that and see what happens? Maybe you are starving in the morning and eat more than usual for breakfast, but notice if you are hungry for your afternoon snack? You might still be, and that's OK too; the point is to notice patterns over time and not to judge yourself.

What happens if I never feel hungry?

Good question! If you've routinely been ignoring hunger or pacifying it with coffee and cigarettes, chances are you may not know what that gentle sensation of hunger feels like anymore. Don't sweat it though, you can recalibrate your hunger and fullness; with a little time and patience those signals will come back – the main thing is to build some routine and consistency. As a guide, try eating every three to four hours. That usually looks like 3 meals plus 2–4(ish) snacks. I usually recommend that clients anchor their day with breakfast at roughly the same time every day (it doesn't have to be as soon as you get up, but when you start feeling the more nuanced signals of hunger as per our body scan). This is because our body's processes are on a 'timer' and respond well to consistency. If you eat a meal at roughly the same time each day, it can help your body know what to expect and help your hunger signals come back online.

If you're only managing two meals a day at the moment, don't go 0–100 (real quick) – work up to it. Start by adding a snack in and going from there. Having regular and consistent meals for a period and building a little bit of structure in sounds like the opposite of intuitive eating, and it is to an extent. But I like to think of it more as stabilizers on a bike. You add a little bit of support, then eventually you'll be able to take it away and do it for yourself. As long as you don't approach it as a rule; instead, try fostering a sense of curiosity.

Likewise, if you've done a lot of exercise your appetite may be artificially suppressed, so make sure you're having regular snacks and refuelling after your workouts. Use the body scan to help you check in with non-stomach sensations of hunger.

How do I balance my snacks?

It's pretty easy to fall into the trap of bullshit snacking: rice cakes, carrot sticks, maybe an apple. These are sometimes a relic of the diet mindset, that voice in your head that says 'snacking is bad', or that you 'can only have "healthy" snacks'. But these types of snacks can be unsatisfying and sometimes even make you hungrier; chances are they're not going to fill you up for very long. You've probably also fallen into the trap of 'they're healthy so I can eat as much as I want'; twenty rice cakes later and you're in this weird place where you feel

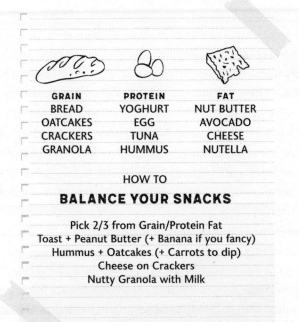

GRAIN	PROTEIN	FAT
BREAD	YOGHURT	NUT BUTTER
OATCAKES	EGG	AVOCADO
CRACKERS	TUNA	CHEESE
GRANOLA	HUMMUS	NUTELLA

HOW TO
BALANCE YOUR SNACKS

Pick 2/3 from Grain/Protein Fat
Toast + Peanut Butter (+ Banana if you fancy)
Hummus + Oatcakes (+ Carrots to dip)
Cheese on Crackers
Nutty Granola with Milk

kinda sick but simultaneously not full or satisfied. That's because these snacks have nothing that will satiate you. Here's a small tip to help you balance things a little. Try and make sure your snacks are also balanced, filling, and satisfying too. A lot of people make the mistake of just having a handful of carrots or a piece of fruit as a snack and, again, that will only nudge your fullness up a tiny bit, so you'll get hungry again pretty quick after that.

Again, this is a guideline, not a rule. The idea is to help you find snacks that are more satisfying, filling, and balanced. Pick two of the following: grain, protein, fat. Sometimes protein and fat come in the same package, like cheese or nut butter, but that only counts as one; you'd still want to add a grain to that to round it out. Remember that grains are helpful to keep your blood glucose levels stable, and letting them dip too low for too long will trigger that ghrelin–NYP cascade to spiral out of control and make cravings take over.

I'M SCARED I MIGHT EAT MORE THAN NORMAL

—

I hear you. Learning to listen to your body and trust the signals it's sending you is scary. And you might very well eat more than you're used to. But that's not necessarily a bad thing. Especially if you have been restricting calories and counting macros and doing all sorts of exercise and still putting on weight. That's a definite sign that you're not eating enough to support your metabolism. Just like a car needs fuel before it can run, without enough fuel in the tank your body will grind to a halt. Giving it enough fuel can help stoke the fires of your metabolism, recharge your hormones, and help everything function normally.

Am I hungry, or is it really just thirst?

This is a question I get asked ALL. THE. TIME. And it's because we've had it drilled into us by diet culture that our bodies are lying to us, trying to trick us and sabotage us into . . . fulfilling a fundamental need. I mean, what the actual fuck? How many times have you heard someone say something like 'Oh, babe, you're probably just thirsty, have a glass of water and wait fifteen minutes.' THANKS, CAROL, BUT I PISS LIKE A RACEHORSE SO I'M DEFINITELY HUNGRY.

What this message does is encourage people to 'silence' their hunger by drinking a shit ton of water/tea/coffee/Diet Coke, when they're actually just hungry and need a meal or snack. Hunger is hunger and it means you should eat. I see this happen a lot in clinic where people are legitimately hungry, but because they've read that it's 'just thirst', they end up drinking more than they need and making their bellies feel artificially full. Because they haven't filled their need for food, they end up raiding the fridge the second they get home at night.

We have a super-complicated system in place to regulate thirst. We lose water through sweating, breathing, pooping, and peeing. Our brains detect the TINIEST shifts in hydration because our cells shrink, sending the signal that we need to drink. A bogus myth is that being thirsty is a sign that we're already dehydrated. Shut the front door. Thirst is a PREVENTATIVE mechanism to stop you becoming dehydrated; it's really sensitive so that when the body perceives a little liquid has been lost, your thirst mechanism kicks in before you can become dehydrated. Biology is smart like that, and from an evolutionary perspective it makes sense. Why would we wait until we were already dehydrated to seek out water? Yeah, doesn't make sense, does it?[23]

We feel thirst in the mouth or throat as dryness and like we need to drink something RIGHT NOW. Only something wet and refreshing will satisfy thirst. We feel thirst in our mouth long before headaches and not being able to focus set in.

Where it gets confusing is when you end up dehydrated (in hot weather, playing intense sports) and you get a headache; this can happen when you're hungry too and they can feel similar. But instead of trying to guess which one it is, there's a really objective measure – your wee. Take a look at your pee, it should be a light straw colour. If it's darker than that you probably need a drink. Otherwise it's hunger; use the hunger body-scan checklist to help you differentiate.

REMEMBER: NOT A DIET

——

Non-diet warrior Isabel Foxen Duke explains how intuitive eating, when used in the context of the diet mentality, is just another diet. It wasn't until she let go of that thinking that she was able to understand the real sentiment of intuitive eating; there are no rules! By respecting your hunger and satiety cues you're less likely to want to eat outside of the parameters of hunger and fullness, but if you do, that's totally cool. There are loads of reasons why we eat (emotional/taste/practical hunger).

Remember, this is a process. Some of you may take to it really easily; for others it might take a bit more work, but that's OK too. In the next chapter we'll build on the hunger thing by beginning to practise food neutrality.

Also, you might feel you're SUPER-HYPER-AWARE of eating right now, and that's also part of the process. You're retraining yourself. When you learned to ride a bike you were super-aware of every turn of the wheel, but now you just get on with it! Same thing here. Remember to be kind to yourself as you're going through this process, and do something nice for yourself every day, every damn day.

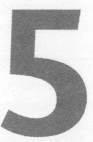

WEIGHT AND BODY
NEUTRALITY

——

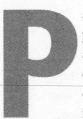art of the reason many of us start dieting in the first place is because we believe that being thinner is more attractive; after all, that's the message we receive from diet culture. The other reason many people get into different diets is because of promises that have been made about health. We are told that fatness is unhealthy, and in order to mitigate the health risk, we need to lose weight. Now immediately you should have alarm bells going off in your head, because we know that diets don't work. Even if you are at the higher end of the weight spectrum. So, in this chapter, there are two things I'd like to explore. Firstly, your relationship with your own body and undoing the notion that you have to be thin to be beautiful or worthy or deserving of love and respect. And secondly, I want to unpack the idea that your weight determines your health. Ready? Let's rumble!

Let's begin with a little bit of science. We've talked a lot about why diets don't work but many of my clients are afraid that if they're not sticking to some highly regimented eating plan, or if they don't monitor their Fitbit 24/7, they'll just get bigger and bigger and bigger until they are the size of the moon.

This won't happen. Because of biology.

Our DNA is our genetic blueprint; it determines key characteristics about our appearance like our hair and eye colour, our height, and, yup, our weight. In fact, it's estimated that approximately 70% of our weight is determined by genetic factors.[1] SEVENTY! To put it into perspective, about 80% of our height is determined by genetics and the other 20% by environmental factors (like making sure you have enough food as a baby to grow to your potential). Ain't no one tryna grow taller.

This genetically determined weight is called your set point weight; essentially, this is the weight that your body will naturally settle at.[2,3,4] It is largely genetically determined but can be influenced by environment and our behaviours, and in general it can only go up, not down. The name set 'point' is a bit of a misnomer, though, because it's more like a small range in which your body feels most comfortable and works optimally; perhaps 10–15lb (4–5kg).

In her brilliant TED talk, neuroscientist Sandra Aamodt describes set point weight like the thermostat in your house:

> There are more than a dozen chemical signals in the brain that tell your body to gain weight, more than another dozen that tell your body to lose it, and the system works like a thermostat, responding to signals from the body by adjusting hunger, activity and metabolism, to keep your weight stable as conditions change. That's what a thermostat does, right? It keeps the temperature in your house the same as the weather changes outside. Now you can try to change the temperature in your house by opening a window in the winter, but that's not going to change the setting on the thermostat, which will respond by kicking on the furnace to warm the place back up. Your brain works exactly the same way, responding to weight loss by using powerful tools to push your body back to what it considers normal.[5]

The great thing about set point weight is that it means when you let go of dieting and disordered behaviours, your body pretty much stays at that weight without you having to micromanage food and exercise. Your body knows what it needs to do to maintain that weight. It's when we start trying to manipulate our set point weight that we run into problems. It's estimated that people who have lost 10% of their body weight burn 300–400kcal less because their metabolism is suppressed.[6]

Let's think of it like this. Imagine you're in a pool and you have one of those floaty pool balls (what are they actually called, because I'm pretty sure it's not 'floaty pool ball'?). So, you have the ball and you try and push it under the water. You push, push, push, but eventually the ball comes shooting back up.

The water level represents your set point weight. When you back off, the ball sits there, effortlessly, you don't need to control it. When you push it down it's like you trying to restrict your eating and push your weight down below where it wants to sit naturally. As soon as you let go of the pressure, the ball (your weight) pops right back to where it is naturally more comfortable.

What if every time you pushed the ball down, though, the water level started creeping up, so that every time you let go, the ball would be at a higher set point? This seems to be what happens through repeated rounds of dieting; our set point weight increases, and it has a tendency to go up rather than down.[7,8,9,10,11,12]

This isn't meant to freak you out though. If you've been on lots of diets in the past, you haven't done irreparable damage to your metabolism or anything like that! This is to help reassure you that by relinquishing a little control over food and eating, your body will figure out a comfortable weight that it can easily maintain. No calorie-counting. No tracking exercise. No drama.

Knowing that your body has a weight it's comfortable at can be a huge relief for a lot of people and help them accept that dieting is never going to work for them; it can help them move on with their lives, diet-free. Others, though, may feel disappointed or frustrated that they may never lose weight and are 'stuck' at the weight they're at now. They feel exasperated because they don't want to diet anymore, but they don't feel good about the body they're currently in. Not only

How do I know if I'm at my set point weight?

There's no way to calculate your exact set point weight, but we can think of it in terms of behaviours that you engage in. You're likely at your set point when you're:

- not restricting food groups
- not bingeing
- regularly moving your body for fun and joy
- getting enough sleep
- managing stress
- not using food to pacify negative emotions
- spending time with people you like being around
- eating according to hunger and fullness (most of the time)
- eating food that makes you feel good

does this feel like purgatory, but it's a major stumbling block on the road to intuitive eating so I'm going to give you some tools and activities to help you feel more comfortable and content about being in your body right now.[13] Because, let's be real, even if you went on a crash diet right this second, you wouldn't lose weight straight away, would you? My goal is to help you feel better in your body regardless of the number on the scales or your body's relationship to gravity.

BODY NEUTRALITY

—

In the last few years, body positivity has taken off in a major way, to the point that brands, advertising, and even Weight Watchers have jumped on the trend. And while this is great in terms of moving the dial towards more diverse bodies being represented and appreciated, it also has the potential to set up a new list of shoulds: 'I should love my body', 'I should appreciate my stretchmarks', 'I should accept my belly'. Then when we're having body-image meltdowns, for whatever reason, we can feel bad for not 100% loving every inch of ourselves. This of course wasn't the intention of the body-positive movement, and many BoPo warriors will point out that they also have rough days, and that's OK too. But sometimes the expectation of having to love yourself when you've come from a place of self-loathing can be too far out of reach for many of my clients. That's why in clinic we aim for body neutrality, which is sometimes used interchangeably with body acceptance. In her book *Body Positive Power*, BoPo hero Megan Crabbe neatly summarizes this concept and the related concept of body respect, which is nested just under body neutrality:

> *Body acceptance is about accepting this is the body you have, and feeling neutral about that fact. It means not thinking that you're flawless and bootylicious 24/7, but also not thinking that you're hideous and have to change. Actually, it's not thinking very much about your body very much at all, just accepting that how it looks is how it looks, and getting on with your days.*

I love Megan's suggestion that body acceptance is actually not thinking about your body all that much. When I'm working with clients I tend to conceptualize good body image as taking care of your body but not obsessing about it or over-thinking it. It's freeing up cognitive resources so you can get more important shit done. Remember that your body is a tool for helping you move around in, interact with and experience the world. It's not an object to be gawked at.

BODY RESPECT

Body respect is the idea that maybe we aren't totally comfortable with our bodies; we might be stuck in a place of cognitive dissonance where we simultaneously understand that diets don't work, but are wrestling with wanting to change our bodies. This is totally understandable given the number that diet culture does on us. But while you are working towards intuitive eating and ditching diet mentality, can you show your body respect? You may not love your body, and you may not even feel OK with your body, but can you show your body a level of care and respect that means it's getting its basic needs met? That might look different for everyone, but here are some ideas for what body respect could be like:

- Regularly nourishing yourself with meals and snacks
- Gentle movement that feels good in your body
- Regular medical and dental check-ups
- Taking care of your body (basic self-care, hygiene, taking medicines)

Here's what body respect is not:

- Restricting food/dieting
- Punishing yourself with exercise/earning food through exercise
- Pinching, poking, or otherwise being cruel to your body
- Judging your own or other people's bodies
- Body shaming (again, yourself or others)

If you've been at an impasse with your body for as long as you can remember, the idea of just being neutral or even just respectful of our bodies can be challenging. The activities and tools that follow are designed to nudge you closer to that, but if you don't get there straight away, no sweat, this work is hard! Come back and read through this section or do the activities as often as you need. Let's think about how to start practising body neutrality.

YOU FEEL BETTER IN CLOTHES THAT ACTUALLY FIT!

How many of you would let your cat or dog wear a collar that was too tight and half-strangling the animal? How about letting your kid go out in shoes that were too tight? Yet we're all going around wearing bras that dig in and jeans that are too tight. Look, shopping for clothes is never easy, but it's especially not fun when you're having body-image stuff going on. It's super-tempting to buy the size too small or the one you 'usually' are as an incentive to 'tone up', and we keep the clothes as a 'reward' for manipulating our bodies. I get it, I've been there too. But here's the thing. Having 'goal' clothes, or wearing clothes that are too tight, pinch, or dig into us, keeps us tethered to diet mentality. They draw our attention to our bodies and away from the moment we're in. Be real, how many times have you covered your belly with a cushion because your jeans were too small? And remember that top you were constantly pulling down? Clothes that are too small make us feel like our bodies are the problem. Your body is not the problem. It never was. Show your body some respect by dressing it comfortably.

CHALLENGE

Go through your closet/wardrobe/cupboard/drawers and clear out any clothes that do not fit you; whether they're teeny-tiny or drown you like a circus tent. Getting some jeans that fit properly makes a huge difference in how comfortable you feel; camel toe isn't a good look on anyone.

If you're uncomfortable about the idea of throwing clothes away, you could donate clothes to the charity shop or to friends and family, or sell them on Ebay. It can be hard to see all that money go down the pan, but there are two things here: one, holding on to clothes that don't fit is basically holding on to the diet mentality (keeping them just in case!), and two, wearing ill-fitting clothes that pinch and rub and that you can't breathe in isn't respecting your body; it draws attention to your body, keeping you focused on it instead of on more important things.

GO SHOPPING
—

Once you've ditched the clothes that don't fit, it's time to re-up your wardrobe with new outfits. Here are my favourite shopping tips to make clothing yourself a fun experience, not a shitty one.

Personal shopper: Book an appointment with a personal shopper/ stylist. Most big department stores will offer this as a free service. You can tell the stylist your budget, and it's literally their job to make you feel good and help you find clothes that look good on you! This has really helped some of my clients turn a shopping trip they were dreading into something they've really had fun with.

How do clothes make you feel? When you're trying clothes on, close your eyes and think about how they FEEL on your body before looking in the mirror. Do they fit? Are they comfortable? Can you sit down in them without them cutting off circulation? If the answer is no, take 'em off and get rid. If they feel good then open your eyes and look in the mirror and make sure you're happy with the way they look.

Clothes sizing is bullshit: Remember that clothes sizes are super-variable and totally arbitrary. They are NOT a reflection of how smart, funny, caring, compassionate, or awesome you are. Last year I bought four dresses on ASOS (my first mistake) for an event I was going to. When they arrived, not a single one fitted me. In the past this could have easily triggered a spiral of restricting and over exercising, followed by bingeing and generally feeling like shit. But on this occasion, I took a step back and said 'FUCK YOU, ASOS, AND YOUR BULLSHIT SIZING'. Then I got mad about the fact that 1 I didn't have anything to wear and 2 I had to pack all the shit back up and send it to wherever the hell it came from. Yes, I was angry, but the difference is that I was turning that anger outwards instead of directing it back in towards myself.

If clothes don't look good on you, it's NOT your fault. You don't have to change your body to fit the clothes. Clothes are mass made, and designed to fit a narrow range of body types. That's awesome if that's your body type, but for everyone else, it's not, and that sucks and it means we have to work harder to find clothes that do look and feel good on us, but buying stuff that's too small and trying to crowbar your ass into it isn't the solution.

If something is too small, resist the temptation to just try and 'make them fit', find clothes that fit and feel good on your body, because those are the clothes that will look and *feel* best on you. You'll feel more confident, comfortable, and most importantly, spend less time internally freaking out about your appearance and self-objectifying. It can be hard to let go of an 'ideal' size and move away from the size you think you should be. It might be worth exploring what's behind that; what does it represent to you? Write down your thoughts in your journal.

'But I can't afford a whole wardrobe upgrade'

Look, I get it, buying new shit is expensive. Especially when you have multiple mouths to feed or you're struggling just to make rent. I get it. I was a broke-ass student for ten years, then I moved to London and was somehow even more broke than when I was a student. If cost is a major factor here, just do what you can, buy some cheap and cheerful new jeans to tide you over until payday, or try the underwear challenge.

CHALLENGE

Time to buy yourself some new undies; it's a (relatively) small cost compared to changing your whole wardrobe but has a big impact.

Often when we are in diet mentality, we put conditions around treating ourselves to nice things. 'I'll buy sexy underwear once I've lost weight', 'I'll replace those skanky panties once I'm a size X'. We believe that we will only deserve pretty underwear once our diet has magically transformed us into this self-assured, sexy, confident person. But guess what, diets can't actually do that. It's just what diet companies want us to think!

So, in the meantime we wear bras that dig in to our sides and give us quad boob. We wear panties that pinch or ride up. If we think about this from a fundamental level, our underwear is what we wear closest to our bodies. What message are we sending to ourselves if we don't even wear underwear that fits. Aside from telling ourselves we don't value our body enough to make it comfortable, we're also drawing our attention back to our bodies (and not in a good way). Think about how many times you have to yank up your bra strap or pull out a wedgie from uncomfortable undies; how often do you blame yourself for being the problem instead of the underwear itself? Remember that, however transiently, body-checking takes us out of the moment (our flow state) and can use up precious cognitive resources that move us away from experiencing our internal cues.

So something as seemingly innocuous as poorly fitting pants could be keeping you tethered to body hate.

Can we show our bodies some respect by investing in underwear that is supportive, comfortable, and makes us feel great? There are amazing options out there that are supportive AND cute, even for those of us who're in the big-titty committee, so you don't have to compromise on feeling sexy either. It's a small thing, but when diet culture teaches us that we can't feel good about ourselves unless we're conforming (aka shrinking away), clothing our bodies comfortably is subversive and defiant; a little act of rebellion every time you get dressed. Plus it can disrupt that loop we play over and over and over that 'we're not good enough', and reinforce the idea that actually, you totally deserve to feel like a rock star in your body. It helps nudge us closer to body acceptance, bit by bit.

When we start taking care of ourselves, right down to what we put on our bodies, it's totally infectious. Try and enjoy this challenge. OK, nobody likes a stranger coming into the fitting room and telling you one boob is bigger than the other (or is that just me?), and fluorescent lighting and 360-degree mirrors are not flattering. Don't let that experience stop you though because it will be over in thirty minutes and you can go back home and try your new undies on in peace (maybe light a candle and set the mood?). Try and make it a special experience rather than letting it stress you out.

STOP PLAYING THE BODY-CHECKING GAME

We've talked about this already, but just in case you're still doing it; when you walk into a room or a party, do you automatically look other people up and down? Do you rank your waist size against other people in the room? Do you rate your attractiveness relative to other people? No judgement; we've all been there. But consider this, how does judging your body against other people's help you feel better about your own? There will always be people who are physically more attractive or thinner than you. Fact. If your self-worth is tied up in your appearance you will always lose out. Remember that you're so much more than your body. Be honest with yourself; does your 'ideal weight' have more to do with health or aesthetics? A US study showed that women's 'ideal' weight was 20% below the range considered to be healthy for them. Be real about what your healthy weight is. Studies have shown that when we are hyper-focused on our body image, we feel worse about ourselves.[14]

BODY-IMAGE ACTIVITIES
—

Ultimately the goal here is to think less about your body and to stop body-image issues from getting in the way of you living a whole and fulfilling life. Some of these activities may feel as though you're hyper-focused on it instead. If this ever feels like too much then come back to this section when you're in a better place. The amount of 'work' people have to do on body image varies enormously, and unfortunately there's no magic formula for feeling more comfortable in your own skin. In this section, you'll find a veritable party mix of challenges and journal activities; you get to decide which ones resonate with and are most helpful for you. If you don't like the look of an activity or don't find it helpful, can it. If there's one that's particularly helpful, come back to it or take it to your therapist, or talk to your mum or a close friend about it.

My body

In your journal, I want you to describe your body. Start at your toes, and build a picture with words, until you reach your head. If you prefer, you can literally draw yourself, using words to describe the parts of your body.

Journal questions

Reflect on how you described your body:

- Did you mostly use positive, neutral, or negative language?
- Did you focus on the parts of your body you liked or disliked?
- How does this description compare to how a friend or partner would describe you?
- How would you describe your body image: positive, negative, or neutral?
- Write down what positive body image means to you.

Your zero-fucks day
(adapted from Kylie Mitchell @immaeatthat)

Imagine what a day would be like if you gave zero fucks about what you looked like, how much exercise you did, or what you ate. What do you think it would be like to be completely at ease with your food choices and have no hang-ups with your body? It can be hard to imagine, so think back to when you were a little kid – you ate when you were hungry and then got back to playing. You didn't obsess about what you ate, you didn't worry about your body size because you weren't judgey about it, and you moved your body because it was fun and playful, not because you were trying to burn calories.

In your journal, write down what your day would look like if you were at peace with your body and all foods:

- Imagine the whole day without worrying about the foods you ate, without negative thoughts about your body size or concerns about food.
- What time would you wake up? What would you wear?
- What would you eat?
- Who would you spend time with? What would you do?
- How many meals and snacks/desserts would you have?
- What would you do for self-care?
- Would you move your body playfully or take a rest day?
- What would you read/listen to/watch?

Journal reflections

Read back what you wrote to yourself and think about the following questions:

Was your day different from a typical day? Did you have extra headspace to think about the things, people, and causes you care most about? Did you eat more or less food than you usually would? How did you feel throughout the day? What were the emotions you experienced? How did you feel when you went to bed that night? Is this a day you'd like to live? What steps could you take to make this day happen?

Goals

In your journal, set yourself two or three goals based on your 'zero fucks' day to tackle over the next week to two weeks.

Maybe in the day you visualized you went for a cycle along the beach front with your family/partner and afterwards you all enjoyed an ice cream together. A goal could be simply to do that in the next week, and not have any feelings of guilt or remorse, simply to enjoy the day. Reflect on your goals. What went well? What challenges did you have? What do you need to do to work through those obstacles?

What are 100 things you like about you?

In your journal, make a list of 100 things you like about you. They don't have to be all physical things (although having some is cool too). They can also be characteristics or accomplishments, skills, special talents, or just simple reasons why you're a badass; 100 things may sound like a lot – because it is – but that's kind of the point. The aim is for you to be able to look at that list and see how superfuckingcool you already are. Without changing a damn thing about your body.

Going through this process will help you internalize it in a way that hearing someone else say it won't. It's also important to physically write this down in your journal, rather than just doing it on your phone or in your head.

Try and come up with as many as you can on your own, and if you're really struggling you can ask family and friends for help. Whenever you're in a body-image funk, whip out this list.

Write a letter to your body

In your journal, I want you to write a letter to your body: you can do this in one of two ways.

1 Write an apology to your body, apologizing for the years of abusive, punishing exercise, or the semi-starvation, for trying to squeeze it into clothes that don't fit, or for hating it for not fitting into society's narrow standards. This is obviously very, very difficult and potentially quite upsetting, so if it feels too intense then start with the second option.

2 Write a love letter to your body thanking it for all the amazing things it allows you to do; from moving through the world to allowing you to be intimate, to having children, swimming, dancing, reading, listening to music, hugging your dog, to just living and breathing.

If you feel up to it, it would be great if you could do both (or maybe they are two parts of the same letter?), it's completely up to you. Reflect on this experience in your journal; were you able to cultivate a sense of gratitude for your body?

Dress to impress

Pick one or two days this week where you dress to impress; rock some bright lipstick, wear a statement necklace, own a bright colourful top or some jazzy earrings, fuck it, wear a flower in your hair! Do whatever makes you feel strong and beautiful and confident. Even if that means taking an extra ten minutes in the morning for yourself – you deserve it and you are worth it!

We know that you are so much more than your appearance (remember the 100 reasons you wrote that make you awesome?) but at the same time respecting your body and putting a little extra effort into your appearance can make a huge difference to how you feel about yourself. Just investing a little time in ourselves and channelling some energy inwards helps us feel better about ourselves without going down the path of self-restriction.

Reflection: how did you feel at the end of the day? Did investing a little extra time in yourself give you a confidence boost?

Touch yourself!

Not like that, I mean, maybe like that, if that's what makes you feel good! This last challenge is intended to help you reconnect with your body. Most of us are used to ignoring it and pretending like it doesn't exist, doing minimal things to care for it other than shower! Through touching our bodies in a compassionate and respectful way, we can find a new appreciation for them, and begin to feel more comfortable in our skin. When I ask clients in clinic to describe their body to me, they have a tendency to tug, pull, and pinch the parts they don't like. Notice if you do that and see if you can touch it the way you would something you care about.

Here are some suggestions:

- Self-massage. Do a quick YouTube search for self-acceptance massages that teach you how to touch your body kindly.
- Use a fancy lotion after a nice bath.
- Give yourself a mani/pedi.
- Do a DIY face mask.

If you feel like splashing out, you could treat yourself to a nice massage at a spa, but if that's not an option for you, or the idea makes you feel uncomfortable, that's completely fine too.

Body-image meditation

This body-image meditation was inspired by one of my clients who developed a similar version to help her work through her own body-image struggles. I thought it was so beautiful that I developed my own version for using with clients. It's such a good way to check in with your body and show it some gratitude, even when you're not feeling great about it. Just before bed read it out loud to yourself or record your voice to play back to yourself. This is just an example, but you can adjust it so that it makes sense to you and your body; the idea is simply to thank the parts of your body that work hard for you every day, instead of being resentful. You could also flip it around and make it about waking up the different parts of your body and getting them ready for the day ahead. You can do this practice in a comfortable seated position with your feet planted on the floor, or lying outstretched on your bed.

Take a deep breath in through your nose, exhaling out of your mouth and sighing away the day . . .

Take another breath in through your nose, and releasing the breath and the day through your mouth . . .

Once more, take another long, deep breath, in through your nose, and sighing out through your mouth . . .

Gently close your eyes.

Today I'm grateful to my body for all the things it has helped me achieve.

I am grateful for my feet, which have helped me move forward today.

I am grateful for my legs, which have helped me stand tall today.

I am grateful for my bottom, which has let me sit comfortably and provided me soft cushioning today.

I am grateful for my hips, which have allowed me to sit and stand, walk and bend.

I am grateful for my belly, which has kept me fed and nourished today.

I am grateful for my chest, which is home to my heart and my breath.

I am grateful for my shoulders, which have carried the weight of my woes and burdens.

I am grateful for my arms, which allow me to embrace those I love.

I am grateful for my hands, which allow me to interact with the world (and pet animals!).

I am grateful for my mouth, which has spoken my truth, kissed, given me breath, and tasted delicious food.

I am grateful for my nose, which has let me smell the richness of flowers, perfume, and fresh baked bread.

I am grateful to my ears, which allow me to listen to music and hear the voices of my loved ones.

I am grateful for my eyes, which allow me to see the world, read books, and gaze upon the faces of those I love.

I am grateful for my mind, which allows me to think deeply, to create, and dream.

Now I rest my body, grateful for all it does for me, appreciative that it gives me life, and that I am safe.

Use the exercises above as much as you need to help you feel good in your body. Chances are they won't be a one-time deal though, so revisit them often until you feel you are beginning to practise body neutrality.

————

Now I want to switch things up a little and talk about weight and health. Some of you might be wondering if it's unhealthy or bad for you to embrace your natural size, especially if being at your set point weight puts you in the 'overweight' or 'obese' category. For a lot of you, health concerns might have been what led you to dieting in the first place. Indeed, weight loss might be one of the first treatment options your doctor suggests to help you manage a particular condition and there's barely a day goes by without something in the news about 'the obesity epidemic' and how the nation needs to go on a diet. So how is it possible that, as a nutritionist, I'm recommending that we give up dieting?

If we look at the weight-science literature (the branch of nutrition and medicine concerned with weight) we see that we have a compelling scientific evidence base that shows a correlation between higher weight and disease risk (such as certain cancers, heart disease, and type-2 diabetes). This is not in dispute. However, because this association is a correlation, we cannot infer causality. What we mean by this is we don't know if it is fat *per se*, or other risk factors that lead to health problems. To give you another example, the number of people who died by getting tangled in their bedsheets correlates nicely with per capita cheese consumption. And the number of people who drowned by falling into a pool correlates with the number of films per year Nicholas Cage appeared in. Clearly Nicholas Cage and cheese aren't causing these deaths, there's some other variable or risk factor not being accounted for.[15] The same may be true when it comes to health. There is an assumption in the weight-science literature that weight, in and of itself, *causes* poor health, but we cannot know that for sure unless we take other risk factors into account.[16]

An obvious and important risk factor that comes to mind is something we've already touched on: weight stigma/bias and fat phobia; when we do research weight and health, these potentially confounding variables are never accounted for, but they could, at least in part, explain the relationship between health and weight.

WEIGHT BIAS

——

The World Health Organization defines weight bias as 'negative attitudes towards, and beliefs about, others because of their weight. These negative attitudes are manifested by stereotypes and/or prejudice towards people with overweight and obesity'.[17]

Judy Swift, a researcher from Nottingham University, conducted a study surveying 1,100 trainee doctors, nurses, dietitians, and nutritionists. She found that only 1.4% of them expressed positive or neutral attitudes towards fat people. That means that 98.6% of the future generation of healthcare professionals are starting their careers with negative or very negative attitudes about fat people.[18] Why does this matter? Because it means that people all along the weight spectrum will receive poorer care. It means that doctors and healthcare providers will assume that thinner people are healthy and fat people are unhealthy. It means that thin people at risk of diseases like type-2 diabetes or cardiovascular disease can fly under the radar and miss being diagnosed, and fat people will automatically be prescribed a diet or weight-loss advice despite the presentation. This leads to worse health outcomes for *everyone*.

Doctors who show high levels of weight bias spend less time with fat patients, give them fewer treatment options and less access to treatment. How does this help improve health? Exactly – it doesn't. Many fat people delay treatment for fear of being judged or shamed by their medical professional.[19] Even doctors who work in 'weight-management' – a euphemism for doctors who put people on diets – show varying degrees of anti-fat sentiment towards their patients, characterizing them as lazy, stupid, and worthless.[20]

Weight bias can lead to **weight stigma**, which is the social sign or label affixed to an individual who is the victim of prejudice.

Specifically, weight bias and weight stigma have been associated with:

- Poor body image and body dissatisfaction
- Low self-esteem and self-confidence
- Feelings of worthlessness and loneliness
- Suicidal thoughts and acts
- Depression, anxiety, and other psychological disorders
- Maladaptive eating patterns (i.e. disordered eating and eating disorders)
- Avoidance of physical activity
- Stress-induced pathophysiology (increases in inflammatory markers like C-reactive protein)
- Avoidance of medical care

In other words, the diseases we often associate with being in a larger body might actually be related to fat phobia and bias from healthcare providers, not just from being fat.

Arguably, 'weight bias' and 'weight stigma' are euphemisms and 'politifications' of the social justice terminology **fat hatred** and **fat phobia**. In her book *Fat Activism*, Charlotte Cooper defines fat phobia as 'The fear and hatred of fat people'. She goes on to explain:

> Social cleansing is central to gentrification and so too to the professionalistion of fat activism. This can be seen through the use of language. 'Fat' is too abrasive and politicized in this context, so the more anodyne and less specific 'weight' is substituted. Instead of fat phobia or fat hatred, which confer some of the emotional experience of being fat, 'weight stigma' and 'weight bias' become preferred terms. No fear, hate, rage, oppression, or other untidy emotion is allowed to clutter these fascinating and dispassionate debates.

I think *fat phobia* more honestly and accurately describes the problem so I will use this term, otherwise the experiences of fat people become gentrified and erased, further compounding the issue.

Many researchers have argued that fat phobia is a consequence of the public-health 'war on obesity', where fat bodies are often dehumanized and portrayed as 'headless fatties' or are told they are a drain on NHS resources.[21,22,23,24,25,26,27] I'm inclined to agree. Between the periods 1995–1996 and 2004–2006, fat phobia increased by 66%, a rate that can't be accounted for by increases in weight alone. This suggests that fat phobia is being driven by other factors. Many have argued that weight-focused public-health policies can lead to unintended consequences, including excessive weight preoccupation, which can lead to body dissatisfaction, dieting and disordered eating, death from extreme dieting, anorexia and bariatric surgery complications or from suicide resulting from weight-based bullying or depression, and finally, discrimination.

Think about how discouraging, demoralizing, and dehumanizing it must be to be in a bigger body and be told that you are a liability? You're a ticking time bomb? What kind of incentive is that to make positive health changes? We know there are so many benefits to exercise, nutrition, smoking cessation, reducing alcohol, and even meditation, that improve health INDEPENDENT of weight, no matter where you lie on the weight spectrum, so why would we do or say anything that discourages positive changes? To quote Cambridge University geneticist Giles Yeo: 'Fat shaming is not an effective tool to fight biology.'

Internalized fat phobia is defined as holding negative beliefs about oneself due to weight or size.[28] In 2017 a small study of black American women was published that suggested that people who experienced high levels of internalized fat phobia (people who perceived that they were discriminated against on the basis of their size) were *three times* more likely to develop metabolic syndrome and *six times* as likely to have high triglycerides than people of the same weight who didn't perceive high levels of internalized fat phobia.[29] Likewise, people who experienced high levels of fat phobia had *double* the risk of becoming ill than those who didn't experience fat phobia.[30]

Fat phobia is related to higher blood pressure, binge eating, bulimia symptoms, negative body image, low self-esteem, and depression in children and adults.[31] Again, fat phobia may contribute to a number of diseases we usually ascribe to being in a bigger body. However, due to unexamined weight bias among researchers, the contribution of weight stigma to disease is rarely controlled for in weight science.

What about IRL?

All this science is great, and having evidence is important. But I also wanted to share a real-life example of what it's like navigating a fat-phobic healthcare system when you are someone in a bigger body. Jenni is a client of mine who I have worked with on and off for a while now. She's smart, sassy, incredibly self-aware, and super-clued-up on weight bias in the medical community, and she herself is a healthcare professional. Here she shares her experiences of going to get help from a physiotherapist for a shoulder problem that was unrelated to her weight, but, as is fairly typical among healthcare providers, she was recommended to lose weight, even though it **1** wasn't what she wanted help with and **2** wouldn't help her condition:

It was 2016 and I was working in a large London hospital, when I began to have severe pain in my upper back. After a few weeks of muddling through, unable to lift my arms higher than my shoulders, I caved and made an appointment with the hospital staff's physiotherapist. I was hopeful that with a bit of manipulation, and some daily exercises to perform, I'd soon be back to 100%.

When I arrived at the physio, I filled in the pre-screening health questionnaire, and waited my turn. The physio systematically examined my upper body, asking me to move, and tested my range of motion. He came to the conclusion that my neck, upper back and shoulders were very tense, and there was a large tight band or 'knot' causing muscle spasms, hence the tightness and pain. He gave me a deep-tissue massage and a series of daily exercises to do. Everything was going well as we scheduled the dates for the next appointment. And then the inevitable moment, as I asked about prevention of future shoulder pain . . .

The physio looked me up and down. 'You're overweight, you need to lose weight.'

'Did my weight cause the shoulder pain?' I asked, a bit confused.

'Will losing weight help or prevent it coming back?'

'No,' the physio said, 'completely unrelated, but you should lose weight. Here's a leaflet.'

The leaflet thrust into my hand was the usual NHS fare, a leaflet that had been photocopied so many times that the words inside were barely legible. But what was clear was that the advice it contained was simple, just eat less and move more. And that was it. No patient-centred care. No conversations about my needs or expectations or previous experiences. Not only was the advice completely irrelevant to my visit, by the physio's own admission, but the advice was neither tailored nor useful.

Due to the nature of my job, I was walking 20,000+ steps a day. I was lifting and moving heavy loads all day (hence the injury in the first place). I ran several nights a week. I ate my 5-a-day. My general health was fantastic – blood pressure, cholesterol, blood sugars and more, all spot on. I ran a busy department, I managed a team of thirteen staff. I was a healthcare professional with fourteen years of experience and a wealth of knowledge.

All of this information was in my pre-screening questionnaire and in my referral. But in that moment, in that consultation, to that physio, it was all irrelevant. I was just a fat woman, and that was wrong and a problem to be fixed.

I went home feeling tired and frustrated. On a whim I posted to Facebook, recounting my experience. I ended with my thoughts on the miracle weightless tool I'd been offered: 'HOLY FUCK, A LEAFLET, THAT'S WHERE I'VE BEEN GOING WRONG ALL THESE YEARS. IF ONLY I'D HAD A LEAFLET.'

Within moments many of my friends – especially women in similar bodies – chimed in, cheering me up. 'Can I read the magic leaflet so we can slim together?', 'Does it have to be a particular leaflet or will any do?', 'How do we use the leaflet? Is it a magic spell?' Laughing, I suggested perhaps we rub the leaflet on three times a day and see what happens.

So, the assumption in weight research is that fat *causes* poor health – but we know that we cannot make that claim based on the evidence we have available, and that weight stigma and fat phobia may account, at least in part, for this risk. Unfortunately, though, it doesn't end there. In 2017 the BMJ published a paper summarizing many more assumptions made by the weight-science literature that don't hold up under scrutiny.[32] I've pulled out a few of the most pertinent ones here to help you begin to dismantle the idea that your weight dictates your health. I know some of these ideas are probably sort of mind-blowing, so if it feels uncomfortable, don't worry, it was hard for me to get my head around at first too. Just sit with it, and go off and do some of your own research; I've shared some further reading in the resources section.

––––

Studies show that long-term weight loss is only possible for a select few, and isn't the norm for most people. Of those who do lose weight long term, many of them are engaged in extreme or disordered behaviours.[33]

Although not everyone can achieve a specific 'goal' weight, they CAN improve their health and well-being with lifestyle interventions, if that is something they want to pursue and have access to. Consistently evidence shows, time and time again, that around 80% of diets fail within the first year and that after five years, most if not all weight has been regained.[34,35,36,37] This can trigger weight cycling, which is associated with an increase in set point weight in animal studies (this is harder to measure in humans, although some human studies seem to suggest it too), increased heart-disease risk in lower-weight individuals, and higher risk of mental-health issues like depression.[38,39,40,41,42]

The point is that the harm caused by weight-focused interventions may outweigh the benefit, and from an individual and a public-health perspective, focusing on developing a healthy relationship to food, body image, and movement is exponentially more beneficial.[43]

I hope this helps to explain why fighting diet culture isn't limited to people in smaller bodies and why it's important for everyone to be included in this conversation.

So what does it mean for your health if your set point weight is in the 'overweight' or 'obese' category by BMI? It's helpful to remember that BMI or body mass index is a crude tool that is simply your weight divided by your height (squared). It was a metric designed to monitor trends in populations over time, not as a measure of health. The cut-offs for a BMI above 25 being 'overweight' and a BMI 30 being 'obese' are also fairly arbitrary. In fact 'overweight' used to be defined as a BMI of 27 or more, but this was reduced to 25 in the 1980s. This meant that thousands of people who were previously 'normal' weight abruptly became overweight overnight. You'd have thought, then, that there must be pretty compelling evidence that having a BMI over 25 conferred significant risk to one's health, right? Wrong.

In 2013, a team of researchers led by Dr Katherine Flegal conducted a meta-analysis, one of the strongest pieces of evidence we have available. Meta-analyses pull together data from multiple studies into one mega-study; the researchers were hoping they could find out which BMI category has the highest death rate. They found that the 'overweight' group (BMI 25–<30) had the lowest death rate, and that those in the 'obese' BMI group of 30–35 had the same risk of death as those in the 'normal' group.[44] Seriously. This isn't a fluke finding either. A large Danish observational study of over 100,000 people published in the *Journal of The American Medical Association* in 2016 found that those in the 'overweight' category had the lowest risk of death from cardiovascular disease and total deaths. Pretty mind-blowing, isn't it?

So can you be fat and healthy?

Lots of factors influence a person's health, and body weight is only a small part of the picture. Epidemiological studies examining the cardiovascular risk at a higher body weight show that it increases relative risk by only about 20% when known risk factors are controlled for. Like I've already mentioned, weight bias and stigma are rarely controlled for in studies, neither are health-promoting behaviours, or past dieting experience, meaning this number could be even smaller. This compares with a roughly 100% increase in relative risk with smoking. Health and well-being can improve even without weight reduction. For example, cardiorespiratory fitness, mental health, and blood glucose control can all be improved with physical activity, even if the person's weight does not change. By using only the surrogate marker of weight loss, we don't recognize the health benefits of a change in lifestyle behaviours. People are labelled as 'unsuccessful' because their health gains are unnoticed. With this sense of failure, people are likely to lose motivation and stop the changed lifestyle behaviour and in doing so lose the health benefits.

In many cases weight loss is *associated* with better health, but again we can't infer that this effect is from weight loss *per se*, or because of an improvement in health-related behaviours such as exercise or nutrition. In order to prove that weight loss causes health improvements we'd have to do a study where people lost weight without improving their behaviours. A study like this is very difficult to do, but one way of testing this is looking at people who have had liposuction; they have lost weight, but haven't changed their behaviours. What we tend to see in these studies is that, when subcutaneous fat (fat just beneath the skin) is removed, there is no improvement in biomarkers of health like insulin sensitivity, total cholesterol, and triglycerides.[45,46]

On the flip side though, the evidence is really clear that we CAN improve health, independent of weight loss. In a study of over 11,000 people in the US, researchers wanted to understand the impact of health-promoting behaviours on disease risk. They measured people's weight, as well as the following four behaviours: eating five or more fruits and vegetables daily, exercising regularly, consuming alcohol in moderation, and not smoking. What they found is that with people who didn't engage in any of the behaviours, the people in the 'normal' BMI category had the lowest risk of disease, followed by 'overweight' and 'obese'. However, even just engaging in one of the four behaviours cut disease risk in half! And engaging in all four behaviours meant that disease risk was the roughly the same, independent of weight.[47]

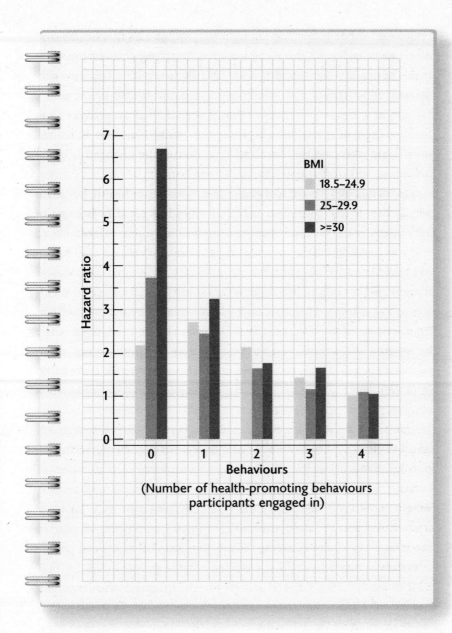

Exercise, independent of weight loss, appears to be particularly beneficial at reducing the risk of heart disease, type-2 diabetes and stroke, especially among people at the higher end of the weight spectrum.[48] The key to this may be cardiorespiratory fitness; a systematic review from 2010 concluded that 'The data indicate that the risk for all-cause and cardiovascular mortality [death rate] was lower in individuals with high BMI and good aerobic fitness, compared with individuals with normal BMI and poor fitness.'[49] This is likely to be because physical activity, and consequently improved fitness levels, help reduce visceral adipose tissue, the type of fat that can cause metabolic issues, without necessarily impacting subcutaneous fat, which is considered to be relatively harmless.[50,51] Aerobic exercise may also have a greater impact on attenuating risk of type-2 diabetes than resistance training for those who are at a higher weight.[52]

———

Compared with our current climate of shaming and judging people into being healthier, imagine a public-health message that focused on the health benefits of engaging in regular physical activity and eating nutritious meals no matter what shape or size? We don't even have to imagine it. The This Girl Can campaign was responsible for getting almost 3 million women between the ages of fourteen and forty moving. What's more, it was created using images of actual women running, sweating, and jiggling, as opposed to the idealized images of women's fitness we're so used to seeing. The campaign showed a diverse range of bodies, including women in hijabs and disabled women, all taking part in activity. There was no mention of weight loss anywhere. Compare this to Cancer Research UK's 2018 campaign: an ominous Hangman-esque campaign reporting that 'OB_S_ _Y is a cause of cancer'. On Twitter the same day the campaign was launched there were horrific fat-phobic comments hurled at fat people, and public shaming of fat bodies in the media. This is a clear case of how public-health messages can contribute to fat phobia and weight stigma. The most frustrating part about the campaign, however, was that it used the word *causes*. 'Obesity *causes* cancer'. But again, that's not what the evidence says – there's an association, sure, but nowhere does the campaign quantify the risk of cancer for people at a higher weight. Ian Olver explained this nicely in The Conversation:[53]

> A woman from a Western country has a 2 in 100 chance (2% absolute lifetime risk) of developing cancer of the endometrium (lining of the uterus) by the age of 85.
>
> If the woman is obese, her risk of endometrial cancer is twice that of a woman of ideal weight. That is, a relative risk of 2 or 100% greater chance of developing endometrial cancer than a woman who is not obese.
>
> This 100% figure may sound like obese women have a very high risk of endometrial cancer. But, in fact, the risk is still quite low, since doubling the 2% population risk still only makes the absolute risk of endometrial cancer in obese women around 4%. This is still a low probability of cancer.

This means that 96/100 obese women won't get endometrial cancer, yet a campaign such as CRUK's that is based on fear and shame, contributes to weight stigma. Remember the issues associated with weight stigma? Weight-focused campaigns like this can lead people to stop engaging in health-promoting behaviours, avoid routine and preventative medical screenings, and jeopardize physical and mental health.[54,55]

Health at Every Size®

Health at Every Size (HAES) is a weight-*inclusive*, anti-diet healthcare paradigm that shifts the focus away from weight loss and instead promotes *health gain*. The idea at the core of HAES is simple: help support behaviours that improve health independently of size. It's a fat-positive movement that aims to eliminate stigma in healthcare (which as we've just seen, is super-fucked-up). Intuitive eating and HAES go hand in hand.

HAES principles

Weight inclusivity: Accept and respect the inherent diversity of body shapes and sizes and reject the idealizing or pathologizing of specific weights.

Health enhancement: Support health policies that improve and equalize access to information and services, and personal practices that improve well-being, including attention to individual physical, economic, social, spiritual, emotional and other needs.

Respectful care: Acknowledge our biases, and work to end weight discrimination, weight stigma and weight bias. Provide information and services from an understanding that socio-economic status, race, gender, sexual orientation, age and other identities impact weight stigma, and support environments that address these inequities.

Eating for well-being: Promote flexible, individualized eating based on hunger, satiety, nutritional needs, and pleasure, rather than any externally regulated eating plan focused on weight control.

Life-enhancing movement: Support physical activities that allow people of all sizes, abilities and interests to engage in enjoyable movement, to the degree that they choose.

Benefits of HAES

Although research on HAES interventions is a relatively new field, there are some potentially exciting benefits of this approach:

- Improved diet quality and increased intuitive eating[56]
- Less eating restraint, less and less disinhibited eating, aka fewer food rules and restriction and less bingeing behaviour[57]
- Improved blood lipid profiles and blood pressure[58,59,60]
- Increased fitness[61]
- Improved psychological well-being[62]
- Lowered risk of heart disease and type-2 diabetes[63,64,65]

Like IE, HAES encourages body acceptance as opposed to weight loss or weight 'management'.

HAES supports reliance on internal regulatory processes, such as hunger and satiety, as opposed to encouraging cognitively imposed dietary restriction, in other words, IE. Finally, HAES supports active embodiment as opposed to encouraging structured exercise; this means moving in ways that feel good in your body as opposed to punishing yourself with rigid workouts, aka intuitive movement, which we'll cover down the line.[66] To learn more about HAES, check out the recommended reading in the resources section.

EXAMINING YOUR OWN INTERNALIZED FAT PHOBIA
—

I would encourage everyone to reflect on the unconscious biases they may hold against people in larger bodies and to consider challenging their own assumptions, or stereotypes they may see in the media, as well as the assumptions listed above. Both thin and fat people harbour anti-fat sentiments, so it's important to check yourself no matter what your phenotype.

Take a moment to reflect on your assumptions of fat people and write them down in your journal. Even if you are a fat person, you may still harbour some anti-fat biases of your own. In fact, for my clients who are fat, this is some of the most difficult work to unpack; after all, we have a propensity to say the meanest, cruellest things about ourselves. So take a moment to list out your associations with fat. Are they mostly positive or negative? If they are mostly negative, can you also list some positives?

It's also important to recognize that just because someone is fat, they aren't obliged to perform 'health' in order to be valued; if you are a living soul, you deserve love and respect.

HOW TO EXAMINE YOUR OWN INTERNALIZED FATPHOBIA

———

Step 1: Educate yourself

Read books and blogs written by fat people. Listen to podcasts and watch vlogs. If you are an academic or healthcare professional, get your ass over to PubMed and do some recon on weight bias and weight stigma in nutrition research. Pay attention to people who are sharing their experiences of living in a society that systematically medicalizes and declares war on their bodies. Do not dismiss their perspectives as being less valuable or valid than your own.

Step 2: Follow fat people

I share a list of fat-positive accounts I love in the resources section at the back of the book; follow these people. Again, pay attention to what they have to say. Really, pay attention to their stories, experiences, and the lessons they have to teach you. Again, it's important that you aren't just following barely plus-size models, but people at the higher end of the weight spectrum. It may feel uncomfortable to view fat bodies, but sit with the discomfort until it dissipates, that's part of the work.

Step 3: Challenge thoughts and judgements

Notice any automatic negative fat-phobic thoughts you have in response to viewing fat bodies, or in reaction to hearing the perspectives of fat people. Come up with three counter-thoughts to help you reframe those automatic negative thoughts. This could look something like this.

Fat-phobic thought: Fat people can avoid stigma if they just ate less and moved more.

Counter-thought 1: Everyone is deserving of respect, independent of their shape or size or any other identity they hold.

Counter-thought 2: Diets don't work and diet culture contributes to a society that is conducive to intolerance towards fat bodies.

Counter-thought 3: Don't be a fat-phobic asshat!

Step 4: Find community

If you are fat yourself, finding a community with other fat people (either online or IRL) can be enormously healing.

THIN PRIVILEGE

—

Quick question – if I were fat, would you be so willing to hear me out on this? I have colleagues who do the same work as me, who have the same level of education and experience, who aren't being listened to or taken seriously when they talk about the same concepts and ideas I do. This is just one of the advantages conferred to me, not based on merit or hard work, but because of . . . the size of my jeans? Yup, pretty backwards, huh? These advantages are collectively termed **thin privilege**. If you are a thin person, you might not have even realized that this was a privilege you held (herein lies the problem with privilege!). You might even feel uncomfortable or resistant to the term. That's understandable, no one likes their privilege being called out; it can feel shameful. But it's important to recognize that privilege is systemic. Yes, we all individually hold different privileges, depending on the intersecting identities we have. But these privileges are reinforced through power structures. Acknowledging your own privilege, and making space for people who are less privileged, is critical in healing the damage caused by inequality and oppression.

Let's take a look at some of the privileges conferred by being thin.

- Not having to worry if you'll fit in the airplane chair.
- Not having to endure the humiliation of people gawking at you when you ask for a seatbelt extender or as the person next to you kicks up a stink about having 'no space'.
- Not having to pretend you just LOVE accessories when you shop with your friends because you know you can't fit into any of the clothes at that store, so you try on 7,000 hats.
- Not living in fear of breaking a chair at a restaurant.
- Not having the doctor prescribe a diet for *literally everything*. Got an eye infection? Diet! Broken your arm? Maybe if you lost some weight ... Brain haemorrhaging from a car accident? You get the point!
- Oh, and if this wasn't enough, then how about not having to deal with weight-based educational and employment-related prejudice?

Nobody is saying that thin people don't face challenges, or have an easy time accepting their bodies – that's categorically untrue; thin privilege doesn't immunize us against the societal scrutiny on bodies, it just means less scrutiny than fat bodies. The conversation is more nuanced than that though. What we mean when we say we have thin privilege is that we recognize that fat people have an extra layer of shit to wade through, making their lives more challenging. And ditto if you have multiple intersecting marginalized identities, then you could have additional layers of shit to wade through.

UNCONDITIONAL
PERMISSION
TO EAT

Research on intuitive eaters has revealed a really interesting phenomenon: intuitive eaters don't have food rules and restrictions; they give themselves unconditional permission to eat all food. But at the same time they engage in less emotional eating, binge eating and disinhibited eating. Why is this?

In chapter 4, we talked about physical deprivation from eating too few calories and not getting enough energy. But a sense of deprivation can also arise from food rules and restrictions. This leads to food preoccupation, obsessing about foods and generally just losing our shit around food. We're placing a cognitive boundary around food, which replaces a more intuitive regulation of food intake; in other words it's like Kanye applying to MENSA every time we want to eat.

An overly cognitive focus on food (being too in our heads about every food choice) reduces sensitivity towards our physiological hunger and fullness cues. Instead we rely on psychological (i.e. stress), cultural (i.e. 'it's lunchtime') or social signs to eat (i.e. 'they aren't eating gluten, maybe I shouldn't eat gluten').[1] It also sets us up to be in a scarcity mindset.

THE DEPRIVATION MINDSET
—

The basic premise of most diets and food rules is cutting something out; restricting, or depriving ourselves of a food that we enjoy eating. Even when diets claim to be about 'abundance', there are usually conditions on foods we love, that satisfy us and fill us up. But the very act of psychologically ring-fencing a food or food group can trigger a sense of deprivation and scarcity that heightens our desire for the thing we can't have.[2] Think about it this way, recall a time when you were flat broke. Financial resources are scarce, and you have to make rent, buy groceries, and pay your bills. Does your lack of funds help you feel chill about money? No way! It's the complete opposite, right? Or let's say you're really hot for someone, like, really into them but they're playing hard to get, and just a bit out of reach. That only makes you want them *more*! OK, maybe that was just eighteen-year-old Laura. Anyway, in my experience with clients, placing restriction around food, whether physically through dieting, emotionally through labelling foods as 'bad' or 'unhealthy', or because of food insecurity and poverty, can result in heightened attention towards food. In psychology, when resources are scarce and needs are unmet we think about them more.[3,4] Here, this extrapolates to food, whether that deprivation is real, à la carbs in the Paleo diet, or psychologically when you label foods you love as 'bad'. It can create a sense of urgency, intensity, and deep desire for the thing you can't have; the forbidden-fruit effect. But of course, you *can* have that food if you really wanted it and if you violate the terms of this cognitive boundary you have placed around food, you might end up triggering the fuck-it effect. Oh, don't play coy with me, you know *exactly* what I mean. 'Well, I've had a cookie now, fuck it, might as well have ten.' In other words, a sense of deprivation not only makes us feel slightly obsessed and preoccupied with food, but it can set us up to make us feel out of control; when we finally do eat a particular food it can result in eating past the point of comfortable fullness, eating in the absence of hunger, or binge eating.[5]

This can reinforce the idea that we have no willpower and can't be trusted around food. Instead, by giving ourselves unconditional permission to eat all foods (yes, even gluten and sugar!) we begin to dismantle the scarcity mindset that can make us feel weird around food. In this chapter, we'll break down that cognitive boundary around good and bad foods and replace it with food neutrality. We'll decimate food rules and restrictions and learn to eat according to what our body wants and needs and what makes us feel good! We'll kick the scarcity mindset in the face so we can make food choices from a place of security and stability, without the threat of future deprivation, to nourish our bodies and souls![6] Getting back to a place where you are no longer restricting foods that you crave and giving yourself full, unconditional permission to eat is a process and can take some time. Think of it this way...

THE 'COW IN A FIELD' ANALOGY

—

Imagine a rolling, verdant pasture full of lush green grass as far as you can see. In the middle of all of this there's a small fenced-off field with a single, solitary cow. The cow can see the tall delicious grass all around her, but she can't get out of the field and is forced to eat the same half-dead grass from the field that she's also stomped and shat all over for months on end. Then one day, a benevolent farmer comes along and lets her out of the field to roam around the pasture. What do you think the cow does? Does she delicately graze and nibble the tips of the grass? Of course not. Baby girl GOES TO TOWN. She has been in a state of deprivation for as long as she can remember, causing her to ignore her satiety cues and eat way past the point of comfortable fullness for fear of future deprivation. But slowly, and very gradually, she begins to trust that she won't be forced back into the crappy dingy field and is free to eat the luscious thick grass. After time, she feels comfortable and content just eating enough grass to satisfy her cravings and respond to her hunger and fullness cues without fear of future deprivation.

I forget where I first heard this analogy, but it sums up exactly what happens when we go from being in a state of deprivation to learning to give ourselves unconditional permission to eat. At first, we might have a lot of fun experimenting with foods that have previously been forbidden and, frankly, eating way past our point of comfortable fullness. But this is a normal response to deprivation. Until we have completely shrugged off the risk of future deprivation, it's unlikely that we'll be able to find that comfortable level of fullness or the amount of food that's appropriate for our bodies. However, this period doesn't last forever, and I'm going to give you tools to handle it like a boss; in a way that's systematic and methodical that balances nudging you up against your comfort zone, without tipping you over the edge. Delicious foods will always always be around. There will always be pastries at brunch, cake and coffee afternoons with friends, and pizza date nights. They're not going anywhere, we need to learn how to handle them without losing our shit every time we come in contact with them. Simply forbidding foods doesn't equip us to navigate these foods in a healthy or sustainable way, but giving ourselves unconditional permission frees up cognitive resources that allows us to truly experience how food will feel in our body. That space allows us to decide if we really want or like that food, and allows us to be curious about how much of a particular food it takes to satisfy us. To begin to give ourselves unconditional permission to eat, we first of all have to examine conscious and unconscious restrictions we have around food.

THE FUCK-IT EFFECT

—

Thanks to years of conflicting nutrition advice from self-appointed Instagram nutrition gurus, women's 'health' magazines, and diets masquerading as 'lifestyles', it's pretty likely you've built up a set of food rules that dictate what, when, and how much you eat. They may even just be there unconsciously. Some of them might be contradictory, some of them kind of irrational, others just straight up weird.

Layered on top of those rules we all invariably have a shit list – a set of foods that are prohibited. Or, if eaten, have to be done in a controlled way – fitting in with points, calories or macros. Alternatively, they might need to be 'made up' for or bargained against running an extra mile, or only having a salad the next day. In other words, they are attached to a set of conditions, and if we violate these conditions, eating becomes loaded with self-judgement and criticism, guilt, shame, and other negative emotions. This can trigger the fuck-it effect – when you've broken a food rule or eaten a 'bad food' so you say 'fuck it, I've fallen off the bandwagon, might as well go all the way'. This can lead to eating past the point of comfortable fullness, bingeing, and feelings of guilt.[7,8] And while you might be giving yourself permission to eat those foods in the moment, you make a promise with yourself never to eat those foods again or never to break that rule again. Instead of obliterating the bandwagon, you're committing to get back on it. This can reinforce the threat of future deprivation and the deprivation mindset. It can make us more obsessive about food, increasing cravings and desire for 'shit list' foods, and, when we inevitably do eat those foods, we eat them with such urgency and intensity that it can feel like we're addicted to them. Illegal foods carry a sense of shame, guilt, and anxiety, and the longer you've been restricting and depriving, the more intensely and deeply you will experience these feelings; this in turn can cause you to eat them past the point of comfortable fullness.

Examining your FOOD RULES

In your journal write a list of the rules you have around what, when, or how much you eat. You may not even be aware of all of your food rules initially, many will be subconscious, so pay attention to what crops up when you go out to dinner or if you have multiple portions of carbs in the same day. Whatever it is, write it down, and then answer the following questions.

- How do these rules help facilitate joy and pleasure around eating?
- How do these rules allow me flexibility in my eating?
- How do these rules give me the space to discover the foods I really enjoy and want to eat?
- How are these rules helping or holding me back from trusting my own ability to regulate the amount of food that's appropriate for me?
- How do these rules stop me from paying attention to my own hunger and fullness signals?
- How do these rules help me become an intuitive eater?

What's on your
SHIT LIST

In your journal write a list of the foods you restrict or, consider bad, beat yourself up for eating, or generally freak you out. These are usually foods higher in sugar or fat like cookies and crisps, but might also be takeaway foods, processed foods, or snacks/desserts.

The foods at the top of your shit list are usually the worst offenders: the most triggering, the ones that you feel worst about when you eat. The bottom of your list are safer foods that don't stress you out as much.

At this point you don't need to do anything with your shit list – I just want you to recognize that you have created a food hierarchy. How can you cultivate food neutrality towards these foods? Can you stop thinking of them in terms of good/bad, healthy/unhealthy?

But these Food Rules and Shit List foods can be so deeply ingrained that we're not really even sure how to begin to dig ourselves out and give ourselves unconditional permission to eat. It can also feel kind of overwhelming and stressful to think about eating without rules and restrictions (or an app!) dictating your every move. So I just want to remind you, that you've got this. It might be buried under years of diets and diet-culture bullshit, but under all of that, you have an internal GPS that will help guide you. It takes time and it takes courage to let your body take the reins, but over time, you'll gain more and more trust in your body's ability to regulate your food intake, making sure you get a good balance of nutrients, without feeling restricted, eating for pleasure and function, and having a healthy relationship to food.

So how do we get out of this mess? Should you just go to the store and grab a bunch of Pringles and doughnuts, order a pizza and go to town. I mean, that's one way of doing it. And I have clients come to me who are so beyond done with dieting that this is pretty much exactly what they do. And that works for some people. But depending on the way you're wired, this sort of immersion therapy might kind of freak you out. I prefer to do things more systematically, so as it doesn't feel too overwhelming. Yes, you will be nudged outside of your comfort zone, and it might push your buttons at times, but hopefully it doesn't feel like it's too much to handle.

FOOD NEUTRALITY

The idea of giving yourself full, unconditional permission to eat *all* foods can feel scary. So there's an intermediate step that I want you to work towards: food neutrality. This essentially means taking foods down off a pedestal, dismantling food hierarchies, and working towards having neutral emotional responses to food. This is where it can get confusing though, a lot of people think food neutrality means that foods are all nutritionally equal. Objectively, that's not true: we all know spinach is more nutrient-dense than, say, ice cream, but neither of them are morally superior to each other. Just because the spinach is more nutrient-dense, doesn't mean the ice cream doesn't have any nutritional value, nor is it a 'bad' choice. But by placing the spinach higher up in the hierarchy, we're more likely to lose our shit around the ice cream or buy into a false sense of security because we ate the spinach. So the goal here is to level the playing field between foods; this means foods are less emotionally charged, and we can begin to feel more comfortable eating a wider range of foods without spiralling or feeling like we're in freefall as you might if you just go on a pizza bender for three weeks.

HOW DO WE BEGIN TO PRACTICE FOOD NEUTRALITY?

Step 1 – Check yourself before you wreck yourself

Check yourself; how are you talking to yourself and others about food? A simple step we can begin to implement almost immediately is neutralizing our language and becoming non-judgey about how we label foods.

The first step is to get rid of food binaries; think about all the dichotomies that exist in terms of how we describe food. Good/bad. Real/fake. Clean/dirty. Junk food/health food.

There is no such thing as a good food or a bad food. Food does not have a moral value; however, when we dichotomize foods in this way and attribute them with a value we internalize that meaning, consciously or unconsciously. When we label a food as 'good', we are good for eating it. When we eat a 'bad' food, we are bad. How many times have you heard people saying 'oh I couldn't possibly, I'm being good today', or 'oh, go on then, I'm being naughty'. CUT THAT SHIT OUT. YOU ARE NOT WHAT YOU EAT. You are so, so much more. Your worth doesn't depend on what you eat. You are worthy no matter what you eat.

And labels like 'clean' or 'real' are totally meaningless when it comes to food. All food is 'real'; you didn't hallucinate the burrito. It's not a figment of your imagination. Terms like 'processed', 'chemicals', and 'nasties' are arbitrary and reinforce a hierarchy of foods.

So how should we talk about food? When I'm working with clients I tend to ask them how they prefer to refer to foods; some people pick positive vocabulary to describe foods like cakes and crisps, like play foods or fun foods instead of 'treats'.

Some non-diet professionals suggest using 'everyday' and 'sometimes' foods, and while it's certainly a lot less emotive than 'good' and 'bad', I still think it creates a dichotomy. Besides, what's an everyday food? What's a sometimes food? Sometimes I eat chocolate every day, sometimes I don't. Sometimes I eat apples every day, sometimes I don't. To me (and feel free to disagree), this sounds a lot like it could easily get construed into a rule if you're not careful.

Call me old-fashioned, but I like to call a food by its name. I know, pretty revolutionary, right? You're eating a carrot, cool. That's a vegetable. You're eating some cheese. Awesome, that's dairy. You're eating a doughnut, sweet, that's dessert (or breakfast, no judgement). This is a far more objective and unloaded way of describing foods that helps reinforce the idea that all foods are on a level playing field. They are not inherently good or bad, clean or dirty, junky or healthy. It's just food.

How about trying these on for size.

To describe an eating occasion: breakfast, lunch, dinner, brunch, brinner, supper, elevenses, afternoon tea, snack, entrée, appetizer, starter, main course, dessert, pudding, afters.

To describe food groups: fruits, vegetables, meats, dairy, beans and lentils, eggs, oils, sweets, grains.

I know a lot of people might gravitate towards nutrition labels like protein, carbs and fats. However, as I've already explained, focusing too much on nutrition at this stage might not be super-helpful. If you find that it's hard not to spend a considerable amount of time thinking about nutrition, then you might want to try non-nutrition food descriptors and see if that helps you move away from a rigid focus on nutrients.

Step 2 – Stop believing in a perfect diet

Say it with me. THERE'S. NO. SUCH. THING. AS. A. PERFECT. DIET.

And you don't need to eat 'perfectly' to be healthy. A healthy diet means having a balance of foods (not too much, not too little) AND having a healthy relationship to food. Honestly, people make such a stink about nutrition, but it's a small part of what makes us healthy; it's helpful to keep that in perspective. Don't get me wrong, I'm a nutritionist, I know that nutrition is important. But so are sleep, medicine, regular check-ups, relationships, community, getting outside and being in nature. The Centres for Disease Control (CDC) in the US point out that around 75% of health is determined by socio-economic variables that we have little control over, as well as medical care. Around 25% of health outcomes are determined by genetics and individual behaviours including: smoking, alcohol, recreational drugs, medicine, movement, sleep, stress management ... and nutrition.[9]

I don't want this to sound disempowering; that's not my intention. There are plenty of things we can do to support our health at an individual level. But I also think it's important to understand the social determinants of health; the social inequalities that give rise to health disparities have a bigger bearing over health on a societal level than nutrition does. Sometimes putting it into perspective like this can help take some of the pressure away from having a **perfect** diet.

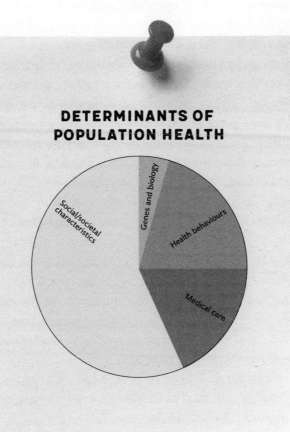

DETERMINANTS OF POPULATION HEALTH

Social/societal characteristics

Genes and biology

Health behaviours

Medical care

Step 3 – Don't think of nutrition in black-and-white terms

As we discussed before, saying all foods are neutral doesn't mean that all food has the same nutritional value. We all know that carrots are more nutrient-dense than, say, a cookie. But it doesn't mean that a cookie has NO nutritional value, or that it's not a valid food choice. Cookies provide energy, white flour is fortified with calcium, iron, niacin, and folate. There's also some fat and protein (from milk and eggs). And even if it didn't have any of that shit in it, food isn't solely there for physical nourishment. Remember that food has a role in emotional nourishment too. The point is that nutrition isn't all or nothing; ALL FOODS PROVIDE SOME NUTRITION. And just because a food is less nutrient-dense than another, doesn't mean it isn't serving a purpose. Remember that shit.

Step 4 – Fuck food guilt

An important step in practising food neutrality is rejecting food guilt, but that's perhaps harder to do when all we hear are messages about 'guilty pleasures', 'being naughty', and 'bad food'. It's hard not to internalize these messages, which manifest as a mixture of sadness and frustration directed at ourselves. Guilt and shame can follow us around for days after a perceived food transgression. But who the fuck decided you should feel guilty about enjoying food? Which asshat told you that you were 'bad' or 'naughty' for nourishing your soul with foods that satisfy you? That's some grade-A, puritanical, patriarchal, fat-phobic, diet-culture BULLSHIT. None of us were born with food rules, but years and years of diets (even the ones masquerading as 'lifestyles'), fashion magazines, and thin-ideal idolization erode our trust in our body's cues and our innate ability to feed ourselves. Diet culture teaches us we cannot be trusted around delicious foods. It teaches us we need to have strategies in place to deal with all the food because YOU CANNOT BE TRUSTED.

Well, guess what? You are a grown-ass adult who gets to eat whatever you like, whenever you like and enjoy the crap out of it! If feelings of guilt, shame, or anxiety creep in, remind yourself those are not your feelings, they were given to you by a culture that preys on your insecurities and vulnerabilities. But you are done with diet culture now, and you are not going to let it walk all over you. Not today. Not next week or next month. And not ever. Eating is a fundamental requirement for life. You would not feel guilty about breathing or sleeping. You should never, ever feel bad about nourishing your body and soul with satisfying and delicious foods that help keep body and mind happy. YOU ARE DONE WITH FOOD GUILT because you deserve to enjoy all the pleasure that food has to offer, there is no space left for feeling guilty, and you will not let diet culture dull your sparkle.

———

It's natural that you will have some concerns about moving through the IE process, and at some point you may feel as though food consumes your every waking second, and 'AAAARRRGGGHHH, this was supposed to help me think less about food, not more'. Chill. The ultimate goal in IE is to think less about food, but there might be a period where we are hyper-focused on food choices. This is totally normal in the early stages of IE. Be curious about it. It doesn't mean you're fucking it up. Here are some common thoughts people have about moving through the process.

I WILL NEVER STOP EATING...

———

After a long period of restricting, there's a good chance that you will routinely eat past the point of comfortable fullness. THIS IS TOTALLY NORMAL. If you have been depriving yourself, the natural response to that is to try to 'make up' for it. Over time, as your body learns that foods are no longer off limits, and as your intuitive eating signals begin to kick in, the feeling of urgency around eating will begin to dissipate. This is because of a process called habituation where we effectively acclimatize to a food (more on that later). In fact, in treatment for binge eating disorders, participants are required to make peace with previously forbidden (shit list) foods, using mindfulness and mindful-eating techniques (which we'll discuss in chapter 8, alongside awareness of hunger and fullness cues.)[10]

I WILL ONLY EAT UNHEALTHY FOODS . . .

—

We all know that different foods have different nutrient profiles and contribute in different ways to our overall health and well-being; whether that's nourishing us physically or mentally, therefore, no foods are inherently healthy or unhealthy. There isn't a single food that will cause or cure disease by eating it once or twice (unless it's gone off). Sure, too much of anything isn't great for you; too much cake might give you a tummy ache, but so would too much broccoli. By allowing yourself to eat a wide variety of different foods, including the ones on your shit list, chances are you will naturally gravitate towards a healthy balance of foods because that's what feels good in our bodies. However, like I've already mentioned, and like I'll keep saying, focusing on nutrition in the early stages of intuitive eating can undermine the intuitive eating process. Remember, making food choices based solely on nutrition (or what you think you know about nutrition) can perpetuate feelings of restriction and deprivation, trigger diet mentality and scarcity mindset, and ultimately prevent you from fully embracing and embodying intuitive eating. No bueno.

It's also important not to have any expectations around when intuitive eating signals will begin to kick in; for some it can happen relatively quickly, for others it can take longer. But it's important not to get too ahead of yourself, even if you feel like you have been eating less 'healthfully' than usual. Be gentle on yourself, chances are you'll gravitate towards a balance of foods without having to force it or feel restricted. Eating less nutrient-dense foods for a while is unlikely to do any harm to your long-term health; but if you're concerned, it might be worth taking a multivitamin in the short term as a sort of safety net to make sure you're getting all your nutritional needs met. Also, remember we all have a negativity bias, we can have a myopic laser focus on the foods we have eaten that we deem 'bad'. If you are stressing about eating foods like crisps, cake, and chocolate a lot, remember that they don't cancel out the fruit, veggies, beans, and oily fish you've eaten too!

I CAN'T CONTROL MYSELF . . .

———

Think back to the baby in their high chair who naturally gravitates towards a balance of foods. They don't need to exert any effort or control over that process, they just do what feels good without over-thinking it. Over time diet culture (and all the other shit within diet culture) erodes this innate ability to regulate our food intake. So, how do we begin to get it back? Once you learn to give yourself unconditional permission to eat, you will slowly begin to learn that foods will always be available. You don't have to wolf them all down; eating previously shit list foods doesn't cause you to self-implode. Over time you'll build trust in your body again. It's all very well telling you this, but you really have to experience it to believe it. Throughout this chapter, I'll teach you how.

Diet culture is a breeding ground for food restrictions. It teaches us that food is the enemy, that you can't or shouldn't enjoy it and to anyone who has had a history of disordered eating, enjoying food can feel like a terrible idea. This is rooted in our fear of food, which is in turn rooted in our fear of fat. Diet culture teaches us that we shouldn't enjoy food; if we have pleasurable foods around, then we will inevitably eat them all at once, get fat, and die. 'KEEP SUGAR OUT OF THE HOUSE', 'only eat dessert at a restaurant (but split it with your friend), and categorically do not have an appetizer, it's one or the other', 'if you absolutely must have them in the house, then at the very least keep them locked up in the freezer', as though a little cold was ever going to stop anyone. I fully admit to having fallen for this trap. Healthy-living blogs and books love to tell you to keep your 'bad' foods in the freezer: cupcakes, cookies, chocolate, even homemade energy balls! The subtext here is that if something tastes good, it's dangerous, so out of sight, out of mind. Right?

Uhhhh, not so much. I remember getting sent a bunch of cupcakes for my birthday one year, way more than I could ever eat in one sitting, or so I thought. I was a diligent diet culture/wellness devotee at this point, so I shoved the cupcakes in the freezer, promising myself I would ration them out. Yeah . . . that didn't happen. Frozen cupcakes be damned.

Habituation visualization: the ice-cream sundae

When confronted by the idea that it's OK to eat whatever you want, whenever you want, it's pretty common for people to *flip the fuck out*.

Typical responses include:

- 'I won't stop eating'
- 'I'll only ever eat ice cream/pizza/brownies'
- 'I'll only eat bad foods'
- 'I'll never eat any vegetables ever again for the rest of my life'

To be completely honest, it's pretty normal to go a bit OTT on delicious foods after a period of restriction or deprivation. It's normal to get excited about foods that taste good. Some people get over this phase pretty quickly, for others it can take longer. Either way, let's explore what it might be like to have full, unconditional permission to eat whatever you like, all day long. In this activity I'm going to get you to visualize eating ice cream all day long, but you can replace it with whichever food you prefer: pizza, tacos, doughnuts, cake, whatever!

Imagine yourself going to the grocery store and stocking up on all the paraphernalia for an ice-cream party. You can pick absolutely anything you like from the ice-cream aisle, buying more than you could ever feasibly eat. Your shopping cart is practically overflowing with pints of ice cream, bags of candies, and bottles of sauces.

ICE-CREAM FLAVOURS

- strawberry
- vanilla
- chocolate
- cookie dough
- mint choc chip
- raspberry ripple
- salted caramel

TOPPINGS

- sprinkles
- mini marshmallows
- gummy bears
- M&Ms
- chocolate chips
- cookie crumbles
- crushed peanuts
- strawberries
- coconut flakes

SAUCES

- chocolate syrup
- strawberry sauce
- caramel sauce
- hot fudge
- espresso
- whippy cream

When you get home with all your ingredients, you get to work designing your perfect ice-cream sundae; a combination of ice creams, toppings and sauces, you can even add a cherry and one of those little paper umbrellas. Remember there are no rules; make it as big as you like, with as many different flavours and textures as you like. Describe or draw it in your journal. Now imagine that you'll be at home by yourself for the whole day and no one will interrupt you. Your phone is on silent, and you're not expecting anyone to come over, not even the Amazon dude. There is no one watching you, there is no one judging you. You realize you've forgotten to eat breakfast and you're hungry; you decide to make yourself the sundae of your dreams, piled high with mountains of sprinkles, sauce dripping down the edge, and whipped cream in a perfect point on top. It's a beautiful warm, sunny day, so you take your creation outside to eat it on the patio furniture in the garden. No one can see you're eating ice cream for breakfast except the birds in the trees. It's cool and refreshing with lots of different flavours and textures; you take your time over every mouthful, enjoying the freedom to eat something you would never usually allow yourself, and savouring each bit. You spoon up every last mouthful of ice cream and feel full and content.

You go back about your day, reading your book in the sunshine, sunbathing, listening to music. You know, summer stuff. A couple of hours pass and you start to feel hungry again. You go back into the kitchen and build yourself another sundae and eat the whole thing, and then again for an afternoon snack, and for dinner, and another snack before bedtime. You continue this for a number of days. Eating only ice-cream sundaes for every meal and snack.

How did you feel after that first bowl of ice cream? Was it satisfying? Did you feel full? How would you describe how you physically felt? Was it pleasant, unpleasant, or neutral?

Now think about how you felt after eating ice cream for the whole day? Were you satisfied? Did you feel full? How would you describe how you physically felt? Was it pleasant, unpleasant, or neutral?

How many meals or days do you think you could eat ice cream for without getting bored? How long would it take you to feel a bit sickly? Do you think you might start craving any other foods? If so, which ones?

There is no right or wrong answer here; you certainly don't have to write down that you will start craving vegetables, that's not the point. All I want you to do is open yourself up to the idea that, eating ice cream, or pizza, or bread all day, every day, no matter how much you love those foods, might not be the most pleasant way to experience food. Sure, those things taste good, and there's no reason for us to exclude or restrict. We also don't have to arbitrarily put them on a pedestal; if we allow ourselves to have them when we want them, we realize that they're just not that big a deal. If we experience a few days of eating more sweet foods than usual, the chances are, we'll gravitate back towards a balance of foods that feels good in our bodies.

When I do this visualization with clients, they often tell me that after eating ice cream for a day, they start to crave a proper meal; they want something savoury. This is sometimes called **meal hunger**. One client of mine had spent a few days at Disneyland with her nephew and when she came to her next session she reported that at the end of the day, after eating candyfloss and caramel popcorn and going on rides, she was ready to have an actual balanced meal for dinner. Not because she was restricting, but because that's what she fancied.

HABITUATION

When we bring foods down off the proverbial pedestal and start to see them neutrally, we begin to lose the urgency and intensity that they once held over us. That feeling of like 'OMFG GIVE ME ALL THE COOKIES' becomes a bit more like 'Ooh, a cookie, yum, I might have that later if I'm in the mood for it when I'm feeling hungry.'

This happens via the process of habituation; when your cookies are way up on that stool, you can't touch them, right? You never really get to experience the cookies, so when you inevitably do (at someone's house or someone takes some to the office), you are going to lose your shit. When you can experience cookies whenever you want, they kind of stop being such a big deal. They're no longer the forbidden fruit. Initially, you might feel drawn towards the cookies, just because you can. Being excited and potentially eating more of something than usual is a totally normal response to restriction and deprivation.

Think of it this way. You partner has been away on a work trip; they're gone for a week or two. When they come back you're all over them, leaving cutesie notes in their lunchboxes and all of that. BUT, after they've been back for a while you start to forget how much you missed them and get back to telling them to make their own damn breakfast. This is the process of habituation. In psychology, habituation is a form of learning in which repeated exposure to a stimulus leads to a decrease in responding.[11]

In a classic experiment, women were given macaroni and cheese every day for a week. Living the dream, right? At the beginning of the week they were all like 'fuck, yeah, mac and cheese' but by the end of the week, they were kind of over it, essentially getting burnt out on the macaroni.[12] Scientists believe that the time it takes to habituate to a food is less when the food shares similar characteristics (for instance, the same flavour and brand of ice cream), which is why I'm going to ask you to get really specific when we reintroduce foods from your shit list.

The point of giving yourself unconditional permission to eat all foods isn't to get so burnt out on a food that you never want to eat it again, though; I don't want you to eat so much pizza or ice cream or bagels that you make yourself sick, because that would result in restriction and deprivation, which would be self-defeating. You'd be back at square one. The point in food neutrality is to really bring those foods down off that pedestal so they no longer have the same emotional pull. You don't have to eat them with such an urgency or intensity, and you can have them when you really want them, as opposed to when you feel compelled or drawn to them.

I CAN'T EAT THIS FOOD

Over the years I've worked with clients, many of them have reported that they can't give themselves unconditional permission to eat because they have food intolerances and sensitivities. Let's explore this a little. Food allergies are reactions to proteins found in food and they can be life-threatening. Immunoglobulin E (IgE) is an antibody produced by the immune system. If you have an allergy, your immune system overreacts to an allergen by producing IgE antibodies. These antibodies travel to cells that release chemicals, like histamine, that cause allergic reactions.

There are three main types of allergic reaction: IgE mediated, non-IgE mediated, or a mixed reaction where both processes are taking place. IgE mediated reactions are *immediate*: these are the things we think of as causing life-threatening anaphylaxis, like in peanut or shellfish allergies. Non-IgE mediated reactions can either be localized to an area (like the skin) or produce a more generalized response, as in coeliac disease. Mixed IgE mediated and non-mediated reactions are things like eczema. In order to test for a true allergy, you'd need to do a special test that measures IgE activity after exposure to a potential allergen. Seems reasonable and straightforward, right?

Just one teeny-tiny catch. The types of tests that you buy over the counter or online don't measure IgE, they measure Immunoglobulin G or IgG. Unlike IgE, IgG measures exposure to a food. In other words, it's a test of whether or not you have eaten a particular food lately; it's basically a measure of tolerance rather than intolerance and is not a valid test for detecting a food allergy, sensitivity, or intolerance. But these tests get peddled by charlatans, and I've seen many clients get sucked into believing they have an issue with a particular food and then cutting it out of their diet. This winds up in them feeling anxious or stressed about the alleged offending food, often compounding the issue more.

I spoke to gastroenterologist Dr Jim Stewart (@leicnut), a consultant and clinical lead of the Intestinal Failure team at Leicester Royal Infirmary about this: 'The problem that I, like many gastro-enterologists face, is patients who have developed GI symptoms, but seek advice from a nutritional therapist and/or IgG testing. The corollary of this is that they put themselves on hugely restrictive diets which can exacerbate the GI symptom (e.g. constipation). The first hurdle is to disabuse them of the notion that IgG testing has any value and then secondly persuade them they do not have an allergy to rhubarb, pine nuts and sorrel (you get my drift). This all takes an inordinate amount of time and it is often very difficult to persuade patients that they have been given misleading information. My main concern is when I look after very sick patients with anorexia and not infrequently they have a history of "wellness" or restrictive diets.'

I've also experienced clients coming to see me who rationally understand that these tests are meaningless but have a lingering fear and sense of anxiety over these foods. I'm not a psychologist, so I don't understand all the cognitive processes at play here, but what I can do is discuss the science and encourage people to slowly reintroduce these foods so they can experience for themselves that nothing catastrophic will happen. Other than a breath hydrogen test for lactose intolerance, there are no validated tests for food intoler-ances. In order to decipher a food intolerance, you'd need to talk to a specialist dietitian who will help you systematically remove and challenge suspected foods. IgE tests are typically used to detect food allergies that can potentially result in anaphylactic shock like milk, eggs, peanuts, tree nuts, fish and shellfish (although some other tests are available) but you should only be diagnosed by a doctor, and not by someone who may use an invalidated test.

If you have had an intolerance or allergy confirmed by an appropriately accredited professional (usually a registered dietitian, GP, or specialist allergy doctor), then you can't go reintroducing foods that cause you problems; fortunately there are tons of great dairy- and gluten-free alternatives available for those who need to be on a medically restricted diet.

'HEALTHY' ALTERNATIVES

The concept of healthy alternatives is rampant in wellness culture; raw cheesecakes made from cashews and dates blended up, sweet-potato brownies, grain-free pancakes made from eggs and a banana, cauliflower pizza, avocado chocolate mousse, fucking courgetti, dehydrated, low-fat, peanut-butter powder that you have to reconstitute with water and tears.

Before you all go angry tweeting me, I know, some people genuinely enjoy these foods, and that's fine; no shade. What I object to is that people feel morally obliged to eat 'healthier' versions of foods that 1 aren't all that different in terms of nutritional value anyway, 2 don't taste as good as the real deal, 3 create a food hierarchy, and 4 promote over-consumption of the healthier version.

Take sweet-potato brownies, for example, how many of you have devoured the whole pan in one go because they didn't quite hit the spot? Or because they're 'healthier' you eat way beyond the point of comfortable fullness, when one regular brownie would have probably left you feeling satisfied and content? If we look at diet ice-cream brands, their business model banks on you devouring the whole tub in one sitting and then going and buying another tub the following day to do it all over again – a behaviour I'd consider disordered for sure. What if you could just have a couple of scoops of regular ice cream instead?

Like it or not, only allowing yourself the 'healthy' version of a food is a form of restriction, and as with the deprivation mindset, when we place a cognitive boundary on what we can and can't eat, our head perceives that as restriction and it can backfire as (subjective) overeating or even bingeing, guilt, shame, and anxiety around food. No part of that is healthy.

YOU ARE NOT WHAT YOU EAT
—

The saying 'you are what you eat' seems fairly innocuous on first inspection. But if we take a closer look, we realize it's healthist bullshit that has been manipulated and bastardized by the clean-eating brigade to justify restrictive and shame-based eating rules.

In his book *The Angry Chef*, Anthony Warner explains that 'you are what you eat' is actually a misquote from French gastronome Jean Anthelme Brillat-Savarin (try saying that after a glass of wine), who actually said 'Tell me what you eat, and I will tell you who you are.' The original intention had very little to do with health and everything to do with how people project themselves to the world through their food choices. If we look at clean eating through Brillat-Savarin's lens, we might infer that clean-eating and wellness trends are a means of social signalling; it has more to do with the symbolic associations of eating this way than about the food itself.

Warner explains:

When it comes to clean eating, creating an association with cleanliness and purity in food is likely to imbue the eater with feelings of a similar nature. To break the rules is to eat something dirty and to become dirty yourself, creating feelings of disgust. It is perhaps this powerful association that has given the clean-eating movement its greatest power to evolve and grow. Tapping into these feelings and creating a strict morality around food choices gives followers the impetus to stick to the rules, to follow the diet and to feel virtue and superiority over those who do not.

This isn't throwing shade at people who have followed clean eating – remember, no judgement – but to show that when people say 'you are what you eat', it's not just a judgement of the food you are eating, but a commentary on who you are as a person; your food choices are wrapped up in morality, in your character, in your social standing. But green juice and turmeric are neither a prerequisite for nor a guarantee of health.

We've already talked about how nutrition plays a relatively small role in terms of our health outcomes but the idea that 'you are what you eat' places a premium on eating 'pure' foods.

Let's be clear, you are not what you eat, you are your genetics, your environment, your thoughts, experiences, ideas, your relationships, emotions, talents, skills, and personality.

And while we're at it . . .

FOOD IS NOT MEDICINE
—

Sure, nutrition can be an important part of our overall health and well-being, and we'll discuss how we can gently apply nutritional concepts towards the end of the book. But quotes like 'every bite you take is either harming or healing you' vastly overstate the power of nutrition.

Nutrition can play an important role in helping prevent and manage certain conditions, but so can exercise, reducing alcohol intake, getting better quality sleep, reducing stress, stopping smoking, being gifted genetically, having strong social bonds/community, therapy, not being poor (as though it was a simple choice), living somewhere that isn't super-polluted (again, like it's a choice), oh yeah, and ACTUAL MEDICINE. Part of the issue with the food is medicine rhetoric is that it can inadvertently put people off seeking pharmacotherapies by creating a culture of shame around prescription medicines. Antidepressants are a perfect example; there is so much stigma around them (and mental health more generally), yet for some people they are lifesaving. The most 'perfect' diet and 'lifestyle' in the world cannot completely eradicate the need for antidepressants, and to be able to argue otherwise is an incredibly privileged position that not everyone who needs these medicines shares.

Here's the other major issue I have: sometimes food is less medicine and actually more part of the problem. We know that orthorexia and other eating disorders are often about control, purity, and perfectionism. 'Food is medicine' can propagate the fallacy that there is such thing as a perfect diet; it can legitimize food rules, restrictions, and other disordered behaviours. If 'medicine' comes at the expense of your mental health, then it's not healthy at all. We also know that people who suffer from orthorexia, people who have very pure, 'clean' diets are paradoxically at risk of malnourishment and deficiency. Prescriptive 'food as medicine' regimens often appear eerily similar to that of someone suffering orthorexia, yet few lifestyle doctors warn of the potential side effects of these types of diets: micronutrient deficiencies, hypothalamic amenorrhoea (loss of menstrual cycle), social isolation, low blood pressure, hair loss, osteopenia and osteoporosis (loss of bone density), constipation, night sweats.[13,14,15]

The problem is that this discourse is often served up with a side of fear-mongering that leads to rigid food rules and exclusions that can lead to stress and anxiety around food. The reality is that there is no evidence to say that if you completely eliminate whole food groups or types of food from your diet and have a 'perfect diet' you will be healthier than if you have a generally balanced approach to eating, which includes having a healthy relationship with food.

The fact is, there's no such thing as a perfect food, and there's no such thing as a perfect diet, especially if thinking about food and eating makes you anxious or stressed out. I am less concerned with the specifics of what you eat at this point, and more concerned with how you eat. Are you responding to hunger? If you eat when you are way past hungry, at say a 2 or less, the chances are it won't be a great eating experience; you're likely to eat with a lot of intensity and urgency, and probably overshoot comfortable fullness too. There are times when life will get in the way and you can't really avoid it, and that's OK, no need to beat yourself up about it. Likewise, there might be times when you have to eat when you're neutral or even a little full; maybe you're going to be in meetings all afternoon or going to a movie before dinner. You aren't exactly hungry in the moment, but if you don't eat now, then you'll end up going over hungry later. It's totally fine to have a snack or something to tide you over. But the sweet spot will be when you're gently or moderately hungry. Food will taste better, you'll be able to eat mindfully and respect your fullness more easily.

A NOTE ON FULLNESS

We have yet to discuss fullness in much detail, and I have deliberately left it out of the conversation because, in order to even contemplate embracing this principle fully, you have to make sure you're adequately nourished (eating when hungry, eating regularly, eating enough) and practising food neutrality, having given yourself unconditional permission to eat (which I'll walk you through soon). Without both of those elements, the chances are that you will continue to eat past the point of comfortable fullness. This is normal as you work to counteract the effects of being in a deprivation mindset. This could last a short amount of time or longer, depending on how long you have been restricting and the degree of restriction; it's important to let this run its course without expectations of how long this phase will last.

WHEN IT'S HARD TO JUST EAT IT

When a thin person, particularly a thin white woman, eats a doughnut or a giant slice of pizza it's labelled as cool, sexy even. It's usually also performative for the male gaze to keep up 'cool girl' appearances (think of Jennifer Lawrence 'where's the pizza?'). It's branded as a treat, a little time out from their (presumed) otherwise strict regimen of salmon and courgetti. They've earned it, right? When a fat person orders a cheeseburger or a cupcake, the assumption is that is ALL they eat; that there is a never-ending conveyer belt of burgers, fries, and milkshakes being delivered straight into the mouths of fat people, despite having no information whatsoever about what they *actually* eat. Aside from the fact that it's nobody's damn business what anyone else eats (except maybe your doctor or nutritionist), society's collective weight stigma poses a real and significant threat to the physical and mental safety of fat people. This in turn influences the degree to which fat people can make peace with food and give themselves unconditional permission to eat; the omnipresent fear of bigotry, abuse, and prejudice. For fat people, it's not as simple as going into a bakery and ordering a box of doughnuts. OK, this might be tough for a thin person who is struggling with their inner food critic, but let's be real, there's a whole other layer of shit that fat people have to wade through to get that box of doughnuts.

I recall a conversation with a client once who had done some great work systematically working through her shit list and was doing an awesome job of giving herself unconditional permission to eat all foods ... until one day, she was stumped by a cheese sandwich and couldn't put her finger on why. We set her some homework: to eat a cheese sandwich with curiosity and non-judgement and see what came up. In our next session, she told me that the anxiety around the cheese sandwich was less about the food itself, and more the circumstances surrounding the sandwich. Cheese sandwiches are often prepackaged convenience foods that you eat on the go. In *public*. As a fat woman, this raised a lot of anxiety for my client; she perceived she would be judged for eating even something as innocuous as a sandwich. She was afraid that people would think 'how dare she, she clearly doesn't need that' or 'she's fat, shouldn't she be on a diet, eating a salad!' I'll even concede that as a nutrition student, I remember having similar thoughts when I saw a fat person eating dessert at a restaurant once; I'm sure you've even caught your brain going there too, perhaps even about yourself. When you are fat, suddenly everyone is interested in your lifestyle, passing unsolicited advice and making all kinds of wild assumptions and judgements about your character and devaluing your humanity; as though 'bad' foods had infected you like a pathogen, turning your soul black. Obviously that's ludicrous.

But the fact remains: fat people still have to eat. And this isn't just a perfunctory act. They *deserve* to eat without the threat of a fat-phobic slur being hurled at them. They deserve pleasure, joy, and satisfaction from delicious foods without the threat of physical abuse, stares, and judgement. However, fat people are forced to make a choice between safety and nourishment, particularly when eating in public, and for this reason it can be especially challenging to make peace with food; not only are you dealing with your own inner food critic, but that of the rest of the world too.

I don't pretend to have any magical solutions to this, but I will share things that have helped my clients. If you hold thin privilege, challenge fat phobia whenever and wherever you see it. Start with internalized fat phobia and then call it out when you come across it publicly. Whether it's a comment, an advert, a social media influencer, whatever. Shut it down. Tell people that fat phobia is a form of prejudice and that by participating they are actively contributing to worse physical- and mental-health outcomes of fat people.

On the flip side, if you are fat, know that it's a radical act to eat in public, to eat foods that people perceive to be 'bad'. You are not weak-willed, self-indulgent, or undeserving of sustenance and nourishment. Buying into this bullshit narrative that society has made up about you doesn't facilitate a peaceful relationship with your body or food. You have the power to rewrite the narrative on your terms. Follow fat-positive babes online, read their books, listen to their podcasts. See them living full, unapologetic lives, not tied down by fat-phobic expectations of how they *should be* or what they can and can't eat. Let them inspire you and teach you (if that's your thing). I'm not saying this is easy, and sometimes it isn't even safe for fat bodies to live in all their glorious fatness (please keep yourself safe above all else), but by casting off these expectations we give ourselves the freedom to walk into the doughnut shop and give zero fucks about what other people think, at least sometimes.

SOMETIMES FOOD IS DISAPPOINTING, AND THAT'S OK TOO

——

When you begin to take foods down off that big, shiny pedestal, we take a lot of the excitement and fun out of them and begin to start seeing them for what they really are. Sure, when you're in a deprivation mindset or have been heavily restricting, a Twix feels like a golden baton that has been handed down from the gods. But when you practise food neutrality, you see it for what it is. A boring, uneventful Twix. Sure, it tastes pretty good. But it's no longer the most sensational food in the world and you don't feel the need to hammer ten of them.

When you are doing Paleo, bread seems like the greatest thing you could put in your mouth, and sure, bread is delicious, especially hot from the oven and slathered in butter. BUT, it soon gets old and it's not the only thing you want to eat. When food stops having such an impossible hold over you, it can feel a little disappointing. Something that you used to think was a heavenly delight is just kinda average. This disappointment can leave a little hole in your heart where that food used to be. I don't mean to bum you out, think of it as an opportunity. Perhaps you can fill the space where food used to be with a new hobby or activity, more time for friends and family, or maybe you can discover foods that you really love and will make you happy but not in an obsessive way. Another thing that can happen when you start treating all foods as equals is that it starts losing its emotional appeal. Again this can be disappointing or even frustrating, it no longer feels great to smash your feels down with bread; you actually have to deal with your shit. We'll get to that in chapter 10, but just know that it's a possibility.

——

For some of you, you'll feel delighted at the prospect of eating foods that were previously on your shit list. For others, it can be scary and intense and overwhelming and frightening to go to the shop and buy previously forbidden foods you thought were 'bad' or had promised yourself you'd never eat again. So, let's move slowly. And if you dip your toe into your shit list foods and it feels too cold, don't sweat it; I don't want you to do things until you're good and ready. If you're ready to cannon ball on it, that's awesome too, let's do it!

GIVING YOURSELF UNCONDITIONAL PERMISSION

—

As I've said in chapter 4, when some people decide to ditch diets, they might do a complete 180 and start eating all sorts of previously forbidden foods, all at once; and that can totally work for some people. Like some people are just really ready to give themselves unconditional permission to eat. But for others, that can feel overwhelming, **1** because they have skipped the food neutrality stage, and **2** because they haven't taken a more systematic approach to giving themselves unconditional permission to eat all foods. They may be stuck in a pseudo-permission battleground. Let's look at some strategies that we can implement to approach unconditional permission in a more methodical way.

Let's just be clear about something here though: the idea of giving yourself unconditional permission, and going through the habituation process, is not to burn out on foods so that you never want to eat them again. It's not to binge on them so you get so sick of eating them you never want to look at that food again. Both of those situations would be setting you up for deprivation again, and that's what we're trying to move away from.

The goal is to learn to get you comfortable with eating a wide variety of foods; it's to help you trust that your body is a reliable tool for guiding what, when, and how much you eat. It's to build up confidence in your innate ability to feed your body. In order to do this, you actually have to experience eating a variety of different foods; you have to learn that nothing catastrophic will happen. Doing this gives us a little more space to be in our bodies and experience how food really makes us feel. I get that the trust in your body thing is a huge challenge, especially if you've been putting more trust in apps and diet plans than your body, so we're going to take it slowly; only do this step when you feel ready for it. Here's what we're going to do.

Step 1 – Select your shit list food

Flip back through your journal and find your shit list; pick one food that you enjoy eating but limit or intentionally restrict, or don't trust yourself around. Depending on your confidence level, you might want to pick something higher or lower on the list.

Feeling confident: pick something higher up the list.

Not sure how this is going to go: pick something in the middle of the list – something that pushes you outside of your comfort zone but doesn't totally freak you out either.

Feeling trepidation: pick something lower on the list; something that is just outside your comfort zone.

Step 2 – Get specific

Once you've selected your food, decide which brand and flavour you want to work towards giving yourself unconditional permission to eat. Say for instance it's ice cream, you might want to start with Ben & Jerry's Phish Food. Then you can go to Chunky Monkey or whichever other flavour you want to get cosy with. Being specific is important; if you just pick chocolate, well there are so many different brands and flavours of chocolate that it will take longer to habituate. Keeping it specific can also feel a bit less frightening.

Step 3 – Make a plan

Decide when and where you're going to have the food; you might want to have it as part of a meal or snack, on its own, or mix it up. You could start by keeping smaller amounts in the house, and then work towards keeping your cupboards stocked. Are you going to have it at home or out (like your favourite restaurant)? Do you need to try this alone or get some support from a caring friend or partner?

Step 4 – Get your head straight

Check in with yourself and make sure you're in the right headspace for this challenge. Are you approaching it with the mentality that you're going to binge and overeat it (which runs the risk of becoming self-fulfilling prophecy) or can you approach it with mindful, non-judgemental awareness? Also pay attention to whether or not you're stressed, overly hungry or tired, as these can all influence how much you eat. If you're experiencing any of these things and feel there's a danger you will have a negative experience with the food, maybe come back to it later when you're rested and feeling good.

Step 5 – Goldilocks that shit

Have the food as per your plan and then start asking questions. Goldilocks that shit: how much is too little, too much, just right for you to leave you feeling content but not so stuffed you feel sick or so restricted you feel deprived? Or maybe you don't actually want ice cream but grilled cheese or a doughnut? How did it go? How did the food taste? As good as you expected or was it slightly disappointing? Was the experiment pleasant, unpleasant, or neutral? Did you eat more or less than you expected?

There's no right or wrong answer. You're just gathering information. The first few times you try this, you might eat a lot of the food, more than is comfortable; remember that's totally normal when you're trying to reverse the deprivation mindset. Notice if on subsequent eating experiences, the amount of food you eat changes, goes up or down. What often happens is that people require smaller amounts of the food to feel satisfied; this can take different lengths of time for different people, so it's impossible to say how many times you need to repeat this activity before you start to feel like you're giving yourself unconditional permission. Remember what we talked about at the very beginning? Patience!

Step 6 – Rinse and repeat

Repeat the experiment until you begin to experience unconditional permission to eat that food. There's no hard and fast test for this, but here are some things to look out for:

- I don't feel guilt/shame/anxiety about this food anymore.
- I don't feel a super-intense desire for this food anymore – I could take it or leave it.
- I could have this food in the house and not feel as though I would demolish it in one sitting.
- I don't need to engage in any compensatory behaviours to 'earn' this food.
- I don't think this food is good or bad, healthy or unhealthy, it's just food.

Don't judge how many times or how much of the food you need to eat in order to feel comfortable with it. If you've been restricting for a long time and are deep in deprivation mindset then it may take longer; this can be frustrating, so remember and approach it with a sense of curiosity, like an experiment. You don't know what the results will be until you've finished the experiment and it may or may not prove your hypothesis.

Giving yourself unconditional permission to eat expands your comfort zone so once you've given yourself unconditional permission to eat one food, it's time to try the next one on your shit list. This time try going a step higher on the list, gently nudging yourself outside the new comfort zone. You'll probably only need to do this with a handful of foods before you start to internalize unconditional permission for all foods. You'll be flexing that intuitive eating muscle, and the more you do that, the less you'll need to be so methodical in your approach to eating; you'll be able to trust that you can eat all foods without conditions, without rules, or without having to justify it to yourself or anyone else.

If you find you're really struggling with this activity, there are some techniques for helping you feel more comfortable giving yourself permission in chapter 7.

DO YOU KNOW ANY INTUITIVE EATERS?

'Normal' eating is subjective and looks slightly different for everyone. What constitutes a healthy relationship with food varies from person to person, but there are hallmarks of what a healthy relationship is not:

- Feeling stressed/anxious around food
- Using loaded or judgemental language around food: good/bad, clean/dirty, 'junk food', 'nasties', real/fake
- Regularly skipping meals in order to 'make up' for eating
- Punishing yourself for eating with exercise, or using exercise to 'earn' food
- Having rigid food rules with little flexibility
- Only eating at specific times or not eating after a specific time
- Avoiding eating in social situations because you don't know what food will be served
- Always choosing the 'healthiest' option on the menu rather than what you really want
- Cutting out whole food groups without a medical (allergy) or ethical reason
- Compulsively counting calories or macros

Intuitive eaters are flexible in their eating, don't have arbitrary food rules, and don't restrict or deprive themselves. Think of someone in your life who is an intuitive eater and recall a meal you shared with them. **In your journal, describe a food or meal experience or experiences you have shared with this person and then answer the following questions:**

How did you know they were an intuitive eater?

What characteristics, traits or behaviours did they have?

How did you know they were eating flexibly?

What did they/didn't they do?

What habits did they have?

How do the food rules you wrote before compare to this person?

Consider showing your food rules and shit list to this person and ask them what they think about them. Ask them how they would feel following your rules and limiting the foods on your shit list.

It's important that this person be non-judgemental and compassionate – if you don't feel comfortable discussing your food rules or shit list then you can skip this activity and come back to it another time. However, if you feel as though the person will be understanding, then this can be a really powerful activity. I've noticed that for many clients I am the first person they have spoken to about their relationship with food. Sure, they've probably talked about diets and clean eating and stuff, but the messy, sometimes contradictory rules that swirl around their heads? Not so much. They tend to suffer through that alone. Getting these thoughts out of your head and down on paper or out in the open can help you see them just as thoughts, and not as facts, and help you realize if there are contradictions or they just straight up don't make sense.

NEUTRALIZING YOUR INNER FOOD CRITIC

—

n recent years, 'clean' eating and myths born out of the wellness guru generation have been thoroughly debunked and chalked up to pseudoscience. There is more scrutiny than ever on nutrition professionals, and the public are holding them accountable by asking for scientific evidence to back up their claims. But even after the 'clean eating' backlash in the aftermath of wellness, we inevitably still have a lot of noise in our heads about good food/bad food and little titbits we've picked up from the media and social media, and weird things our mum said to us about when it was OK to eat carbs. Layered onto that we have the ghosts of clean eating, haunting every food choice we make.

The corollary of all of this is that our inner food critic launches a diatribe against us every time we want to eat something. And not only at the time of eating! The inner food critic gets off on making us feel guilty about what we ate, even days after we've eaten it. Anyone who has been on the dieting merry-go-round or dabbled in wellness will know the judgey voice that lives in our head, second-guessing every food choice we make, bargaining and negotiating with us about 'making up' for foods we've eaten, or telling us we don't deserve to eat a particular food. The inner food critic isn't rational, they don't make choices in your best interest or based on nutritional sciences. They get their kicks from making you feel worthless for eating a piece of chocolate cake, they tell you that you are nothing because you had a takeaway, they make you think you're just one bite away from cancer or diabetes. They focus on those cookies you ate last week, even though, on balance, you've eaten a good variety of different foods.

From the perspective of my clients, the food critic is a huge stumbling block to making peace with food; it prevents them from tuning in to what their bodies are telling them because they're always so in their head about food decisions. It prevents them from giving themselves full, unconditional permission to eat any food. But it's not easy to quieten these judges, especially when disordered thoughts are seemingly backed up by media headlines and this or that 'expert' touting their bogus claims.

In this chapter, we're going to focus on bringing down the inner food critic, and replacing it with a gentler, more nourishing, and compassionate voice that encourages you to approach foods with curiosity and non-judgement. We're going to learn how to let go of all-or-nothing thinking, and do a little rewiring of our brains so we can deal with imperfect eating, and tell the inner critic to pipe down.

BLACK-AND-WHITE THINKING

—

Our inner food critic doesn't get nuance – they think in black-and-white, all-or-nothing terms. 'If you eat sugar, you will get fat.' 'If you eat carbs after 6pm, you will get diabetes.' 'Dairy causes acne.' And so on. But hold up. Your food critic doesn't have a degree in nutrition. And that's also not how nutrition works. No individual food or nutrient is inherently 'good' or 'bad'. We don't eat foods or nutrients in isolation. And nutrition isn't zero sum. You can eat the cookie *and* eat the carrot (if you want to!). Eating a cookie doesn't negate the benefits of the carrot. Eating a carrot doesn't detract from the pleasure, satisfaction, and joy of eating cookies unless you make some weird carrot cookie in which case all bets are off. I joke, but that is essentially how ludicrous sweet-potato brownies are. The judgemental, disordered voice of the inner critic, however, will make you believe that there's no point in eating a carrot if you're also going to have a cookie. They will lie to you and tell you that you have to 'earn' the cookie. In order to quash the food critic, we *need* to get comfortable with shades of grey. Food and eating is messy and imperfect – a bit like, oh, I don't know, life! We need to adapt to different food situations without having a complete and total meltdown.

ACTIVITY

Take a moment to reflect on your inner food critic. What do they sound like? Are they all-or-nothing thinkers? Do they make you feel guilty for eating particular foods? Or try and convince you that you have to 'earn' foods? Write your thoughts down in your journal.

Is your inner food critic saying things that are grounded in fads as opposed to something widely accepted and supported by scientific consensus? Did it come from a social media guru, or can you fact-check it on the NHS choices website? While there are always new studies and flashy headlines, promises of new superfoods and miracle diets, and anecdote upon anecdote of people online who claim to have cured themselves from all sorts of chronic conditions, credible nutrition advice hasn't changed that much, and isn't likely to do so. Check out Pixie's Bullshit Detector later in this chapter for more on how to spot pseudoscience.

NEGATIVITY BIAS

Humans have an inbuilt bias towards catastrophizing situations in our brains. From an evolutionary perspective, this makes complete sense; the world was dangerous, predators and starvation and other scary things were omnipresent threats. But in the relative safety of the modern world, our brains going to the worst-case scenario isn't always super-helpful. Particularly in the case of food. When I help clients examine their shit lists, we discuss why certain foods belong there, and what beliefs they hold about that food. Inevitably, clients will gravitate towards the 'bad' stuff in the food. I have one client in particular who had a thing with Nutella. She loved Nutella, it was one of those foods that she remembered from her childhood that gave her the warm and fuzzies. But of course there was no way she would allow herself to eat it as an adult. Something about 'nasties', and sugar, and not trusting herself not to eat the whole jar. We discussed taking Nutella down from the pedestal and why placing a restriction on it was making it into a bigger deal than it was. We decided to set her a homework so that she could have a little Nutella every day, and see how she felt about it. Halfway through the week between our appointments I got a panicked email signed by 'Nutella Natasha'. Fake name, but you get the point. My client was *spiralling* over this damned Nutella. I got on the phone to her to help get the swirls out of her head and into the light of day so we could examine them rationally. She was adamant that Nutella was the worst food on the planet: processed, full of 'chemicals', high in fat and sugar. She was focusing on what she perceived were the negatives of this food. Now, sure, if all she was eating was a couple of jars of Nutella a day, I'd be worried. But the reality is she was having a few spoonfuls. Slathered on a freaking banana. I think we can all agree, objectively, that's a solid snack. But her negativity bias and her inner critic were colluding BIG TIME to make her feel out of control. So, here's what we did, we shut down the food critic, and focused on the more positive aspects of the food, like, oh I don't know, her *enjoyment* and *satisfaction*.

Let's be clear, the inner food critic has been trying to sabotage our relationship with food for, well, pretty much forever. It's not like you can just shut it off. It's going to try and rebel. But what if every time it makes unhelpful comments or criticisms about what you eat, you pushed back? Eventually it'll back off and make more space for a gentler, more supportive voice instead. We can begin to flip it on its head by reframing those negative, judgey thoughts. Here's how we can do it: in your journal, describe or draw the food that's causing you to freak out a little, it can be one from your shit list or just one you've eaten recently or are about to eat. Write out all the words the food critic was filling your brain with, thoughts that were making you fearful of eating this food. Here's what I did with Nutella Natasha to give you an idea what it looks like (you can draw the food out or cut out an image from a magazine). Now cross out the negative associations and replace them with more neutral or positive ones. Now you can think about the nutrients that food provides you (if that's helpful), but I want you to think more in terms of the pleasure, satisfaction and feeling you get from eating this food. For my client, Nutella was associated with the conviviality of eating, meaning the celebratory nature of foods. What a beautiful sentiment; think about the role that food has played in your life, as love and as celebration, as history and tradition! Helping yourself reframe the foods in this way shuts down the inner food critic and helps you give yourself unconditional permission.

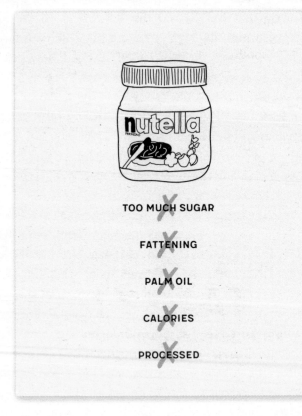

TOO MUCH SUGAR

FATTENING

PALM OIL

CALORIES

PROCESSED

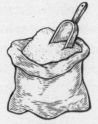

Sugar
to satisfy my
sweet tooth

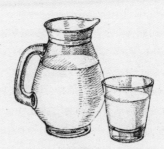

Milk
protein, calcium, iodine, B12,
potassium, etc

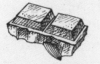

Delicious chocolate
restricting leads
to bingeing

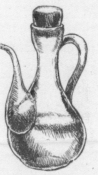

Hazelnuts
essential fats,
protein, vitamins
and minerals

Some protein + fats + carbs = balance

HITS THE SPOT
TASTY!

**REMINDS ME OF SHARING NUTELLA
WITH MY BEST FRIEND**

A NOTE ON NUTRITION

—

At the beginning of the book I asked you to put nutrition concerns to the side. Not because I don't think nutrition is important; it's definitely important, but there's a time and a place for nutrition. But focusing on nutrition too early on just fuels the inner food critic. If you are still in diet mentality, your inner food critic will seek out 'nutrition information' to support their disordered beliefs, making their voice louder and stronger. That said, bringing some myth-busting and very basic nutrition can help blow the lid off your food critic. Your thoughts, beliefs, and attitudes guide your behaviours. If you believe that sugar is 'poison' (it's not!) you're not going to mess with it. But that can also leave you feeling deprived, socially isolated (nobody is going to invite you out if you don't do cake), and might lead to bingeing or overeating, or just plain being fearful of foods. To help I've given you a few key facts about foods and nutrients that you can use to combat that inner food critic.

What to say when your food critic talks shit about . . .

Sugar – satisfies my sweet tooth and keeps my cravings from taking on a life of their own. I deserve some sweetness in life.

Fat – a component in all cell membranes and wrapped around nerve cells allowing messages to be carried throughout my body. Fats also make up 60% of our brains. Fats are responsible for carrying flavour molecules and making food taste delicious, as well as for helping absorb important fat-soluble nutrients like vitamins A, D, E, and K. Makes foods more satisfying and satiating.

Protein – essential for growth and repair of wounds, plus also makes foods more satisfying and satiating.

Carbohydrates – give us energy and stop us feeling hungry ten minutes after our meal. Foods with carbohydrates may also have other important nutrients like fibre, B vitamins, and minerals.

White flour – foods made from white flour, like white bread or pasta, in the UK legally have to be fortified with calcium, iron, and other B vitamins.

Dairy products – contain lots of nutrients like protein, calcium, iodine, B12, and potassium and help support bone health.

Calories – calories are not evil monsters hidden in our food, but a unit of energy; we need energy to carry out almost every single process in our bodies!

Cholesterol – cholesterol from the food we eat is unlikely to make much difference to blood cholesterol levels, so don't sweat it!

Fructose – fructose is a sugar that is usually found in things like fruit and vegetables so it's packaged up with other nutrients like vitamins and fibre.

'Unhealthy foods' – healthy is what we eat over long periods of time, not individual foods or nutrients. No single food can make you unhealthy and no single food has magical health properties.

AUTOMATIC NEGATIVE THOUGHTS

—

Another way to deal with our inbuilt negativity bias is to reframe automatic negative thoughts (ANTs) – those thoughts that reflexively go to the worst-case scenario; whether it's the voice of the food critic, diet culture, or that self-doubt that tells you you're doing it 'wrong'. These thoughts are rarely based on actual fact or evidence, but we let them rule our actions and dictate how we feel about ourselves and the food we're eating. While I'm suggesting this as a strategy to combat the voice of the inner food critic, I've found that going through the IE process brings up a lot of ANTs along the way, so this might be a useful strategy to deal with negative body image or when your brain is telling you 'you can't possibly be hungry again'. We've actually already used this tool in chapter 4!

If we can mindfully identify thoughts as an ANT, then we can put a little distance between ourselves and the thoughts and look at them a little more objectively. We do this through 'the power of three' – three sentences or counter-points to balance out the ANTs and help reframe them. For example:

The 'cookie will make me fat' ANT becomes:

1 maybe this cookie will satisfy my cravings, so I can stop thinking about food

2 eating a few cookies won't harm my health

3 if I eat the cookie, I might realize it's not that big a deal

The 'sugar is addictive' ANT becomes:

1 cutting foods out makes my cravings more intense

2 all foods can fit as part of a healthy diet

3 sweet foods give me energy and nourish my soul

Your turn: pick an ANT that you've had playing on repeat in your head. Writing it out on paper or as a note in your phone can be really helpful, but in a bind, just do it in your head. Now write out your *power of three* – your three counterbalance points. Like I said, it might take some time to shush that voice in your head, but over time, if you can identify and combat ANTs, you'll slowly begin to rewire unhelpful thoughts. Use this as often as you need.

Your food critic says	Your rational brain says
'Food is addictive'	There's very little scientific evidence to support the concept of food addiction; many researchers believe that what people perceive to be food addiction is actually a backlash effect from restriction and deprivation (ahem, dieting). In studies where they witness rats compulsively eating sugar, the rats have usually been starved for 12 hours beforehand, whereas this effect is not seen in rats who have free access to food, meaning it was the restriction that led to bingeing. Studies in humans don't control for dieting either, so we can't rule out the idea that what may feel like compulsive eating, is actually just our bodies making up for being really hungry. And yes, delicious foods make the pleasure centres in our brains light up, but so do our favourite music, our favourite people, and kitties! We are supposed to find pleasure from the food we eat, otherwise we wouldn't have any incentive to eat![1,2]
'Gluten is sandpaper for the gut'	The only people who can diagnose me with coeliac disease or non-coeliac gluten sensitivity are my doctor or my dietitian. Cutting out gluten-containing foods can lead to a lower fibre intake, which in turn can reduce the diversity of micro-organisms in our guts, and may increase our risk of heart disease and even death in those who don't have coeliac disease![3,4,5]

'This are so many scary chemicals/ nasties in it'

EVERYTHING IS CHEMICALS! Literally everything. Air, water, our bodies. It's all made from chemicals. People like to scaremonger on the internet about nebulous and frightening-sounding chemicals, but the reality is that EU law is very strict on what can and can't be added to our foods. If there is any concern over human health, it will be pulled from the food supply. The European Food Safety Authority rigorously tests food additives on the basis of metabolism, toxicity, carcinogenicity, genotoxicity, reproduction and developmental toxicity and, if required, other studies.[6] In 2011 they commissioned a revaluation programme to test the safety of all the additives currently in our food supply, and to date, only three additives have raised concern, and even then, it was not enough to outright ban them. Rather, an upper limit was imposed.[7] Unless you have a diagnosed sensitivity to a food additive, they're not worth worrying about, and ultimately they make our food supply safer and less expensive, help reduce food waste, and make our lives more convenient.

'There are too many pesticides in this'

Scientists have found that the health risk posed by pesticide residues on our food is equivalent to drinking one glass of wine – every three months.[8] If you prefer to buy organic because you have environmental concerns, then that's great, but they're not more nutritious, and they're not 'better' for our health either.[9]

'Your body can't process it'	Your body can process all foods – some people eat non-food substances like clay and washing powder, but this is an eating disorder called pica. Your body is really adaptable and can digest a wide variety of different food – this allowed us to evolve by eating whatever we could get our hands on. We're basically just scavengers! Unless we have an allergy or intolerance (diagnosed by an actual doctor!) we can process all foods, but sometimes it's the inner food critic that gets in the way.

How to be a bullshit detector

Pixie Turner @plantbased_pixie

Thanks to social media, misinformation has allowed to spread further than ever before, and it's never been more important to be sceptical about what you read. Here are my five steps to becoming a bullshit detector and protecting yourself, especially online:

1 Be sceptical – don't take anything you read at face value, and don't assume someone is right just because they sound convincing or have a great set of abs. Even if the person is someone you admire or get on well with, or have followed on Instagram for ages, you still never know.

2 Check qualifications – are they qualified to talk about this subject? Do they have qualifications to back them up? Just because someone looks a certain way or has a lot of followers on social media doesn't mean they know what they're talking about. You don't suddenly gain a degree when you reach 100k followers. There is zero correlation between how many followers someone has and whether they know their shit. And even if someone does have qualifications, are they talking within their area of expertise? I would always recommend being wary of doctors talking about nutrition, as generally they receive very little training, and be especially wary of American doctors with crazy diet books and supplements for sale.

3 Ask for evidence – if they respond with their evidence that's a good start; if they shift the burden of proof (i.e. ask you to prove them wrong) that's bad; if they become rude and defensive that's a clear sign they got nothin'. Any credible person will be able to back themselves up with peer-reviewed science, not just YouTube videos.

4 Check for red flags: 'detox', miracle cures and conspiracies, appeals to ancient wisdoms (just because something was done for a long time doesn't make it right), advocating restriction without a clear medical reason, black-and-white absolutist statements . . . these are all red flags that should make you especially wary from the start. That doesn't mean immediately discounting or ignoring what someone is saying, more that the previous two points (checking qualifications and asking for evidence) are even more important.

5 Beware of fear-mongering language – if someone make you feel bad, guilty, or afraid of food or the way you eat, shut them out. Either they don't know how to communicate their message and so are doing harm or they're trying to scare you into buying something. Whichever one it is, the result is negative for you.

If, after going through all this, you're still unsure about something, ask an expert. Or, even better, ask two. It's your body, your physical and mental health that's potentially at stake, so don't be afraid to ask.

SETTING THE RECORD STRAIGHT

—

Thanks to fear-mongering in the media and unqualified people claiming to be nutritionists, there's a LOT of vilification of single foods and nutrients, and myths and misconceptions are ubiquitous. People have written entire books that critique #nutribollocks (many of which I've shared in the resources section at the end of the book), but I just wanted to quickly dive through some common myths to help put your mind at ease when the inner food critic pops off. Let's start with sugar; when I ask clients why they think sugar is 'bad', they often tell me it's because it causes big swings in our blood sugar levels; a huge surge of sugar, followed by a massive crash that leaves us curled up in a pile under our desks. But this is another example of diet culture pulling a fast one on us and misleading us about how food and nutrition really works. My mate and specialist diabetes dietitian Nichola Ludlam-Raine (@nicsnutrition) explains it like this:

'Sugar crashes' are made up

'People often talk about having a "sugar crash" after eating something sugary; referring to a feeling of lethargy and a craving for more sugar to perk themselves back up again. Sugar though isn't broken down by the body very quickly as it actually has a medium- rather than high-glycaemic index (GI); the GI is a scale of how quickly carbohydrates (including starches and sugars) are digested into glucose. To put this into context, pure glucose, which is found in Lucozade or jelly babies, has a GI score of 100; which is very high, whereas foods containing more fibre, protein and/or fat have a lower GI because the rate at which the carbohydrate is broken down is slowed. Low GI foods include oats, pasta, basmati rice, most fruits and vegetables as well as chocolate! The GI scale isn't a scale of health though as jacket potatoes, which are brimming with vitamin C and fibre, happen to have a high GI. Most people don't eat jacket potatoes by themselves though; they'll eat them as a part of a meal containing some protein, fibre, and fats (e.g. tuna, salad, and mayonnaise) which means the entire meal actually now has a low to medium GI.

'More interestingly though, it's actually the amount of carbohydrate that has the biggest effect on blood sugar levels and not the type or GI; this means that eating five slices of white bread will raise blood sugar levels much more than eating a packet of sweets because the former has more carbohydrate in it. The amount of carbohydrate that a food contains, in relation to its GI, is known as it's glycaemic load (GL).

'It's a myth therefore that eating a couple of biscuits will result in a "sugar crash" because a) the amount of carbohydrate that you're eating isn't that great and b) the added protein, fat, and fibre slow down the rate of digestion. This means that a steady release of insulin is triggered, which helps to move the broken-down carbohydrate (sugar/glucose) into the cells (including brain and muscle cells), where it is used as energy. Isn't the body just brilliant?!

'The only way to get a true "sugar crash" is to eat a family-sized bag of sweets or jelly babies or drink a litre of Lucozade all at once, and the only way that this could be problematic is if it happens on a regular basis at the expense of more nutritious foods.'

So, if your custard creams with your cup of tea aren't to blame for your 3pm slump, what is? Recent research into our body's circadian rhythm, aka our 'body clock', shows that we naturally have a dip in the stress hormone cortisol around mid-afternoon that could explain why we feel sleepy. But don't blame it on the biscuits, it's just biology doing its thing!

Here are a few more myths that, although they have been thoroughly debunked, still persist today. Let's quash them once and for all. Repeat after me:

People of the world, myth-bust your life. Every boy and every girl, myth-bust your life

- Juices and cleanses and special supplements can't 'detox' you, your liver and kidneys do that all on their own. Every time you poop or pee – that's a detox.
- 'Unrefined' sugar isn't a thing – chemically speaking, sugar is sugar – it doesn't matter if it comes from sugar cane, honey, maple syrup or coconut sugar. It all behaves the same way in the body. While things like coconut sugar may contain marginally more nutrients per 100g than table sugar, the amount you'd need to eat to get any significant benefit is entirely negated by how much sugar you'd have to eat, thus defeating the point entirely.
- The 'alkaline diet' is whack – the foods we eat cannot change the pH of our blood, if they did, we'd either be critically ill in hospital or dead.
- 'Superfood' is a marketing term, not scientific terminology! The nutrients contained in so-called 'superfoods' can be found in a variety of other foods. For instance, there's nothing special about kale; rocket, spinach, and broccoli all contain similar nutrient profiles. Likewise, claims about 'superfoods' are spurious fake news: 'oxygenates blood', 'adaptogenic', 'immune booster', 'energy booster' etc . . . are all made up. Side note: all food 'boosts' energy, that's the whole entire point in food and a 'boosted' immune system is one that overreacts to foods or other substances resulting in inflammation.

As my mate The Angry Chef points out in his book of the same title, 'pseudoscientific beliefs are born out of misunderstandings of science, based on grains of truth that are over-extrapolated many times to become vast monsters of unstoppable woo'. Myths are scary, but like monsters, they're not real; by exposing the truth we can help shush the voice of the inner food critic who is keeping us fearful of nourishing ourselves. Having a little understanding and appreciation for the scientific process will give you some insight into how nutrition information can easily get misconstrued in the wrong hands.

The hierarchy of evidence
The Rooted Project @rooted_project

The problem with nutrition science is that it's messy. It's complex, nuanced, and rarely black and white. In fact, being able to really understand it and interpret it takes a really long time. Even nutrition scientists are continually learning to hone their skills years after leaving university with undergrad degrees.

This complexity is the main reason nutrition science is easy to exploit and sensationalize. It's the reason we see all the confusing and conflicting headlines in the media, and why people with good intentions (but little by way of qualifications or training) can get things wrong. In all honesty, you can probably find a study to back up any viewpoint in nutrition, but stating single studies to 'prove' that you're right is bad practice in nutrition science (and most science, in fact).

What matters when it comes to interpreting evidence in nutrition is quality and context. This means questioning the quality of the evidence we're being presented with and looking at how it fits into the bigger picture.

Scientists rate evidence by what information it can give us and how reliable that information is likely to be, which (crudely) involves using what is referred to as the hierarchy of evidence.

This hierarchy starts at the bottom with the least reliable source of information: 'anecdotes'. Anecdotes are stories based on personal experience. They are interesting and can be used to form the basis of scientific research, but as humans, we are prone to making connections even when there are none, so as a source of info they are unreliable. This means that when you hear health bloggers talking about how changing their diet cleared their skin or cured their tummy woes, you need to remember that although the diet or product they're plugging may have helped them, there are a million other things that could've played a part too. So take testimonials like this with a pinch of salt.

Next on the ladder are expert-opinion pieces, these can be useful (if they are written by someone with expertise and clinical experience in the area they are talking about), but keep in mind that academics, doctors, and experts are also not immune to bias. This is why scientists have developed methods to collect and review all the scientific research on a topic, which helps to reduce the effects of bias and give us a better overall picture of a topic (these are the systematic reviews and meta-analyses, sitting pretty at the top of the pyramid).

Observational studies are up next. These are not experiments, but exactly what they say on the tin – studies that track and observe the habits of large numbers of people over time. They are fantastic for showing us patterns and trends, but as health and disease can be affected by lots different things, they can't be used to show that one thing causes another. To do this, we need to conduct an experiment or a randomized controlled trial that tests an intervention (e.g. intuitive eating) against a control group (e.g. people who are put on a diet) to see if it has a meaningful effect.

Intuitive eating is actually a relatively new idea, but an exciting and proudly expanding area of research. The evidence base for intuitive eating is interesting because it draws not just on studies and systematic reviews for its effectiveness, but also on the body of research that shows us that weight-loss diets have risks, and that for many people they are ineffective in the long term, not just for long-term weight loss, but for promoting physical and mental health.

CHALLENGE ACCEPTED

—

This is a little challenge that I've been using lately with my clients that seems to be helpful when trying to shut down the inner critic when it pops up and second-guesses every choice you make about food. It's usually a hangover from the diet mentality that insists that every single food choice should be of the highest nutritional benefit, and it usually causes us to feel anxious or guilty if we eat something less than 'perfect'.

So, whenever a sneaky diet-mentality thought or food rule pops into your head, write it down and alongside it write 'CHALLENGE ACCEPTED' and go ahead and break the rule.

Afterwards reflect on how the experience was:

- Did you enjoy the food?
- Is it a food you'd like to eat again?
- Did anything catastrophic happen?

POST-IT PERMISSION

—

Another tool for giving yourself permission to eat all foods when the inner food critic is giving you a hard time is the humble Post-it. Sometimes you rationally know that it's cool to eat a food from your shit list, but it can be hard to break old habits and you can feel trepidatious about reintroducing that food into your life. This is where it can be helpful to have some external reinforcements that reiterate that it's OK to have these foods.

Use the Post-it note outline below to practise writing out permission and override the food critic. Then if you feel a bit weird about actually sticking Post-its to your lunchbox and in your fridge, this can be a sort of proxy. Otherwise go ahead and write them out and stick them to everything!

You are a grown-ass adult and you can eat what you want, when you want

Carbs are cool!

It's OK to eat the cookie!

Whenever you want! It's OK!

TUMMY TROUBLES... OR DISORDERED EATING?

———

Gut health is hot right now, and like all good trends, there are pros and cons (#leakygut) and tbh I think we all need to calm down. Because what I'm wondering is, is this trend yet another way to legitimize disordered eating? Another way to legitimize the voice of the inner food critic? One of the big problems of this trend is the over-pathologizing of normal bodily functions. Guys, a little bit of bloating and gas is TOTALLY FREAKING NORMAL. It happens to most people. It may feel a little uncomfortable, but check in with yourself every half-hour after a meal and notice if it goes down – eventually you'll start to make space and get hungry again (check out the checklist from chapter 4 if you're still struggling to feel hunger in your belly). Being hyper-focused on every teeny-tiny toot leads to unnecessary food exclusions and restrictions that may in and of themselves lead to MORE GI symptoms. Did you know that the average woman farts fifteen times a day? And for dudes it's twenty? The point is that bloating, gas, burping, and feeling full after a meal are all totally normal bodily functions; don't let the voice of the food critic try and label that as a food intolerance (if your symptoms are severe, worsen over time, or interfere with daily life, then please go to your doctor and if they can't help then ask for a referral to a specialist allergy dietitian; don't try and self-diagnose).

With trends in gut health and clean eating, there has been a lot of focus on cutting out and excluding certain foods: dairy and gluten are usually the main culprits, despite little evidence that they are related to digestive issues in the absence of coeliac disease, non-coeliac gluten sensitivity, or lactose intolerance. In many cases, cutting out foods unnecessarily can exacerbate or worsen the problem. When we restrict foods, a few different things can happen.

Gastroparesis

First off, food can stay in our stomachs for longer due to gastroparesis – this literally means a partial paralysis of the stomach muscles, leading to the stomach being unable to empty in the usual way, meaning food stays in the stomach for longer. Our stomach is functionally split into two parts: the fundus is the top part of the stomach, responsible for relaxing and stretching to accommodate food during a meal, a bit like a balloon. In case you forgot, it's the stomach's job to act as a food reservoir; it holds the food and slowly releases it a little at a time into the small intestine for digesting. If it didn't do this, and food was dumped into the small intestine all at once, you'd have bigger problems, trust me. In the lower part of the stomach, the antrum, muscles move over one another to 'grind' and mix food with digestive 'juices' until it's pretty much liquidized. This food and digestive juice concoction is called chyme, and this is what gets released into the upper part of the small intestine to be further digested by enzymes and absorbed into the blood stream. If the stomach has partial gastroparesis, it can leave us feeling fuller for longer, bloated, and kinda gross as it takes longer for the chyme to leave the stomach. If you have been very restrictive or have habitually ignored feelings of hunger and fullness, or cut out food groups (like grains) it can take your stomach a while to, well, stomach again the way it should. If you are experiencing early satiety (fullness), bloating, and feeling uncomfortably full, you can help yourself by eating regularly and consistently (every 3–4 hours) to help your gut get back 'online'; little and aften is best to help manage symptoms.[10]

Changes to the microbiome

The other reason cutting out foods is unhelpful is because removing foods can shrink our microbiota (the healthy bacteria living in our guts), making it less diverse and changing the composition of the bacteria that live there. When we do then eat a different food (like bread) it can stimulate the growth of bacteria causing them to react by producing more gas. A totally normal reaction. But we interpret that as 'abnormal', our food critic labels that food as 'bad', and we continue to restrict the food: this is called a conditioned food aversion.[11] Speaking of which...

The nocebo effect

Clients often ask me: 'If it's bad to restrict this food, how come I feel better when I don't eat X?' Typically, when someone makes a lifestyle change, like going gluten-free, they're not simply removing gluten from their diet. They're also sleeping more, getting more movement into their days, eating more fibre and vegetables, maybe they even start meditating. Any of these changes are likely to make you feel good in your body, but they have nothing to do with gluten! So I always check what else people did when they gave up gluten. I then always ask clients what they believe to be true about gluten and examine any underlying beliefs; most of the time they've read that it causes 'inflammation', 'leaky gut' and various other scary-sounding problems. Cue our brains playing crazy tricks on us! If I told you that green juice was 'detoxifying', will give you healthy skin and improved energy, or that a turmeric latte was anti-inflammatory and immune system-boosting, you might actually feel better when you drink them; not because they are actually detoxing anything (only your liver and kidneys can do that, remember), and as we've discussed a 'boosted' immune system is what happens when you trigger an allergic response. So what's actually going on here?

Basically, it's a trick of your brain; the placebo effect. Because I tell you something is good for you, it may actually cause you to have a positive physiological response to that food. The placebo effect is a really well-established phenomenon in science, and people are generally pretty happy to accept it. If we consider the top tier of evidence, placebo controlled trials can tell us if the result is due to a real effect or just a fluke. What we're less willing to accept though, is the phenomenon called the nocebo effect, essentially the opposite of placebo. If I tell you that gluten is sandpaper for the gut or that dairy is the devil, then you may actually experience a negative physiological response from eating that food – WTF? In his book The Gluten Lie, Alan Levinovitz describes the nocebo effect like this:

> The placebo effect occurs when expectation of benefit – not therapeutic value – produces positive results for a particular kind of treatment. Acupuncture, painkillers, antidepressants, even some kinds of surgery: studies have shown that people respond well to fake versions of these interventions, reporting alleviated symptoms when the acupuncture needles don't pierce the skin, the pills are sugar, and the surgery is a sham. The nocebo effect is the placebo effect in reverse. It was first documented when patients receiving sham pills ended up suffering negative side effects – because they expected the pills would make them feel bad. Now scientists recognize the nocebo effect must be taken into account when people report physiological food allergies. This applies even to people with documented allergies.[12]

One 2009 study on milk found that fourteen out of fifty-four patients with documented intolerance to lactose reported symptoms after ingesting sugar pills. They were lactose intolerant, but it was their expectation of the symptoms that made them sick.[13,14]

This shows how, even when there are no underlying issues, the beliefs we have about food can produce strong negative consequences.

The inner food critic latches on to sensationalist headlines and titbits of pseudoscience, which can actually make us feel ill. Always make sure your nutrition information comes from qualified and reliable sources, and don't believe the inner food critic when they pander to pseudoscience.

———

OK, so let me be totally clear. There are legitimate reasons you need to be on a medically restrictive diet and if you're experiencing weird GI symptoms you need to go to your GP and get any underlying organic disease ruled out. We've already discussed why over-the-counter and home 'food allergy' testing doesn't work; the only person who can diagnose a genuine food allergy is your doctor, and intolerances need to be systematically eliminated and rechallenged with the help of a registered dietitian. If your doc gives you the all-clear and you are STILL experiencing tummy troubles, here are some suggestions (not intended to replace individual medical advice) that DON'T involve food restrictions.

I always try and work from the least restrictive place possible because food restrictions can trigger disordered eating and we need to be really real about how they might be totally contraindicated in people with disordered eating.

- Eat regular meals, not 'by the clock', but don't let yourself get over-hungry. Digestive enzymes are partially controlled by circadian rhythm (your 24-hour 'body clock'), so if we can eat at vaguely regular intervals our digestive juices will be flowing, as it were. Yum.
- Try and eat when you're peaceful (i.e. not super-stressed out) and bring a level of mindfulness to it (phones down, laptop shut). We'll discuss mindful eating in chapter 8.
- Chew your food. I'm not going to specify an amount but until it's liquid-like. This will make it easier to pass through the tum (mastication = mechanical digestion).
- Cut down on your La Croix/Prosecco habit – adding gas to your tummy, makes you, uhhh . . . gassy!
- Try meditation and other relaxation techniques (and stop

comparing yourself to the shit you see on social media). It's not as easy as cutting out gluten, but stress management is super-underrated for helping with digestive issues, even getting a CBT referral may help.[15,16,17,18] Recent research has shown that mindfulness-based stress-reduction programmes can help reduce the severity of irritable bowel syndrome (IBS) symptoms.[19]

● Try adding a probiotic – there are a few different probiotics that may be beneficial in IBS so it's best to check with your GP or registered dietitian.[20]

● Don't try a low FODMAP diet on your own – this is an incredibly restrictive approach to eating and can trigger disordered eating in certain people. There are lots of less restrictive approaches you can take, and a low FODMAP diet should be a last resort if nothing else is helping. It's designed to be a short-term diet to help identify potential triggers, you're not supposed to stay on it forever. A specialist gastro dietitian can help you navigate a low FODMAP diet and help you reintroduce foods to find your own individual level of tolerance.[21]

In clinic, I see a lot of women who self-identify as having gastro-intestinal problems but who have had the all-clear from their doctor. They've usually embarked on a whole bunch of restrictive diets, cutting out grains, dairy, sugar, and so on and nothing really helps. But when we dig a little deeper, it's pretty apparent that their issues are probably a lot more straightforward than they first think. Not to put too fine a point on it, but the reason they ain't poopin' is because they ain't eating enough. You gotta put the goods in to get the goods out. If you're underfeeding yourself, not only will you experience issues with gastroparesis, but you might just simply not have enough substrate to work with. This is especially true if you've been restricting carbohydrates in your meals. Carbs add bulk, but they also add fibre, and fibre's pretty important for keeping things moving. Look, I get it, carb phobia is rampant. So we'll work up to including more carbs; don't go freaking out on me just yet.

CARB PHOBIA

—

I don't think I've ever had a client who isn't just a little bit afraid of carbs and restricting them, even on a subconscious level. This also seems to be the one thing the food critic can't let go of. Whereas low-fat diets are like, so nineties, carbs are the new supervillain of the nutrition world, and, chances are, you've had a little freak-out about eating carbs along the way. But here's the thing, carbs are a really important nutrient; they're broken down into simple sugars, like glucose, which is the preferred fuel source our brains, central nervous system, and red blood cells run on. They're also an important source of other nutrients like fibre, B vitamins, calcium, and iron. They provide energy; I can't tell you how many times a client has told me they have no energy and I tell them to eat more carbs and after an initial meltdown, they're like, 'whoah, carbs give me energy'. They're also versatile (think potatoes, bread, pasta!), cheap, and taste fucking delicious. And I mean, this isn't based on actual science, but there seems to be a direct correlation between being on a low-carb diet and being a complete prick on Twitter. Life's way too short not to mess with carbs.

As a little reminder

Here's a list of all that's awesome about carbs, and why you should not cut them out if you are generally healthy. It might be helpful to write these out in your journal or snap this list on your phone for when you need reminding:

- Carbs help keep our moods even – they don't call it hangry for nothing, and the theory is that you need to feed your brain regularly for it to go at full speed. Unlike other organs, your brain relies on a steady supply of glucose (from carbs) as its primary fuel, and without them you risk becoming a mega bitch.

● Simple carbs from sweet stuff can help improve our mood in the short term (which is why a bit of cake or a cookie can help us feel better if we're having a bad day).

● And complex carbs from beans, pulses, legumes, and whole grains (bread, pasta, quinoa) can help our mood longer term.

● Carbs in the evening can help us sleep.

● Carbs are satiating and delicious and without them we're hungry again in, like, five minutes or our meals feel super-unsatisfying.

● Carbs are a great source of energy. I've noticed that when clients are eating very low-carb diets they are super-tired – no shit, Sherlock.

● Cutting out carbs can cause massive cravings, leading to binges – do not recommend.

● And if you're doing any kind of endurance sport, you're going to hit the wall so much sooner without enough carbs in your diet.

● And, carb-rich foods like whole grains and beans have the nutrient fibre; which I think it's fair to say is pretty essential for pooping, and feeding your gut microbiota. Seems like kind of a no-brainer, no?

● AND, even though whole grains and beans are great and they help us poop and stuff, it doesn't mean that foods made from simpler carbs like cakes and cookies are inherently bad or unhealthy, or that eating them cancels out the fibre or other nutrition we also eat – nutrition isn't all or nothing like that, it's cumulative.

● Plus, wheat flour in the UK is fortified with calcium, iron, and B vitamins. So you don't need to sweat when you eat that stuff!

WHAT'S THE DEAL WITH PROCESSED FOODS?

———

Let's just get something straight: unless you're picking food straight off a tree or digging it up from the earth, it has undergone 'a process'. We could even argue that fruit ripening over time is 'a process'. And certainly, cheese ageing or beer fermenting is 'a process'. Chopping tomatoes is 'a process'. Cooking beans is 'a process'. Baking a cake is 'a process'. How helpful is it then to classify foods as processed versus unprocessed? To me, it creates another unhelpful food dichotomy (remember we're done with black-and-white thinking). All food is processed to one degree or another. Cooking, chopping, blending, and pasteurizing are all processes and, as the NHS points out, processed food is 'any food that has been altered from its natural state in some way, either for safety reasons or convenience'. It does not mean bad, unhealthy, or avoid altogether; something that self-styled Insta-nutritionists are yet to grasp. Maybe they hate efficiency and not getting infected with pathogens? Processing foods has made our food supply safer, it reduces food waste and allows us to eat tinned peaches in February, giving us a fleeting taste of sunshine to get us through until the warmer months. Processed foods aren't necessarily bad. In fact, they might just *make* a meal (personally I couldn't live without a bottle of super-processed hot sauce). Where would we be without tinned beans, pasteurized milk, and frozen veggies?

In fact, a 2012 study from Newcastle University compared the nutritional value of shop-bought ready meals with from-scratch meals made using celebrity chef cookbooks (your Jamie Olivers and the like). The researchers found that the home-cooked meals, which most people would consider to be less 'processed', contained more energy, protein, fat and saturated fat, and less fibre per portion than the ready meals.[22] Now, I'm not saying that one is better than the other. What I am saying is that perhaps 'processed' food doesn't deserve the bad rap that it often receives. For so many, convenience foods are a lifeline. Consider an older adult living alone, a person with chronic fatigue or a disability that prevents them from cooking from scratch. Or just a busy working mum who needs to get some chicken nuggets on the table so she can go out and work a second job.

There has been a lot of attention in the media recently on 'ultra-processed' foods, linking them with cancer and other disease; if you're anything like my clients, this can set off major food-critic alarm bells.[23,24] But the term 'ultra-processed' isn't particularly helpful and the definition is so vague that it includes everything from Haribo to margarine, hummus to oatcakes, and even brown bread. These foods are all obviously very different and objectively don't belong in the same category, but can all be part of a balanced nutritious diet. Whereas foods such as lard, on the other hand, are only considered to be 'processed' as opposed to 'ultra-processed'. There are some other limitations on the studies of ultra-processed foods, which I won't go into here, but suffice to say, as long as you're eating a variety of foods, this really isn't something worth stressing over.

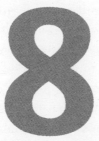

MINDFUL EATING
AND
THE PLEASURE
PRINCIPLE
___

All right, fam, remember way back in chapter 3 I asked you to do a little gentle experimentation with mindfulness? Well, I hope you know I wasn't fucking around. The reason I asked you to do it way back when, is because we're now going to start applying it to food and eating. If you didn't do your homework, then take a time out and go get your meditate on. I'm not kidding. If you come to mindful eating without having established a bit of a mindfulness practice you might inadvertently shoot yourself in the foot. Mindful eating, without any actual mindfulness, can become just another way to control what you eat, and mindfulness and mindful eating are not about control. Don't believe me? Maybe you'll listen to our spiritual leader and chosen one, Fiona Sutherland, aka The Mindful Dietitian (she didn't get that name for nothing):

> Mindful eating is not a way to control, fix or avoid. Mindful eating is not another diet. Mindful eating is not forcing us to do something. It's not about forcing, fixing, controlling ... It's being with it all, including the shit stuff. Like for example if we have an eating experience that's unpleasant, whether that's because we eat beyond the point of comfortable fullness or whether that's because the only food available to us ended up that we didn't like it, and it wasn't satisfying for whatever reason, whether that's taste preference or satiety factors or whatever. Mindful eating also isn't a guarantee of anything. It's not a guarantee that all the foods you're going to eat you're going to love, or that you're always going to get it "right", it's not about being perfect and it's certainly not about certainty, it's about embracing uncertainty actually, and doing the best you can, with a shit load of self-compassion.

Establishing a solid mindfulness practice can help us bring a level of non-judgemental curiosity to the eating experience. There's a lot of 'mindful eating for weight loss' going around, but mindful eating is not a tool to make us eat less. Yes, it absolutely can help you gauge what is an appropriate amount of food for you. But that shouldn't come

Components of mindful eating

Increased pleasure

Mindful eating can help us really heighten the pleasure and the satisfaction we get from meals. Instead of being on autopilot when eating, we gently bring our awareness to the multisensory eating experience: sight, sound, taste, touch, smell, temperature, texture. This in turn can help us find the amount and type of food that will give us the most satisfaction from our eating.

Alimentary alliesthesia

Mindful eating brings awareness of how the perception of pleasure and palatability changes over the course of a meal. You know when you take the first couple of bites of something when you're gently hungry it tastes like pure heaven, but towards the end you can kinda take it or leave it? This is called alimentary alliesthesia, and if you are paying attention, this diminishing pleasure can give you a clue as to when you are edging towards fullness.

Non-judgemental awareness

Approaching the eating experience with a sense of non-judgemental awareness allows us to get in touch with whether or not we are actually enjoying the eating experience, and helps us stop the voice of the inner food critic. Instead of saying 'this cake is so full of fat and chemicals', positive, negative and neutral responses to food are made with curiosity: 'this cake is dry' or 'this cake is fresh and tasty'.

Fostering gratitude

Bringing mindfulness to the eating experience can also help us foster a sense of gratitude for the food we are eating; that could mean just being grateful that we have something to eat at all (so many don't have enough to eat, even in the UK), it could mean being thankful to whoever prepared your food, it could be gratitude for Cadbury's consistently releasing their magical purple and red foiled eggs every year. Or for that ready meal that was a total lifesaver because your disability prevents you from being able to cook meals from scratch and without it you'd go hungry or have a packet of crisps for dinner. It could be to the farmer who grew your food. Or to Tesco for staying open late enough for you to pick up some bread and cheese on the way home after a long day at work. It could be gratitude for a safe food system that means we don't regularly suffer foodborne illness. Or for food technology that allows us to keep milk in the fridge without it going off and curdling after a hot second. Maybe it's to the Uber Eats driver who pedals his bike so hard to get your takeaway to you in the pouring rain despite working for less than minimum wage (give that guy a tip!). There are so many reasons to be grateful for the food we have to eat – even if it's a humble cheese toastie and Heinz tomato soup. Take a second to appreciate it before you swoop in and gobble it all down.

with the expectation of eating less. That is diet mentality, my friend, and you are done with that shit.

Mindfulness can be applied to almost any aspect of the eating experience, whether that is growing your own herbs or tomatoes, chopping veggies, scooping ice cream, opening a delivery-pizza box, or the actual eating experience. Mindful eating is mindfulness specifically related to our experience with food and eating.

SO HOW DO WE DO IT?

I've noticed that people like to go really hard into this mindful eating thing, and while the enthusiasm is great, it doesn't always set you up for forming sustainable habits. My best advice would be to start small and build up from there. The whole idea here is to work on minimizing distractions (phones, tablets, laptops, etc). A lot of us are living pretty frenetic lives, usually multitasking as we eat. Mindful eating is about lessening the distractions (when we can) and gathering information about the eating experience.

Let's break it down into steps.

Step 1 – Set an intention

Before you embark on mindful eating, it's helpful to check in with your intention for the practice; are you treating it like an experiment, with the aim of curiosity and intrigue as to what you might find? Or are you coming at it as a way to control what you're eating and possibly eat less? It's important to be really real with yourself – are you coming at this as another diet? It's OK if that's where you're at, as long as you're being honest with yourself about it and not trying to trick yourself that it's something that it's not. Then set an intention to come at this from a place of curiosity and non-judgement; you are simply bringing awareness to the eating experience and collecting information.

Step 2 – Start small

Later on in this chapter we're going to discuss the various sensory aspects of a meal and try to narrow down your preferences for taste, flavour, texture, temperature, and so on. In terms of mindful eating, begin by focusing your attention on just one of these aspects of the eating experience. Notice if and when you get distracted, and gently bring your awareness back to that aspect of the food you were focused on.

Step 3 – One mindful meal

I would encourage you to set an achievable goal for your mindful-eating practice – maybe it's one mindful meal three times a week; maybe it's one mindful meal or snack a day. It could even be just one mindful bite at the beginning of each meal. In fact, that's a pretty good place to start if you're new to mindful eating or a whole meal feels like too much. I try to aim for one mindful meal a day, usually lunch, where my focus is entirely on the meal I'm eating. That doesn't mean I'm not bringing aspects of mindfulness to other meals, but this is the time I designate for really minimizing other distractions. Speaking of which . . .

Step 4 – Be realistic

It's easy for mindful eating to become another thing to beat yourself up with if you don't nail it every time, but having the expectation that every single eating experience will be perfectly mindful and free from distraction is totally unrealistic for most people. Some of you will have busy family lives, others will eat lunch with colleagues, and others will only manage a piece of toast in the car on the way to work. Think about ways you can gently apply aspects of mindfulness to these experiences, and if it doesn't always work out that way, that's OK too.

Step 5 – It doesn't have to be perfect

Like I said, people have a tendency to want to perfect this mindful eating thing, but here's the thing: it doesn't have to be perfect. You're allowed to read a magazine or listen to a podcast. It's your call!! Gently incorporating mindfulness when you can is the key here. If you get lost in thought or distracted by your phone, no worries, just gently come back to the meal or snack when you notice your attention has wandered.

Step 6 – The elements of mindful eating

John Kabat Zinn famously described the 'raisin meditation' – a mindful-eating practice using a shrivelled-up old grape. Here I'm outlining the components of this meditation to give you a sense of the elements of mindful eating you may want to place your attention on and to give you a sense of things you can think about.[1]

You don't have to use dead grapes; use whatever works for you to get a feel for mindful eating and use the outline opposite as a guide. We'll practise with chocolates, too.

Holding	First, take a raisin and hold it in the palm of your hand or between your finger and thumb. Focusing on it, imagine that you've just dropped in from Mars and have never seen an object like this before in your life.
Seeing	Take time to really see it; gaze at the raisin with care and full attention. Let your eyes explore every part of it, examining the highlights where the light shines, the darker hollows, the folds and ridges, and any asymmetries or unique features.
Touching	Turn the raisin over between your fingers, exploring its texture, maybe with your eyes closed if that enhances your sense of touch.
Smelling	Holding the raisin beneath your nose; with each inhalation drink in any smell, aroma, or fragrance that may arise, noticing as you do this anything interesting that may be happening in your mouth or stomach.
Placing	Now slowly bring the raisin up to your lips, noticing how your hand and arm know exactly how and where to position it. Gently place the object in the mouth, without chewing, noticing how it gets into the mouth in the first place. Spend a few moments exploring the sensations of having it in your mouth, exploring it with your tongue.
Tasting	When you are ready, prepare to chew the raisin, noticing how and where it needs to be for chewing. Then, very consciously, take one or two bites into it and notice what happens in the aftermath, experiencing any

	waves of taste that emanate from it as you continue chewing. Without swallowing yet, notice the bare sensations of taste and texture in the mouth and how these may change over time, moment by moment, as well as any changes in the object itself.
Swallowing	When you feel ready to swallow the raisin, see if you can first detect the intention to swallow as it comes up, so that even this is experienced consciously before you actually swallow the raisin.
Following	Finally, see if you can feel what is left of the raisin moving down into your stomach, and sense how the body as a whole is feeling after completing this exercise in mindful eating.

MINDFUL-EATING PRACTICE

—

Similarly to the hunger body scan in chapter 4, I want you to record this mindful-eating practice on your phone and play it back to yourself. I've written this to be used with chocolate; an individual Quality Street or Celebration would be perfect. But if you're not a chocolate person, you can write out your own script using the following as a template but mixing it up to describe the food you're going to eat. Pizza, yoghurt-covered almonds, ice cream, crisps, cherries, whatever.

Get yourself nice and comfortable . . .

Take a few deep breaths, in through your nose and out through your mouth . . .

Now look at the chocolate in your hand, notice the shiny foil . . .

Are there any patterns or designs on the wrapper?

Gently closing your eyes, move the chocolate around in your hands. Rub your fingers over the foil and feel the textures and shape of the chocolate underneath . . . can you trace any ridges or designs on the chocolate itself? Feel the weight of the chocolate, is it dense or is it light? Imagine what's inside the foil . . . Smooth rich chocolate that will melt when you put it in your mouth . . . Maybe there's caramel in the middle or maybe it has notes of orange or vanilla . . . perhaps there are some nuts or crunchy pieces inside . . . For now just imagine what it's going to taste like as you bite into it . . . Is it hard or soft and melty? Is it solid or filled in the centre? . . .

Now open your eyes and gently peel back the foil . . . listen to the sound of the foil crinkling as you unwrap it . . . Take a look at the chocolate underneath . . . Gaze at it as though you've never seen a chocolate like this before. What do you see? How would you describe the chocolate? Is it textured or patterned, or completely smooth . . . What colour is it? . . . Is it rich and dark or milky and creamy? . . . Anticipate the flavours in your mouth . . . Are they smooth or are they sharp and bitter? . . .

Now lift the chocolate up to your nose and take a deep breath in . . . What do you smell? . . . Just notice all the different scents that go into the chocolate . . . What does it smell like? . . . Does it smell sweet or bitter? . . . Can you pick out the different scents? . . . Vanilla, cocoa, maybe butterscotch or honey, brown sugar, orange blossom or mint . . . Notice any sensations that you might experience in your mouth, stomach, or elsewhere in your body.

Now it's time to take a bite of the chocolate, but don't chew it yet . . . Let the flavours melt into your tongue . . . What do you taste? . . . What flavours are present? . . Is it the same as what you expected? . . . What are the textures you feel? . . . How does it feel on your tongue as you slowly roll it around your mouth? . . . Does the flavour change over time or as you slowly begin to chew? . . . Does it get stuck on your teeth or on the roof of your mouth? . . . When you're ready, go ahead and swallow. Notice the sensation on the back of your tongue travelling down towards your stomach. How does it feel in your stomach and elsewhere in your body? . . .

Now take a second and third bite. Does the chocolate change flavours? Is it as good as the first bite? . . .

Of course it's not practical to do this at every single meal, but it can be nice to repeat this activity every now and then with your favourite snack. I often tell clients to think of it as some self-care-alone time and to find themselves some peace and quiet, even just for five or ten minutes to have a cup of tea and a bite to eat.

WHAT DO YOU ACTUALLY WANT TO EAT?

—

One of the biggest problems people have when they stop restricting themselves is knowing *what* to eat. For the longest time you might have been going along with eating the same old wellness or diet foods. If your usual rotation consists of variation on a theme, you know, smoked salmon, quinoa, broccoli, avocado, and sweet potato . . . well, it might just be about time to start mixing things up. Not that there's anything wrong with those foods, they are all delicious in their own right. But if you're essentially eating the same things, day in, day out, with little variation, it's easy to get bored, and that can feel like restriction.

I remember one client in particular who kept complaining that she was 'picking' in the evenings. I asked her to describe what she would typically eat in a day and she reeled off a bunch of same-y, boring-sounding meals. No freaking wonder she was trying to find something delicious to eat in the evening; her meals throughout the day were uninspired, monotonous, insipid, and mundane. What she was really looking for in the evening was something to infuse a little excitement into her meals, but by not keeping things interesting throughout the day, she was putting a ton of pressure on getting a pleasure hit at night, and because she was in a deficit, it took more chocolate, crisps, and cookies to get that hit than if she'd allowed herself a little more excitement throughout the day.

People have a tendency not to eat anything they perceive to be 'bad' throughout the day, which, if you've had a crappy day, can trigger the fuck-it *effect*. So even if you are eating enough to satisfy *physical hunger*, and you are well nourished, you may still find yourself picking, raiding the fridge, or elbow-deep into a can of Pringles. We'll talk about emotional eating in chapter 10 as this could very well indicate a deeper problem. BUT, before we get there it's really important to make sure you're allowing yourself pleasure and satisfaction from the foods you're eating *across* the day. Don't put that all on a piece of chocolate cake you're saving for Netflix time.

And no, I don't mean you have to have chocolate with every meal either (although that's cool too). What I mean is make sure your meals are interesting, appetizing, something you're actually looking forward to eating, not just some sad soggy salad or sandwich. Make sure they have some colour, variety, spice, texture, flavour, sweetness, crunch – anything to make eating a little more fun. Food is meant to taste good, it's meant to be pleasurable.

This can be the difference between full and *satisfied*. It's what Tribole and Resch call the **satisfaction factor**. It seems so basic and obvious that people don't even really think about it. But if you are eating a box of dry crackers when what you really want is a bowl of crunchy, nutty cereal with ice-cold milk, you can see how you'll feel totally underwhelmed. This increases the chance that you're low-key depriving yourself, meaning it will be a lot harder for you to stop when you reach comfortable fullness; if you're not satisfied with what you're eating then the chances are you'll be more inclined to pick or graze outside meal or snack times.

ACTIVITY
The pleasure principle

The basic premise of diets, meal plans, and 'clean' eating is to have someone else to tell you what to eat. It can be hard to know what you actually like to eat or what you want to eat! Let's start by doing a thought experiment. In your journal, write out the following headings: flavour, texture, temperature, variety, aroma, appearance, experience. Now answer the following questions to help you identify the foods you really enjoy eating and that give you pleasure and satisfaction. There's no right or wrong answer, and you might want to redo this activity periodically to see if things have shifted. The idea is just to help you get more in tune with what you like and want to eat; this can help take the pressure off making food decisions at restaurants or at the supermarket. It might be helpful to do it when you're slightly hungry (but not over-hungry) as your senses will be heightened. Once you have tuned in to your preferences, you can let those help guide your food choices.

Flavour

Think about the flavours or combinations of flavours you enjoy: sweet, spicy, bitter, umami, sour, salty, briny, or pickled. Does that change throughout the day? Do you like to mix flavours or do you prefer plain food? Which type of cuisine do you like to eat? Mexican, Italian, Japanese, Indian. Do you like bold or more subtle and nuanced flavours? Do you like combos or contrasts of flavour like of sweet and salty? Or do you like one unifying flavour? Are there any flavours you really don't like?

Texture

Crunchy, smooth, creamy, hard, soft, puréed, mashed, crispy, chewy, toasted. Which textures do you prefer? Crusty bread or soft pillowy rolls? Which do you dislike? Does your texture preference change over time or even throughout the day? Do you get a variety of textures in each meal? Crunchy foods or puréed? Different textures can appeal at different times of the day.

Temperature

Piping-hot stews, steaming mugs of tea and bowls of soup are great in the winter; but what about when the weather is hotter? Do you like ice cream, watermelon, and bean salads? Do you like freezing-cold food straight out of the fridge? Or does it taste better once it has come to room temperature? Or do you like your food sizzling hot? Do you prefer hot or cold breakfasts? What about lunch and dinner? I *hate* cold food from the fridge and have to eat leftovers at room temp.

Variety

Do you tend to eat the same thing day in, day out? Or do you like to mix it up and get creative? Not every meal can be mezze or tapas style, but think about how you can change things up throughout the week. Also think about how you can add a little interesting variety to your everyday meals with some different sauces, toppings, and garnishes. Variety is good nutritionally speaking, but having options means your taste buds won't get bored! How could you add more variety to meals?

Side note: people seem to get really hung up on eating the same thing for breakfast every day; I am constantly being asked for breakfast ideas, so here are a few for when you're caught in a breakfast rut:

- breakfast burrito/tacos: eggs or tofu scramble with avocado and salsa
- baked oatmeal with cinnamon and shredded apple and raisins
- pancakes or waffles (make these ahead and freeze if you don't have a lot of time, then you can just pop them in the toaster and top with fruit/yoghurt)
- frittata with veg and cheese on toast

- muffins (sweet or savoury)
- English muffin with bacon, lettuce and tomato and a dollop of mayo or mustard
- bagels with cream cheese and salmon
- sweet-potato hash with baked eggs and smashed avocado
- shakshuka – you can swap out the eggs for chickpeas if eggs aren't your bag, or add chickpeas to the rich tomato sauce to add more interesting texture

Aroma

This is another great one that can give you clues about what kind of food you really want. If it smells good then chances are it will taste good to you too. The yeasty smell of baking bread or the richness of fresh coffee. If a food doesn't smell appealing, chances are it won't taste good to you. Which foods do you love the smell of? Which ones smell kinda gross or uninteresting?

Appearance

OK, so it doesn't have to be Instagram-worthy, but putting a little effort into presentation can help with the satisfaction factor. Think about colourful garnishes, pretty bowls for different sauces or condiments on the side, breaking up 'samey' foods with a little something to jazz it up. Think about how you can make meals a bit more interesting to look at. Here are some ideas:

- Do you have a variety of textures and flavours? Imagine a plate of chicken, mashed potatoes, and cauliflower; it's all the same boring beige food. You could make it fresher by swapping the cauliflower for some crisp salad. You could roast the potatoes or make wedges with some tasty seasoning.
- Garnishes are really quick and easy and can make a big impact: herbs like chives or coriander, black sesame seeds, spices like sumac or chilli flakes, a good-quality finishing salt like Malden, cracked black pepper, sauerkraut or pickled veg.

● Sauces/dips: tahini dressings, guacamole, hummus, wholegrain mustard, hot sauce like Cholula, tzatziki.

Dishes: think about how you serve your meals too – I like to use a shallow bowl rather than a flat plate; that way you can show off all the components of a meal and they don't look flat and boring. What can you do to make your meals look a little bit prettier?

Experience

Are you eating standing up, straight out of the fridge? Or do you take time to set the table and sit down and eat mindfully? Are you eating at your computer? With the TV on? Or while aimlessly scrolling through your phone? How many of your meals are eaten while distracted? How can you make sure you're not distracted while eating (with the goal of increasing the satisfaction or pleasure of a meal and knowing when you're full and ready to stop eating).

––––

By applying the mindfulness skills you've been developing, and using them to foster a sense of non-judgemental curiosity to the eating experience, we can start to narrow down what it is we *really* want to eat; this is **the pleasure principle**. It simply means not being afraid to eat food that also brings you joy and pleasure, and yes, foods that bring pleasure can also support your health, as we'll discuss in chapter 12. Over the next week or so, pick a few meals where the goal is to eat them mindfully, and really pay attention to the different sensory qualities of the meal. In your intuitive eating journal, reflect back on what you liked and what you didn't like in the notes section. This can help give you clues as to what to buy when you do your supermarket shop or what you will enjoy eating at a restaurant.

SUPERMARKET VISUALIZATION

(adapted from Susie Orbach's
Fat Is a Feminist Issue)

If you've been in diet mentality for a long time, then you might have no clue what you really like to eat. Hey, maybe you genuinely love rice cakes and celery sticks. Then again, probably not. Going to the shops without a meal plan or without the guidance of good and bad food lists might feel a bit too much at this stage. So we're going to go on a hypothetical shopping trip. This activity allows you to get a sense of what you'd buy at the supermarket without actually spending any money, or having a sense that you won't be able to trust yourself around all that food.

Make sure you're sitting somewhere comfortable where you won't be disturbed; have your journal and a pen nearby to make notes.

Imagine yourself standing in your kitchen. You open up the cupboards and the fridge; there isn't much there apart from a packet of rice cakes and some kale that's starting to go off. Your kitchen is bare. How does this make you feel? Are you comforted by the thought of having no food around you or does it trigger a deprivation mindset?

You decide you need to do a shop and fill the kitchen up with delicious and satisfying foods; you have an unlimited budget and you need to make sure the kitchen is really well stocked. You go to your favourite high-end grocery store that is made up of a series of smaller speciality stores/counters; it has everything you could ever want to eat under one roof. There's a bakery where everything is made fresh each day, a butcher with high-quality meat and fish, a deli counter with delicious prepared foods, a cheesemonger, an ice-cream counter, a smoothie bar, a pizza oven, fresh sushi, a greengrocer, a make-your-own-burrito stand, a salad and hot food bar, and everything in between. You don't need to know the exact meals you're going to make or quantities or anything like that, this is just a low-stress way for you to imagine all the food that you might like to try.

You grab a cart and start working your way around the store, stopping to pick items up and examine them before putting them in your cart. You start in the bakery section, there are fresh sourdough breads, still hot from the oven, flaky croissants, and Portuguese custard tarts that are gently browned on top. There are eclairs with fresh cream, and a whole chocolate fudge cake. There's rosemary and olive oil focaccia with sea salt, and onion and sesame bagels. There are cinnamon buns drizzled in icing and everything else you'd expect from a quality bakery. Stop and note down in your journal what you pick up in the bakery section.

Now move on to the meat counter (unless you're veggie, then skip this part): tender steaks, wild-caught smoked salmon from Scotland, pork and apple sausages.

Next it's the deli counter: smoked hummus, caramelized onion hummus, beetroot hummus, any kind of hummus you can imagine, golden falafel and pickled turnip that has turned bright pink, garlic-stuffed olives, chorizo, sun-blushed tomatoes, artichokes, honey-roasted ham, salami, prosciutto. List what you're going to pick up at the deli.

On to the cheesemonger: Brie, Parmesan, Camembert, Gruyère, Morbier, mature Cheddar and aged blue cheeses, halloumi, Jarlsberg, Stilton and any other type of cheese you can imagine. Pause and reflect on what you pick up from the cheese counter and add it to your list.

Next up is the greengrocer: bright-red cherries on the stem, soft juicy peaches that smell like heaven, soft, ripe avocados, vine-ripened tomatoes, tenderstem broccoli, bright-pink radishes and ruby-red strawberries, perfectly spiralling Romanesco, golden-yellow corn still on the cob, emerald-green leaves, sunny sweet potatoes and humble white ones. List the items you pick up in the greengrocer section.

Continue through the whole shop like this section by section, adding foods to your cart. Dry goods, frozen foods, the salad and hot food bar, the sushi counter, the smoothie and juice bar, the pizza oven, where you can pick your own toppings and take home a hot, fresh pizza, the taco and burrito station, and the ice-cream and gelato bar, plus anything else you can imagine; make sure you write everything down.

Now imagine making your way home and stocking your cupboards, pantry, fridge, cookie jar, fruit bowl, freezer, everything. Take a look around at your kitchen now. How does it feel to have an abundance of foods? Do you feel content knowing that there are plenty of delicious foods available? Or does it feel overwhelming? What would you need to feel safe? Can you relax, safe in the knowledge that food will always be available to you? If it still feels a little scary, can you think of anything that is comforting or soothing about being around the food? Do you feel the scarcity mindset loosening its grip?

IT DOESN'T HAVE TO BE PERFECT . . .

In an ideal world, we'd always eat exactly what we wanted at every meal, something satisfying that totally hits the spot. But that's unrealistic. Sometimes you need to neck a granola bar in between meetings, sometimes you only have the energy to make toast for dinner, sometimes you have to go to your in-laws and they're really terrible cooks. Intuitive eating doesn't mean eating the thing that perfectly satisfies you at every meal. Sure, we want the majority of our eating experiences to be positive, but sometimes you just have to cobble together whatever leftovers are in the fridge; they might not even go together, but in the grand scheme of things, it's better to eat something than to go hungry. I get a lot of messages from people who feel like they were totally nailing this intuitive eating thing, but then life got busy and they don't have time to cook and they basically grab whatever they can to keep themselves going. Yeah, no shit, it's called life. Remember that the goal of IE is not to be 'perfect', there's no such thing. The goal is to be flexible and easy-going when life gets messy. Case in point: I have lost count of how much peanut butter on toast I've had since I've been writing this book. Objectively there's nothing wrong with PB on toast, I especially enjoy it when it comes loaded with a sprinkle of cinnamon and a drizzle of maple syrup. However, clients often come in saying they've been 'eating like shit', grabbing what they can on the go, not doing a weekly shop or cooking things at home and maybe don't feel their best. But instead of taking a step back and looking at the bigger picture, they tend to internalize the blame as their fault, and that manifests as 'I'm fucking up this intuitive eating thing.'

I get that it can sometimes feel like you're screwing up. But I promise you, you're doing better than you think. The problem is probably a lot less about the food you are or aren't eating and more about self-care. Chances are that if you're mega-busy, you're also kinda stressed out, not sleeping well, maybe skipping a yoga class, and don't have much downtime to just kick back. Food becomes the scapegoat, but clearly the issue is much more complicated than that. We'll talk about self-care in a lot more detail in chapter 9 but for now, just let yourself off the hook a little. You're doing the best you can right now. It doesn't have to be perfect, and in the grand scheme of things, you're doing fucking great. Remember, it's way more important to honour your hunger by having something to eat – even if it is beans on toast or hummus, crackers and baby carrots from Tesco Express, or even a Dominos – than it is to let yourself go hungry.

If we're feeling like a hot mess, consider this: are you getting enough sleep? Are you bringing mindfulness and stress management into your day? Or are you frantically running around trying to get shit done? Have you skipped out on yoga for work drinks the past few nights? The point is that when shit hits the fan we like a simple solution to help us feel like we have things under control. Often that manifests as trying to conquer or master what you're eating, which can perpetuate a restrict/binge cycle or lead us to start arbitrarily cutting things out, which we know will backfire long term. Try to keep the bigger picture in mind, because all of these things play into how we feel, not just what we eat.

LET'S TALK ABOUT DARK CHOCOLATE
—

So, we've established that in order to even contemplate stopping at comfortable fullness, we need to not only be physically nourished, but also satisfied. Sometimes this means recognizing when a meal or snack isn't meeting your expectations, and perhaps stopping and getting something else instead, or rounding your meal out with something tasty. I mean, this could literally be anything, a spoonful of Nutella, some cheese and biscuits, a bunch of grapes, a cup of tea and some cookies, a yoghurt, *whatever*. But, there's a theme I've noticed. People invariably tell me that to round out a meal, they just want a corner or two of dark chocolate. 'cue internal eye roll' And before you all @ me saying how much you *love* dark chocolate, just let this percolate for a second. Do you *love* dark chocolate because you *love* its bitter complexity on your tongue? Or do you *love* it because diet culture has taught you it's *healthier*, better for you, and something about antioxidants?

Fine, some people genuinely love dark chocolate, and that's cool. But when a client tells me this, I like to push them a little. Do they *really* love dark chocolate that much? Or has diet culture convinced us it's somehow superior? I'm using dark chocolate as an example here, but you could apply this to almost any diet-y/wellness food. Be really honest, do you get your kicks from rice cakes and skinny popcorn? Or do they leave you feeling short-changed and less than satisfied? I'm not here to tell you there's anything wrong with these foods, no judgement, remember? Whatever flips your shit, I'm cool with. But what I want to help you get to the bottom of is do you legitimately enjoy these foods or has diet culture convinced you that you *should* like them? Try doing a side-by-side comparison of some of these foods, or better yet, get a friend to help you orchestrate a blind-taste test. Be honest with yourself about which one you really prefer. When I've done mindful-eating meditations with groups using dark chocolate, invariably half the group think it's the best piece of chocolate they've ever eaten, and the other half don't finish because they realize they didn't actually like dark chocolate. But often we end up eating foods we actually don't like all that much – what's the point? If you don't like it, don't eat it! And if you like it, really savour it.

FEELING YOUR
FULLNESS

___

ll right, by now you should hopefully be fairly comfortable with recognizing all the subtle aspects of hunger, and by and large, responding to those initial sensations in your body. You'll be practising food neutrality and treating all foods equally, and you'll be giving yourself full, unconditional permission to eat, and with a little practice, you'll be bringing some mindful awareness to the eating experience.

With all of these aspects locked down, you might naturally have started to honour your own subjective feelings of fullness without much help from me. If you're not totally there yet, then no worries either; it really takes some time to work your way out of the deprivation mindset caused by dieting and restriction and to learn that food will always be available, without conditions or restrictions, and it may take some time to internalize that. Don't force yourself to respect your fullness, as this can easily exacerbate the deprivation mindset and feelings of scarcity.

Remember, it's important not to have expectations about how long this should take; don't compare yourself to other people. If you are still regularly eating past the point of comfortable fullness, go back and make sure you are getting enough nourishment and sensory variety throughout the day. If you are, and are still eating past comfortable fullness regularly, i.e. at most eating experiences, then it might be worth taking a look at chapter 10 and considering if there are any underlying emotional reasons as to why you might be unable to respect your fullness.

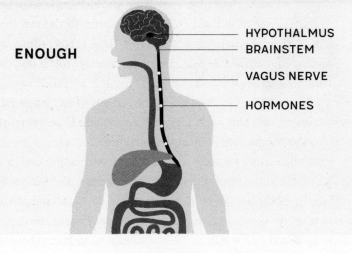

ENOUGH

HYPOTHALMUS
BRAINSTEM
VAGUS NERVE
HORMONES

HOW DOES FULLNESS WORK?

—

Similarly to hunger, fullness is orchestrated by complicated pathways in the body. Let's take a look at the biology.

As we've already talked about, the stomach is designed to hold a lot of food; it acts as a reservoir that slowly releases food into the small intestine. As we eat, food gradually fills the space in the stomach and fills it up like a balloon.

There are a few different ways we perceive the sensation of fullness:

1 Nerves wrap intricately around the stomach, and as it stretches in response to food, those nerves send a signal to the brain stem and hypothalamus via the vagus nerve to register the fact that the stomach is physically full. However, this isn't the only mechanism involved; you'll know yourself, if you try and trick your brain by only drinking water or coffee, it won't keep you full for long.

2 Receptors in the small intestine detect changes in pH from the products of digestion, like fatty acids from fat and peptides from protein. Endocrine cells throughout the gastrointestinal tracts release hormones in response to these products of

digestion, which are then circulated in the blood to the hypothalamus (the brain's food control centre), where they cause a reduction in the feeling of reward you get from eating, and the feeling of satiation begins to kick in, letting you know it's almost time to stop eating.

3 There are over twenty hormones involved in this response; some of them also cause the stomach to relax even further, and slow down the rate of food emptying from the stomach to the small intestine. An important fullness hormone is called leptin.

4 Leptin acts on receptors in the hypothalamus that inhibit the feeling of hunger and stimulates the areas of the hypothalamus that drive the feeling of fullness. However, leptin can be suppressed due to dieting.[1,2] It's no surprise then than some people struggle to feel their fullness cues post-dieting or restricting. Be patient with yourself while your body readjusts and use the exercises below to help you tune back in.

HOW TO FIND YOUR FULLNESS LEVEL
—

Fullness is subjective from person to person, and the amount of food it might take you to feel full can vary from day to day or meal to meal. Some days you'll be inexplicably insatiable, and others you might get full on less food than usual. The key is to go with the flow and not judge yourself for how much you need to eat.

With that in mind, people sometimes get fixated on finding the exact specific point at which to stop eating, and if they go over that line, then they must be failing. Remember all that you've learned from your mindfulness and mindful-eating practices and, if you do eat past the point of comfortable fullness, don't freak out. It's not a failure, it's simply information. What can you learn from that experience? Had you let yourself get *over-hungry*? Are you tired, stressed, anxious, or otherwise upset about something? Regularly eating past the point of comfortable fullness is simply a clue that something else might be going on with you. Read on to chapter 10 to learn more about that.

WORK BACKWARDS

—

I think the easiest way to help determine your fullness level is actually by working backwards; as we did with hunger, try visualizing fullness as the fuel tank in your car. How long after you've topped up the tank does it take you to feel hungry again? I've found this is really helpful to clients who perceive themselves to always be overeating (thanks, diet culture). Working in reverse can help us see that actually we got hungry again a few hours after our meal or snack, so we probably ate an appropriate amount of food. Try it for yourself and experience the tank getting emptier over time. It's best to do this on a day where you won't be too distracted and you can regularly check in with yourself; it may take a while to find the sweet spot for you too, so don't freak out if it takes a while to get it. I'd recommend printing a few copies of the hunger and satisfaction wheel we first used in chapter 4 so you can scribble all over them and keep adjusting until you feel comfortable with your physical sensations of fullness. After a meal or a snack notice how you physically feel in your stomach, but notice the sensations in other parts of your body too. Just like with hunger, you can check if you've had enough to eat by paying attention to cues in other parts of your body too, like your ability to focus or concentrate, or your energy levels (which may dip slightly after a meal as you're digesting, but should increase and leave you feeling energized). Here's what to do:

1 After a meal or a snack, try and gauge where you are on the wheel, note down any words from the list below, or use your own words to help describe how you feel.

2 Set a timer on your phone for every 20–30 minutes after your meal to check in with yourself.

3 At each time point, notice where you are on the wheel.

4 How quickly do you get hungry again? Did you eat an appropriate amount of food to keep you 'topped up' or did you get hungry again quite quickly?

5 If it's helpful, you can start keeping track of your fullness level in your journal (see page 20 for a reminder of how to keep this).

Notice if there's a pattern between how hungry you get when you eat and how well you can respect your fullness level.

HUNGER AND SATISFACTION GUIDE

HANGRY	STUFFED	EMPTY	HEADACHE	COMFORTABLY FULL
HUNGER PANGS	THINKING ABOUT FOODS	DISTRACTED	CONTENT	SATISFIED
SICK	CRANKY	LIGHT-HEADED	SHAKY	STOMACH ACHE
EATING SLOWS DOWN	HEADACHE	SENSE OF WELL-BEING	STOMACH GROWLING	NEUTRAL
NEITHER HUNGRY OR FULL	HAPPY	LOW ENERGY	UNSATISFIED	NAUSEA

Fullness body scan

Just like the hunger body scan in chapter 4, you can use this quick checklist to help you judge your own subjective sense of fullness.

Mood	Energy	Head	Stomach	Body
content	recharged	improved con-centration	comfort-able	not interested in food
calm	energized	focused	gently full	food no longer makes you salivate
happy	sleepy	clear	slightly bloated/burpy	reduced cravings
satisfied			gurgling/digesting	eating slows down
sated				

THE MID-MEAL PAUSE

—

When you are learning to feel your fullness, it's a good idea to check in with yourself about halfway through a meal; take a little breather for about 10–20 seconds. This is not a commitment to stop eating, it's simply a little pause to take a break and visualize where you might be on the hunger and satisfaction wheel. You might like to check:

- Am I still enjoying this food as much as I did at the beginning?
- Is this food satisfying or might I want something else to bridge the gap between full and satisfied?
- What are the physical sensations I am feeling? Pleasant, unpleasant, or neutral?

Again, taking a pause doesn't mean you have to stop eating; as you're about to see, just because you're no longer hungry, doesn't mean you're full yet either!

MIND THE FULLNESS GAP

—

If you have been in diet mode for a relatively long period of time or you are fearful of fullness, it can be tempting to stop eating at a point where you are no longer hungry, but not yet full. I call this the fullness gap; it's essentially the zone between a 4 and a 6 on the hunger and satisfaction wheel, that neutral area. If we expect to be eating again in a few hours – for instance if you're having an afternoon snack to tide you over to dinner – then stopping in the neutral zone might be totally appropriate. However, if you stop there after every meal and snack then there's a chance you aren't allowing yourself the opportunity to properly fill up, meaning you could risk getting over-hungry later.

I remember one client in particular who was complaining that she couldn't stop eating chocolate a little while after a meal. When we retraced her steps from earlier in the day, we discovered that she had only eaten half a sandwich for lunch. When we dug into it a little bit more, I realized that there were two separate but related things going on.

1 First of all, this client was trying really hard to be a 'perfect' intuitive eater. To her that meant that she would intuitively only eat half of her sandwich, and that she would be full and content based on that. This is a pretty common phenomenon, so be aware of that and let go of any expectations of how much you should eat as you could be inadvertently shooting yourself in the foot.

2 The second thing that was happening here was that this client was only eating until she was no longer hungry, but not yet full. She stopped in the fullness gap, meaning that an hour or two later, she was ready for something else to eat, at which point she reached for a bar of chocolate instead of finishing her sandwich (by this point the sandwich was already in the bin).

This is an easy mistake to make, so just keep reminding yourself that your stomach is designed to be a reservoir for food, that's literally its job! Sure, eating to the point of stuffed doesn't feel great, and stopping too soon will leave us feeling hungry again a little while later. Try and find that sweet spot of comfortable fullness. Don't worry if you over or under shoot the mark to begin with, it takes practice, so be patient!

JUDGING OVEREATING

Once a participant from one of my online courses told me she found it REALLY hard to stop when she was full/satisfied. She went on to say that led her to 'overeating'. She said she wasn't restricting, and was no longer fearful of not being able to eat that food again, she just really enjoyed how something tasted. She then asked other members of the group how they were getting on and how they prevented themselves from 'overeating'. She explained how she felt she was 'still eating too much', and then detailed how she had been out to the cinema where she ate . . . wait for it . . . a whole entire brownie. Dun, dun, dun! *Quel horreur*. In fact, she said that she had eaten half, and then gone back for the other half.

I pointed out to her how, objectively, by most people's standards, a brownie was not 'too much', a brownie is a perfectly reasonable amount of food to have as a snack. Sure, some people may need more, some may need less. But it's not exactly overdoing it either, is it?

Another client once emailed me after our first session in a total fluster because she had binged at lunchtime. I asked her to explain what she'd eaten, and she described lunch: a shop-bought sandwich and a chocolate bar. Again, objectively, this was a totally appropriate amount of food for this person to eat for a meal.

What was really going on for both of these women were three things:

1 Being self-critical of how much food they were eating. A common phenomenon in intuitive eating is the expectation that your intuition will tell you to eat less. Therefore, there is a disconnect between how much your rational brain (which is steeped in diet culture) thinks you should eat versus how much your body really wants to eat. That results in a whole load of judgement.

2 Diet culture skews our idea of what should be an appropriate amount of food. Whereas dudes are commended for eating fully loaded man-sized 'dirty' burgers, women are taught how to eat less and somehow feel fuller for longer. This totally distorts our idea of how much we should eat; we are socialized to eat 'ladylike' portions, eat less than our partners eat, avoid snacks, split desserts. Again, this results in a disconnect between how much we perceive we should eat, and how much we may really need to eat.

3 And lastly, we judge ourselves for wanting to eat foods that taste good, as though it was abnormal to want to eat sweet or pleasurable foods. It's not, in fact, it's normal; it can be part of self-care and looking after ourselves. Restriction and deprivation are what's really problematic.

WHAT IF I EAT PAST THE POINT OF COMFORTABLE FULLNESS?

Guess what, you guys? Overeating isn't bad. It's not going to kill you. It's not a fucking crime. It basically happens to everyone. Sure, we might feel a bit uncomfortable for a while but, bigger picture, it's not that big a deal. In fact, I don't really even like the term 'overeating'; it's pretty judgey and reinforces the idea that it's wrong or somehow bad when it's actually totally NORMAL. If a food tastes good, we want to eat a lot of that food. This happens to people who have a totally healthy relationship with food too.

The problem arises when we label it bad or judge ourselves when we eat past the point of comfortable fullness. This can lead to restrictive eating (skipping meals, counting calories) or over exercise in order to 'make up' for the food you ate. This compensation is the real issue as it just exacerbates the problem by getting you stuck in a binge/restrict cycle. What happens when you let go of the judgement? Does your appetite naturally balance out by being less hungry at the next meal? Instead of effortful restriction, can we notice how our bodies respond to the mistakes we make in eating?

Next time you eat past the point of comfortable fullness, try this instead

1 Have some self-compassion. Ditch the self-judgement and remind yourself that you're still a badass boss bitch.

2 Think about what happened. Are you restricting, over exercising, or dieting? Even 'sensible' or 'balanced' diets/ lifestyles can backfire as overeating. Or are you having a tough time? Eating for emotional reasons isn't bad (in fact, it's also really normal), but think about what's likely to make you feel better. Twenty sugar cookies? Probs not. A couple of sugar cookies, a hug, and a walk with the dog? Think about how you can build up your emotional coping toolkit so that food's not the ONLY thing in there. P.S. sometimes food IS the only coping mechanism we have, and that's OK too. How are you talking about it? 'OMFG, I TOTES BINGED ON THE PARTY BUFFET. I'M SUCH A PIG' **1** pigs are smarter than your average gym bro so don't talk crap about them and **2** it may seem like semantics but bingeing isn't the same as eating past the point of comfortable fullness. Bingeing usually feels very out of control, is ritualized, and involves a larger amount of food than an average person will eat in a single day . . . But just that subtle shift in mindset can help you put things into perspective. And if you do find yourself truly bingeing, please seek advice from a Registered Dietitian or Registered Nutritionist or therapist.

3 Remember that diet culture skews what we perceive to be an appropriate amount of food. If you identify as a woman and you eat anything more than a salad then you're basically 'out of control', when actually, no, you're just feeding your damn body.

4 Visualize the food being digested. Something my clients find helpful if they eat past comfortable fullness is to imagine the food moving down from your stomach, to your small and large intestines and out the other end. Visualizing things moving through your body helps reinforce that your body is working the way it should and gradually the levels of fullness go down and hunger comes back up. Don't over-pathologize your body. Remember that a bit of bloating is normal and OK. If you feel uncomfortable, the NHS recommends that rubbing your belly in a clockwise motion for 10–20 minutes may help, especially if you have wind or are constipated. Your body occasionally does weird shit; doesn't mean there's something wrong or that you're broken.

5 If you do eat past the point of fullness, compensatory behaviours may make you feel better in the short term, but long term they're more likely to exacerbate the problem. Try to break the cycle by doing away with restrictive behaviours. The act of compensation mentally, physically, and emotionally reinforces that cycle that keeps us stuck. Find activities that aren't related to food/exercise to help you instead.

6 I'm going to say this again, because it's easier said than done: have some self-compassion, do something nice for yourself, give yourself a compliment or say three things you're grateful for.

BE AWARE OF EMOTIONAL RESTRICTION

—

A super-common question I get asked goes like this: 'I'm not restricting, in fact, I'm eating *all the foods*. But I'm still eating past comfortable fullness. What should I do?'

OK, so the first thing is *don't* panic. Remember that if you've been restricting for a long time it can take a while to work off the sense of deprivation, and begin to trust that you won't be forced back on a diet at some point in the future; even the threat of future deprivation can be enough to trigger the fuck-it *effect*. So be gentle with yourself and give yourself time.

From my experience working with clients, something else that can hinder the process is emotional restriction. OK, you may be physically embracing all foods, but is there a part of you that still believes that certain foods are 'bad', 'unhealthy', or you're afraid will make you gain weight? If so, you might be unconsciously restricting these foods on an emotional level and undermining your sense of unconditional permission. This in turn can reinforce the scarcity mindset that causes you to feel deprived and so eat past comfortable fullness.

How to identify emotional restriction

Perhaps you already have a sense of if and where emotional restriction is taking place. But if not, don't sweat it. There are ways of figuring it out.

Go back to your food rules and your shit list – redo them and notice which foods or rules are still lingering, what are you still holding on to?

In your journal answer the following questions:

- What feels scary about this food that I can't give myself unconditional permission to eat it?
- What is the worst thing that would happen if I stopped micromanaging what I ate?
- Are there any potential positive outcomes that could come from releasing the emotional restriction I have over this food(s)?
- What do I need to do to allow myself unconditional permission to eat this food?

Go back to chapters 6 and 7 and work through giving yourself unconditional permission to eat and neutralizing your inner food critic. If your inability to grant yourself unconditional permission is tied up with a fear of weight gain, then head back to chapter 5 and see if there's more work to be done around body image.

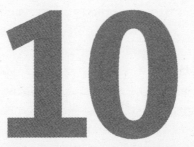

EATING YOUR
EMOTIONS

——

First of all, let's drop this idea that emotional eating is bad or out of control. It's really not as big a deal as most people make it out to be. We could even argue that outside of the context of diet culture, emotional eating wouldn't be vilified the way it is now. In fact, I'd go so far as to say that emotional eating is actually kind of useful. Hear me out. Emotional eating is just your body's way of letting you know something is wrong. It's pretty clever when you think about it. It's a clue, it's your body's way of telling you something is up and you need to address it; it's a coping mechanism.

Food is inextricably linked to emotions from a really young age. When babies cry, parents offer them milk. When you're a kid and you win a dance competition you go for pizza to celebrate. There's cake at birthday parties and weddings. And ice cream when you break up with boyfriends. There are sandwiches and sausage rolls at funerals when we're grieving. Using food to help soothe uncomfortable emotions isn't inherently a bad thing; it's probably healthier than getting blind drunk and going home with a dude whose name you won't remember (not to say some of us haven't been there!). The point is, relative to drugs or alcohol misuse, gambling, self-harm, or sex addiction, food is pretty benign. Not to shame those behaviours either, we're all just doing what we have to do to get by (and if you're suffering with any of those issues, please seek out the help you need and deserve). The point is that food is a coping mechanism, and an important one at that.

The thing that is concerning though, is when food (or lack of it!) becomes your ONLY coping mechanism: if you don't know any other way to process your emotions and just go head-first into a bucket of Ben & Jerry's every night or, on the flip side, you restrict your food intake to help you cope. A bowl of Chunky Monkey is totally cool, as long as it's part of a wider strategy to deal with your shit. In this chapter we're going to take a look at the reasons behind why we eat to soothe uncomfortable emotions, and then start building our emotional-coping toolkit.

A *note on emotional undereating or restriction:* For many people, myself included, when we are facing difficult or challenging emotions the tendency might be to undereat in response. In many ways this response is similar to eating in order to pacify negative emotions; emotional over- and undereating are opposite ends of the same spectrum. The underlying reasons may be similar (unmet needs, lack of self-care), but how they manifest is slightly different. Often when people undereat in response to difficult emotions, it can be a form of control; the world around them is messy, unfair, and unpredictable. But you can leverage control over what or how much you eat. In the same way as being overly full, the physical sensation of hunger can serve as a distraction from more painful feelings and therefore help cope with stress.[1,2] In this sense people who undereat can also benefit from some of the activities in this section and by building up their emotional-coping toolkit. Feeding our bodies is quite literally one of the most fundamental things we can do to show we care about ourselves; withholding food, on the other hand, can be indicative of a lack of self-worth; going back to the list of 100 things you wrote about yourself in chapter 5 can be a gentle reminder of how awesome you are.

———

Before that though, let's consider what emotional eating has done to help you. I know that sounds weird. For most people, emotional eating is bad news, it's something that they want to get rid of immediately, if not sooner. But, here's the thing. If emotional eating wasn't serving an important purpose, you'd have ditched it by now, right? Emotional eating isn't inherently bad, it might have been the best we could do at the time to deal with whatever difficult or challenging things were going on in our lives. Maladaptive coping mechanisms are simply an expression of unmet needs. If we can try and figure out the *purpose* that emotional eating was serving in your life, then we get powerful clues into what your needs really are.

Think about a time when you used food to soothe an uncomfortable emotion or deal with a challenging situation, what *purpose* did the food serve?

For instance, you might have felt lonely and food helped distract you from the loneliness or soothe that uncomfortable emotion. Maybe you were dealing with something very difficult like divorce, illness, or bereavement and needed some sweetness in your life. Maybe you were really angry about something and you needed to take it out on some food.

I know this can seem contrived, but just go with it. In your journal, write out all functions that food has served: numbing out, distraction, comfort, to pacify uncomfortable feelings. Write down your reflections alongside it. Did this give you any clues as to your own unmet needs? For instance, if you've been very sad, perhaps food has provided some pleasantness and pleasure. By reframing how we think of our emotional eating in a more neutral, non-judgemental way, we can begin to build an emotional-coping toolkit that includes tools other than just food on its own.

The point I'm trying to make here is that using food to cope with your emotions is a totally normal response.

There are three main reasons why someone might eat for emotional reasons:

- biology
- self-care is lacking
- pure emotional 'maladaptive' needs; an emotional need that isn't met

BIOLOGY

We've already discussed that sometimes what we identify as emotional eating is actually just hunger.

I'm reiterating it here because I see it happen time after time in clinic; clients don't offer themselves enough nourishment to get through the day, so by the time they get home in the evenings they feel compelled to eat. Then that judgey voice in our heads labels it as 'emotional' or 'comfort' eating, which it also judges as 'bad'. This can so easily trigger a compensatory behaviour, such as restriction or over exercise to 'make up' for it, which will only exacerbate the cycle of binge/restrict. If you're not sure if you're eating enough throughout the day, it can sometimes be worth adding a morning or afternoon snack to see if this helps abate some evening fridge raids. If it doesn't then that gives you a clue that it's something else going on.

You may also be physically eating *enough*, but maybe the food you're eating is monotonous and uninspired, which can also trigger a deprivation mindset. I call this the low-key scarcity mindset; this could be related to emotional restriction or it could be a result of not identifying foods that truly satisfy you.

HOW TO DETECT
LOW-KEY SCARCITY MINDSET
—

All right, so you think you've ditched the diet mentality, you're practising food neutrality, and giving yourself unconditional permission to eat whatever you like, whenever you like.

If you still find yourself regularly eating past the point of comfortable fullness, it might be that you're only giving yourself pseudo-permission to eat shit list foods or that you aren't fully embracing food neutrality. This means you might still be low-key restricting, resulting in deprivation mindset. You might try to 'make up' by eating more food than is appropriate for you when you give yourself temporary permission or are in full on fuck-it mode. Take this quick quiz to find out if you still have residual deprivation mindset:

- I eat three balanced meals per day
- I eat at least two snacks per day
- I get a variety of textures and flavours in all my foods throughout the day
- I include at least one food I'm looking forward to eating at each meal/snack (think fun food!)
- I switch up my meals so I am never eating the same thing more than once in a row
- I don't label foods as good or bad

- I practise food neutrality
- I have given myself unconditional permission to eat all foods, at any time, without having rules around when or how much I can have
- I keep my kitchen well stocked so I have access to a wide variety of different foods

If you disagreed with any of these statements, you may not be eating for emotional reasons at all. Instead you might be low-key restricting or depriving. That's OK! Don't try and rush this process. Take a beat, go back to chapter 6 and chapter 7, and remind yourself of the steps you need to take to practise food neutrality and unconditional permission to eat.

SELF-CARE

OK, so what if you're eating enough throughout the day? The next step is to check in with your self-care.

Listen, I get it, 'self-care' has become this super-annoying, Instagram-aspirational, bubble baths and pedicures bullshit. And while those things are great, what we're talking about here is basic. Like pumpkin spice latte basic. According to researcher Catherine Cook-Cottone[3]:

> Self-care is defined as the daily process of being aware of and attending to one's basic physiological and emotional needs including the shaping of one's daily routine, relationships, and environment as needed to promote self-care. Mindful self-care addresses self-care and adds the component of mindful awareness. Mindful self-care is seen as the foundational work required for physical and emotional well-being. Self-care is associated with positive physical health, emotional well-being, and mental health. Steady and intentional practice of mindful self-care is seen as protective by preventing the onset of mental health symptoms, job/school burnout, and improving work and school productivity.

When our self-care is 'off' it can lead to disruptions in our ability to respond to our internal cues, our interoceptive awareness. Things that throw off our interoceptive awareness are called 'attunement disruptors'. Basically, they make it hard to perceive the other sensations in our body. You'll know this yourself; when you haven't had enough sleep, the next day you might feel extra-hungry or make food choices that don't make you feel your best. Likewise, for some people they don't feel hunger when they are stressed out and might end up undereating in response.

MINDFULNESS SELF-CARE CHECKLIST
—

Look at the following chart adapted from Catherine Cook-Cottone, and see how many statements you agree with.[4]

Positive behaviours	Physical care	Supportive relationships	Mindful, non-judgey awareness
	I drink enough water	I spend time with people who are good to me (support, encourage, believe in me)	I have a non-judgey awareness of my thoughts
	I eat regular meals and snacks	I feel supported by people in my life	I have non-judgey awareness of my feelings
	I move my body in a way that feels joyful	I have someone I can call when I'm upset	I have non-judgey awareness of my body

	I make time for rest	I feel confident that people in my life would respect my choice to say 'no'	I carefully select which of my thoughts and feelings I use to guide my actions
	I get adequate sleep to feel rested and restored	I schedule time to be with people who are special to me	
	If I am unwell I visit my doctor or take time off work		
Positive behaviours	**Self-compassion and purpose**	**Mindful relaxation**	**Supportive structure**
	I'm cool with my own challenges and difficulties	I do something intellectual (using my mind) to help me relax (e.g. read a book, journal, write, do puzzles)	I keep my work/school areas organized to support my work/school tasks
	I don't trash-talk myself ('I'm doing the best I can')	I do something interpersonal to relax (e.g. chill with friends, IRL or virtually)	I maintain a manageable schedule

I remind myself that shit hitting the fan is normal and part of being human	I do something creative to relax (e.g. draw, play music, sing, write creatively)	I maintain balance between the demands of others and what is important to me
I allow myself to feel my feels (e.g. I allow myself to cry)	I listen to relax (e.g. to music, a podcast, radio show)	My home environment is comfortable and welcoming
I experience meaning and/or purpose in my work/school life (e.g. it's for a cause/the greater good)	I seek out images to relax (e.g. art, film, nature, Netflix)	
I experience meaning and/or purpose in my private/personal life (e.g. for a cause)	I seek out smells to relax (lotion, nature, candles/ incense, smells of baking)	

Attunement disruptors	Physical care	Supportive relationships	Mindful, non-judgey awareness
	I don't drink enough water	My friends are emotional vampires (they suck my energy and leave me drained)	I am judgey of my thoughts
	I regularly skip meals and snacks	I don't feel supported by the people in my life	I am judgey of my feelings
	I use exercise as a form of punishment/ compensation or I avoid it altogether	I don't have anyone to call when I'm upset	I am judgey of my body
	I feel guilty for resting	People in my life don't respect my boundaries	I make decisions without checking in with my thoughts and feelings
	I don't get enough sleep to feel rested and restored	I don't prioritize spending time with people who are special to me	
	If I am unwell I keep pushing through	I withdraw from people when I'm stressed out	

Attunement disruptors	Self-compassion & purpose	Mindful relaxation	Supportive structure
	I'm very hard on myself and rarely give myself a break	I don't allow myself any downtime	My living space is disorganized and chaotic
	I talk shit about myself	I don't know how to relax	I overschedule and over-commit myself
	I have to do everything perfectly; if something goes wrong it means I have failed	I feel as though I always have to be productive	I let other people dictate my schedule
	I push my feelings down and try to ignore them	I have a tough time managing stress	
	My work/school doesn't fulfil me	I regularly want to zone out (using food/TV/ napping)*	I am a people pleaser and too often put my own needs second
	My personal life doesn't fulfil me		

* Sometimes you need to veg out after a stressful day, that's totally normal and can be part of self-care too, what I mean here is more a habitual zoning out so you don't have to deal with real life.

JOURNAL REFLECTIONS

Answer the following questions in your journal

→ Which areas of self-care are you pretty much nailing?

→ Which areas need some prioritizing?

→ Which areas need more continuity or consistency?

→ Have you noticed any pattern between self-care and body image or intuitive eating?

When you find yourself freaking out about food or body-image concerns, come back to this chart. I find that when my clients are having bad body-image days or food concerns, it's often a problem with self-care.

Let's take a closer look at some areas where your attunement to physical cues may be off.

SLEEP

Recent estimates suggest that over half (56%) of Americans and 31% of Western Europeans suffered from sleep problems over the previous year. Sleep problems refer to anything from poor sleep quality, taking a long time to fall asleep, waking up after falling asleep, or short total sleep length.[5,6] Why is this a big deal? Sleep problems are considered to be a risk factor for the following:

- impairments in motivation, emotion, and cognitive functioning
- increased risk for diabetes, cardiovascular disease and cancer
- increased death rate

And these associations are found even when the symptoms are below the threshold for clinical sleep disorders. The Sleep Council in the UK has identified that adults aged 18–65 need between seven and nine hours sleep a night. So what can we do? A lot of the research around sleep hygiene is very mixed and so it's hard to give any hard and fast advice, so if you're struggling with sleep, consider this to be a menu of suggestions to experiment with to find the options that suit you best.[7]

Be conscious of caffeine intake – a lot of the effects of caffeine on sleep have been blown out of proportion. What we know is this: caffeine consumption close to or at bedtime disrupts sleep, fact. Caffeine has a half-life of around three to seven hours; that means, theoretically if you have a coffee with 200mg of caffeine in it at 6pm, three hours later at 9pm, you would have a minimum of 100mg of caffeine floating around in your blood plasma. However, the half-life of caffeine is influenced by differences in sensitivity, metabolism, and accumulation. For instance, the half-life of caffeine has been shown to increase with age, in other words, it remains active for longer in older adults. The effects of caffeine on sleep show a dose-response relationship, meaning the more you have, the worse it will affect your sleep (when consumed close to bedtime). However, the impact of morning and afternoon caffeine use is less clear and studies suggest that the harmful effects of caffeine on sleep may be limited to caffeine-sensitive individuals.

Bottom line: if you suffer from sleep problems, it might be worth investigating your coffee habit. Limit your caffeine intake in the late afternoon and evening; it's not just coffee either, chocolate (especially dark chocolate), black teas, like English Breakfast and Earl Grey, and green tea, and cola all contain caffeine too.

Cool off – there's a dip in our core body temperature right before we fall asleep. Some studies have shown that you can recreate this effect by taking a hot bath or shower right before bed. As soon as you get out of the bath or shower, your body temperature begins to drop again, signalling to your brain that it's bedtime.

Keep the blues away – blue light that gets emitted from devices like smartphones, tablets, computers, and TVs can intercept the production of melatonin, the sleepy-time hormone, and lead to sleep issues. If you can, avoid electronic devices for a few hours before bed (bonus points for keeping them out of the bedroom altogether). But, because I'm a realist, also consider apps that reduce blue-light exposure by applying an amber filter to your screen. Night Shift mode is great for iPad/iPhone, and f.lux is a programme you can install on your computer. Some people suggest amber-tinted glasses for watching TV but I think that's too far, even for me.

Got the swirls? – If your brain suddenly pops into action the second your head hits the pillow, it might be worth keeping a pen and paper next to the bed. That way you can do a brain dump onto paper, which might help you fall asleep instead of percolating on all the shit you have to do tomorrow.

STRESS

—

The biological response to stress is to down-regulate our appetites. This makes complete sense from an evolutionary perspective; if you're getting hunted by Direwolves or whatever. When we perceive danger (real or, you know, just gluten), blood is directed away from out gastrointestinal tract and towards our extremities so we can run the fuck away. This is known as the fight-or-flight response. Next time you feel as though you are stressed, anxious, or nervous about something – where do you feel that in your body? For a lot of people they experience it as butterflies or belly flips in their tummy. This is the sensation of blood moving away from our guts towards our arms and legs. When we are running from the threat of predation, we generally don't want to be distracted by thinking about our next snack, so our hunger mechanisms are temporarily shut down. However, scientists believe that humans have adapted and learned to ignore this mechanism, which is why people tend to eat more when they are stressed. When we are calm and relaxed, the opposite of 'fight or flight', this state is referred to as 'rest and digest'. If you experience IBS symptoms (and have had anything else more sinister ruled out by your doc), this might be why. When we are incredibly stressed out, it can affect how we digest food. It can also do weird things to our appetite (making it either non-existent or in overdrive).

EMOTIONAL HUNGER VS PHYSICAL HUNGER

—

Physical hunger: By now you should hopefully understand the signs and symptoms of physical hunger, but just in case, here's a recap:

- builds gradually
- low energy
- is satisfied by eating something
- hangry/irritable (relieved by eating)
- time has passed since your last meal or snack

We also have **taste hunger**, which is the sensation that you want to eat something just because you like the taste of it; this is usually satisfied by having a couple of spoonfuls of Nutella or peanut butter, a few handfuls of chips, or a bowl of ice cream, a few slices of cheese, that sort of thing. If you feel as though you need a much larger amount of food to satisfy that craving, then you might be looking at emotional hunger.

Emotional hunger:

- No physical hunger cues
- Very specific cravings
- Food doesn't completely satisfy (or you feel as though you need more food)
- Occurs shortly after your last meal or snack
- Looking aimlessly in fridge/kitchen

So if you've identified that you're 100% not physically hungry, it's not taste hunger, and that no amount of food will fill you up, then it's likely that you're experiencing emotional hunger. The tricky part now is identifying what you're feeling. This can be tough if we're used to eating our emotions and trying to stuff them down instead of feeling them.

Ask yourself if the emotion you are feeling is related to your desire to eat. Here are some common emotional-eating triggers and the purpose food is serving in that particular situation.

Abandonment – food is always there, it's a reliable constant in your life

Anxious – using food to calm nerves

Bored – using food as excitement

Commiseration – 'I deserve this because I had a shitty day'

Frightened – food is comforting and soothing

Empty – food helps fill the void you feel

Inadequate – making and preparing food gives you a sense of purpose

Joy – food is celebration

Pride – 'I earned this treat because I got the promotion'

Loneliness – food reminds you of happier times with friends, or even acts as a friend

Sadness – comfort foods can make you feel happier in the short term – carbohydrates can give you a serotonin boost

Reward – 'I earned this'

Emotions word wheel

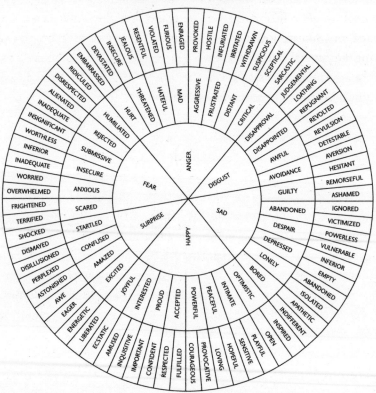

Used with permission from Geoffrey Roberts.

It can be difficult to recognize what emotions we're feeling, especially if we're used to using foods to numb ourselves out. There are two ways we can try and connect with how we're feeling; the first is using the wheel of emotions opposite[8] to help you put words and language to what you might be feeling. It might be easier to identify the emotions in the middle and then work outwards to narrow it down from there. The emotions around the outside are a bit more nuanced.

If you find it difficult to name your emotions, you can use the outline of the person below to identify where you feel emotions in your body. Each emotion has a physical sensation; similarly to body states like sleepiness or biological eating cues like hunger and fullness, emotions are a component of interoceptive awareness.[9,10] Next time you are experiencing an uncomfortable emotion and find that you want to use food to help, take a second to locate on the outline where you feel the emotion. It might be in more than one place. Allow yourself to get a little creative; you could give the emotion a colour, shape, or indicate intensity by making it bigger or smaller. You can print out several outlines to map your emotions over time and see if there are any patterns. You can also note if there was a precipitating event, such as a fight with your partner.

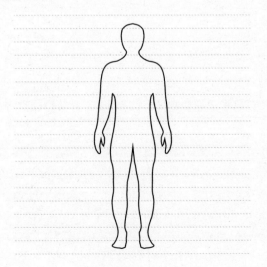

UNDERSTANDING FEELINGS IN THE BODY

Using the outline of the figure above (you can print a copy on the website and stick it in your journal), note where in your body you are experiencing an emotion; there may be multiple emotions present at the same time.

For each sensation think about the following dimensions or characteristics of the emotion:

Physical location: i.e. head, heart, chest, stomach, shoulders, neck, jaw, lungs, etc . . .

Shape: circle, triangle, amorphous blob, squiggle, spiral, zig-zag, octagon, etc . . .

Colour: this is entirely subjective, choose a colour that best reflects the emotion

Size: how intensely you are feeling the emotion might be reflected in the size

Once you have determined the form the emotion has taken, draw it on the figure above.

Now you can see a visual representation of your emotion, can you use a word from the word wheel to name it?

Are you able to identify the trigger for the emotion?

Can you identify what purpose food might be serving to soothe that emotion?

Does this give you any clues as to what you *need* and how to meet that need?

DON'T BE AFRAID TO FEEL YOUR FEELS

Feelings are there to be experienced, not solved. If you are used to pushing your feelings down with food, it can feel overwhelming to let them bubble up to the surface. But by acknowledging them, feeling them, you'll have less need to push them down. Learn to sit with your emotions and experience them, and learn that they may feel painful, but they can't actually hurt you, they are just trying to communicate something to you. Here are some ideas of how to feel your feels:

- journal it out
- call a friend
- allow yourself to cry
- practise meditation or deep breathing
- map them out on the diagram above
- listen to music that helps you express the emotion (yes, I was an emo kid back in the day)
- go for a run, dance, or any other kind of expressive movement

Once you've identified what it is you're feeling, it's time to take action and consider how to meet emotional needs without using food. I want to be clear here though: it is OK to go and cry into a piece of cake! I totally do that, but I also think about what else might be helpful for me. Ditto for my clients. Using food is appropriate if you think it will best meet your needs in the moment. Remember the ways in which it might have been helpful for you or served a purpose; the goal here is not to go cold turkey on emotional eating but to build up your emotional-coping toolkit so that food isn't your only option.

I like to think of physical hunger being filled by food going into your stomach. Physical hunger can only be met by regular meals and snacks. Once you've had enough to eat, it satisfies physical hunger. Emotional hunger can't be met with just food. In order to determine how to meet our emotional needs, we have to consider all the things that fill our hearts.

In your journal, draw an outline of a heart and a stomach. Write out the things that fill your stomach and satisfy *physical* hunger versus the things that fill your heart and satisfy your *emotional* hunger. There are some ideas listed below to help you get started.

Things that satisfy my physical hunger:

- regular meals and snacks
- eating a wide range and variety of foods
- being flexible in my appproach to eating
- no food rules!
- no restrictions!

Things that satisfy my emotional hunger:

Self care and getting needs met: naps, rest, enough sleep, setting boundaries and saying 'no', getting hugs and physical touch, having fulfilling work, being valued in my community, being me

Expressing emotions and being heard and understood: journalling it out, calling a friend, feelings your feels, crying, dance or expressive movement, going to therapy, creative writing, making art, talking and not keeping things bottled up, poetry

Relationships: having regular friend dates, spending time with special people in my life, checking in with family

Things that feed my soul: faith, spirituality, community, being in nature, meditation, yoga, travel, going to museums, learning new things, spending time with animals

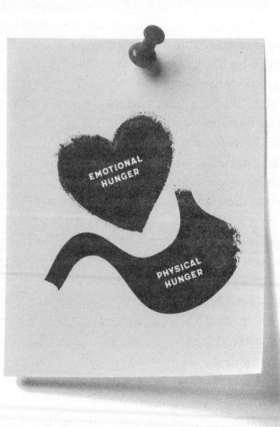

Things that nurture me: listening to music, buying myself flowers or small gifts, getting a manicure, putting together a killer outfit, reading books, listening to podcasts

Self-acceptance: Knowing I am worthy of love and respect, knowing I am more than my physical appearance, knowing I'm not here for other people's viewing pleasure, I'm feelin' myself

Obviously, the list above is not exhaustive and it also assumes that you're having your basic needs met (security, safety, housing), so feel free to add more things that make up who you are. I sometimes like to ask clients to think of what makes them them. Like if there was a recipe or a formula what would it be? Equal parts obsessing about food and exercise? Or would it be a long, complicated recipe with dozens of ingredients? If you prefer to conceptualize it this way, then in your journal, write down your formula. Then, like in chemistry class, check to see if it's balanced, or is there a discrepancy between what makes you you and what you're doing currently?

It may look a bit like this:

- 2 parts kitty snuggles
- 1 part alone time to 1 part friend dates to 1 part time with your partner
- a heaped cup of meditation and therapy
- a pinch of dancing around your room to Queen Bey
- a lot of crying and feeling feels with Drake
- a generous dose of career fulfilment
- a bunch of yoga
- a creative project

It can be whatever you want, but you get the gist, right? Try and notice if anything feels off kilter or where you need to redress the balance. Think back to the values versus goals activity we did in chapter 3 to help you here too. You can also make this into a pie chart of things that make up you. One small slice might be nourishment and movement, but what else makes you whole? Draw out a pie chart in your journal and label all the slices that represent your other interests, talents, and skills.

DEALING WITH THE *REAL* SHIT

—

When we work through our food issues and begin to take the power out of food, we might start to notice that it no longer satisfies us emotionally in a way it did before. When you can have a cookie whenever you like, somehow it just doesn't feel as special and there isn't the same urgency to use it to push down our feelings. We start to realize, it's not really about food. It was never about food. It was about the relationship we have with ourselves; our ability to accept ourselves and offer ourselves compassion. Or perhaps it was about control or perfectionism. Maybe it was about something difficult from your past. Obviously not all of these things are easy to identify or process. If this is the case, I really strongly recommend going to see your GP and asking for a referral to mental-health services. There you can learn tools and a language for helping you understand and process your stuff. There are also suggestions for books and resources that might be helpful in the resources section.

INTUITIVE
MOVEMENT

———

This section is about learning to enjoy movement; intuitive moment is more sustainable than intense exercise routines that you can't keep up with. It will help you differentiate between punitive exercise regimens and moving for fun and enjoyment and for the mental-health benefits, rather than for aesthetics. If you're anything like my clients, you fall into one of two camps: you either do a ton of exercise or none at all. Movement, like food, seems to be another expression of the all-or-nothing mentality and black-and-white approach that so many people get caught up in in relation to food. In this chapter, I want to help you explore all the shades of grey and find joyful, sustainable movement.

IS 'STRONG' JUST 'SKINNY' REBRANDED?

For so many people, workouts are about punishing themselves for eating, 'earning' food, 'shredding', burning calories, and 'sculpting'. They are generally coming from a place of hate for their bodies or at least a desire to want to change their body (sort of antithetical to body neutrality or acceptance, no?). Exercise is seen as a way to manipulate body shape and size and not as a tool for being in your body, caring for it, celebrating it, or making it feel good. The recent explosion of wellness and fitspo has been self-styled as empowerment and liberation for women, but there's still a distinct whiff of creating new body standards to fall short of. No one has written more eloquently on the topic than Anna Kessel, author of *Eat, Sweat, Play*. This is what she has to say on the subject of #fitspo:

> Because with the explosion of fitness for women has come a new preoccupation with our bodies: the quest for muscle – also known as 'fitspo'. It's all delivered under the banner of being good for you, buoyed by the now ubiquitous slogan: strong is the new skinny. But if strong really is the new skinny, then why do the #Fitspo and #SheSquats images show us flat stomachs? Is 'strong' just 'skinny'

rebranded? And why does it all come loaded with this weird front-facing pressure? By its very nature, fitspo wants you to show your muscle off: to tweet it, Instagram it, Facebook it, Snapchat it. Women, once again, are being put on display. What is so pernicious about this movement is that feeling bad about our bodies is being dressed up as female emancipation, wrapped up in the idea of self-control. If you want to look good, you just have to work harder. You'll feel pain now, but you will feel great tomorrow. Look at her! Do you think she just woke up like this? No! She sweated in the gym. (Remember, ladies, 'sweat is just fat crying'.) Rather than 'strong' paving the way to female liberation, it all just smacks of new pressures to look a certain way, to conform to a new body trend. Skinny was bad enough, but now we need a six pack and a tight booty that looks like it's been implanted with beachballs. Plenty of sports at least offer the possibility of inclusivity – but this exercise trend feels entirely elitist. It's expensive, it involves tight-fitting Lycra and revealing crop-top outfits: just how many women are we further alienating in an already alienated section of the population? Sport should move us further away from thoughts about how we are supposed to look, not chain us into a lifetime of butt-taming burpees.

For all the talk of empowerment, #fitspo looks suspiciously like self-objectification; it's no longer enough to go to a Barre or spin class, but there's an expectation to perform, to be on. Workouts apparently don't count unless you are wearing the latest leggings trend, hair braided in 'boxer braids' (and the cultural appropriation tied up in that), then documented on Instagram, recorded on your Fitbit, which also should be documented on Instagram. Performing fitness uses up so many valuable resources: financial, mental, time, and so on. But more importantly it distracts us from grounding down into our bodies and forces us to relentlessly critique our physical appearance; recall that one of the facets of self-objectification is an interference with our ability to tap into interoceptive awareness and distract us from the experience of being in our bodies. Instead of being in our bodies, and using them as a tool for feeling, they are a source of conflict and frustration; a problem that can only be solved momentarily until the next meal presents yet another challenge.

We all know exercise is great for us, that's a given, but having a focus on aesthetics can so easily tip the balance of healthy exercise to an unhealthy, compulsive, or obsessive need to exercise.

Among the general population, exercise addiction is thought to affect anywhere from 0.3–0.5% of the population. BUT, among people who identify as 'regular exercisers', that number shoots up to between 1.9% and 3.2% of the population. I know that doesn't sound like much but that means that regular exercisers are six times more likely to suffer from compulsive exercise than the general population. Different types of exercise might be more at risk too, with as many as 25% of runners and 30% of triathletes having an addiction to exercise.[1]

What are the risk factors for exercise addiction?
- addiction to other behaviours like shopping or internet addiction
- strongly identifying as an exerciser
- low self-esteem
- people who suffer from anxiety or impulsiveness
- extroverts
- men and women appear to have an equal risk

What are the symptoms of exercise addiction?
- overuse injuries (stress fracture and tendinopathy)
- anaemia
- amenorrhoea (loss of menstruation)
- indicators of overtraining: unexplained decrease in performance, persistent fatigue, inability to sleep
- inability to stop exercising even when injured or ill
- social withdrawal (i.e. not going out for dinner with friends because you would have to skip your workout)
- restlessness, anxiety, sadness, or irritability when you can't exercise

WHAT ARE THE CONSEQUENCES OF EXERCISE ADDICTION?

Exercise addiction may put people at risk of eating disorders, osteoporosis, injuries such as stress fractures, cardiac fibrosis and irregular heartbeat, amenorrhoea (loss of menstruation), and even greater susceptibility to infection.

Just like disordered eating, what really sets exercise addiction apart from a healthy attitude towards a health-promoting behaviour is the emotional response to it. Does the thought of cutting back on the level of activity you do cause you a negative emotional response such as stress, anxiety, or guilt? If so, it might indicate that your relationship to movement has tipped the balance from being healthy to unhealthy. Do you flip out at the thought of skipping a workout? How about when you go on holiday – do you prioritize workouts over your sightseeing schedule? Or what if you have a little niggling injury or a cold – can you give yourself a few days for R and R? The following quiz can help you figure out if you're at risk of exercise addiction.

Are you addicted to exercise?

The Exercise Addiction Inventory is a screening tool used to help detect people who are at risk of exercise addiction.[2] It cannot diagnose exercise addiction, but it can help determine if it's worth getting further help or trying to pull back from the level of activity you engage in.

1 Exercise is the most important thing in my life
1. Strongly disagree 2. Disagree 3. Neither agree nor disagree
4. Agree 5. Strongly agree
2 Conflicts have arisen between me and my family and/or my partner about the amount of exercise I do
1. Strongly disagree 2. Disagree 3. Neither agree nor disagree
4. Agree 5. Strongly agree

---

3 I use exercise as a way of changing my mood

1. Strongly disagree 2. Disagree 3. Neither agree nor disagree
4. Agree 5. Strongly agree

4 Over time I have increased the amount of exercise I do in a day

1. Strongly disagree 2. Disagree 3. Neither agree nor disagree
4. Agree 5. Strongly agree

5 If I have to miss an exercise session I feel moody and irritable

1. Strongly disagree 2. Disagree 3. Neither agree nor disagree
4. Agree 5. Strongly agree

6 If I cut down the amount of exercise I do, and then start again, I always end up exercising as often as I did before

1. Strongly disagree 2. Disagree 3. Neither agree nor disagree
4. Agree 5. Strongly agree

If you scored <12, you probably have a healthy relationship with exercise.

If you scored between 13 and 23 it indicates that you are at higher risk and should work on developing a healthier relationship with exercise.

If you scored 24 or higher, it suggests you might have a problem with exercise addiction. The best course of action would be to go to see your GP and seek their advice.

If you suspect your relationship with exercise might be unhealthy then your doctor may refer you to cognitive behavioural therapy or dialectical behaviour therapy.

REPROGRAMMING THOUGHTS

If you get your exercise advice from Instagram, you'd be forgiven for thinking that you should be exercising 24/7, even on your rest day. ESPECIALLY ON YOUR REST DAY. After all, train insane or remain the same. Insert major eye roll here. We've talked about how, by and large, a lot of #fitspo is just diet culture repackaging #thinspo and self-objectification as empowerment. But when the conversation is still centred on bodies we're really only perpetuating an age-old problem; women, people, as objects. As Beauty Redefined have said: 'If your idea of empowerment is indistinguishable from the sexist objectification that has always been used to devalue and degrade women, it might not be all that revolutionary.' The point here being that fitness today has so little to do with how we feel, or our health, and so much more to do with our physical appearance and how we present ourselves to the world. Look at the cover of any women's 'health' magazine:

- 'Get Abs' – uhhh, pretty sure you already have those, bud.
- 'Score a hot core, ASAP' – remind me how self-objectification increases my self-worth and improves my health again?
- 'Torch fat for good' – yeah, no.
- 'The workout that built my body' – that's DNA, babe.

I love how fitness 'grammers are always talking about sculpting this or that body part, as though we were made of clay and can just be moulded whichever way we see fit. Problem is though, DNA.

Here's the funny part, some studies have found that exercising for aesthetic reasons (toning, shaping, and weight loss) is associated with *less* physical activity.[3,4] It seems as though the underlying motivation for movement and exercise may determine the level of activity women engage in as they get older, with women who cite having a sense of well-being and stress reduction as their goals more regularly participating in movement than those who have weight-loss goals.[5]

In the same way that diet culture has duped us into believing that worth = aesthetics, it's also convinced us that health = aesthetics. This hyper-focus on appearance and women's bodies fosters a culture where we derive our self-worth from how much we exercise, how intensely we work out, how hard we push ourselves, if we can achieve a thigh gap. This extreme idea of exercise is disordered.

There are a bunch of myths and misconceptions about exercise, what 'counts', how much is 'enough', and what the benefits are. Getting these things straight can help us reprogramme thoughts and behaviours that might have been twisted.

Go hard or go home

So many of my clients believe that to get the benefit of movement, they have to torture themselves. Nah. You don't have to go hard, beast mode, turbo, or become an ultra-runner to get the benefits of movement. If you've been stuck in diet mentality though and only using exercise to try and control your weight or for aesthetic reasons, it might be hard to untangle that. I remember a client who came back from being away at a wedding one weekend saying she felt the urge to move her body, so she did a HIIT workout in her bedroom. When I asked her why she decided to do that instead of going for a walk or doing some stretching, it hadn't even occurred to her that gentle movement was an option. She'd had an all-or-nothing approach to food too, and it was trickling into her attitude to movement. We experimented with toning down the activity until we found a place that was sustainable and realistic for her.

If you don't sweat, it doesn't count

Not only do you not need to 'go hard', but you don't even need to break a sweat for it to count. Say whaaaat? You heard me. According to Public Health England, moderate-intensity activity is where your heart rate rises, you breathe a little faster, and feel warmer, but you can still carry on a conversation. That's it. No mention of vomiting, passing out, dying, or even breaking a sweat. Getting sweaty and getting your heart pounding can be fun, exhilarating, and exciting, but it's not a prerequisite to get the benefits of moving. So, if you've been inclined to think it only counts if you're close to becoming a heap on the floor, try experimenting with gentler movement like walking, yoga, or Pilates, or even just dancing round your room or playing with the kids.[6]

Earn it

Pay attention here, this part is important, OK? You *never, ever* have to 'earn' the right to eat. You never have to use exercise as penance or punishment for eating. Eating is a fundamental need; you have earned the right to eat by being a living, breathing, sentient being. That's it. That's the only prerequisite for eating. Are you alive? Congratulations, you have 'earned' the right to eat! You've also earned the right to love, respect, safety, compassion, and freedom to be who you are. Just sayin'.

No excuses

Ugh. UGH. UGHHH. Where to start? This little quip is potentially so harmful. There are literally thousands of legitimate reasons why you might want to skip a workout, I don't need to list them all here. But suffice to say, if you're not feeling it, you're not feeling it. Maybe you are coming down with something and you think that an extra hour in bed might be more beneficial for you than an hour at the gym. Don't pay attention to other people's expectations of what will go on in your body. Extra sleep instead of going to the gym? Who's to say which one is better for you? Only you get to make that call. There can be a lot of pressure and expectations from other people to just push through because it will make you feel better. Yes, sometimes exercise can make us feel better, but sometimes it can make us worse. This is your call, you get to decide. You don't need an excuse; if you can't be bothered or just don't want to, that's OK too.

EXERCISE AND DIET MENTALITY

If you've only ever started a new exercise routine at the same time as starting a new diet or lifestyle programme, then you might only be interested in exercise as a tool for weight loss, meaning that exercise and movement is all or nothing for you. This usually means that you go balls-deep into a new routine, fully leaning in, and usually burning yourself out pretty quickly with an unrealistic and unsustainable level of activity. This inevitably leads to exhaustion, injury, or getting sick, which triggers the fuck-it effect. You may only miss one or two sessions, but it can be enough to make you feel as though there's no point and exercise goes out the window.

If you've also been combining hardcore exercise with a diet, *especially* a low-carb diet, you might feel super-low on energy, turning exercise from joyful movement into a living hell.

Because you're not eating enough to cover the extra energy you're using, you burn out really quickly. You ditch your exercise routine and it's no different from an all-or-nothing diet mentality. Carbs are muscles' preferred energy source during exercise; if you don't have adequate carbs you'll start burning protein as well as fat. This leads to a loss of strength, loss of endurance and performance, and increased risk of infection and injury.

Even elite athletes who restrict their carb intake don't perform as well compared to when they do eat carbs![7,8,9]

EXERCISE ≠ WEIGHT LOSS
—

For many of us, it's really difficult to untangle exercising for pleasure, joy, fun and play, from punitive exercise that's just about burning calories. It can take time, and I can pretty much guarantee you'll still have those sneaky diet-mentality thoughts at first, but with time and a little bit of brain-rewiring, that noise will get quieter and quieter, making it easier to tune in to how you want to work it out. To help reframe the motivation to move, below is a list of all of the benefits of moving your body that have been shown to improve health outcomes, *independently* of weight loss. In fact, research consistently shows that exercise, unless fairly extreme (i.e. disordered) doesn't actually result in significant weight loss for the majority of people.[10] If you have to force your body into extremes of exercise and engage in disordered eating behaviours to maintain your weight, then it's not the weight your body was intended to be at. It's just not what our genetics have in store for us. Lucky for us, the benefits of exercise aren't contingent on weight loss.

BENEFITS OF EXERCISE

—

- reduced inflammation
- reduced blood pressure
- improves 'good' cholesterol, reduces 'bad' cholesterol, and decreases triglycerides
- improves skeletal muscle function
- lowers mortality risk (death rate)
- may help improve IBS symptoms
- reduces the risk of:
  - dementia by 30%
  - hip fractures by 68%
  - depression by up to 30%
  - breast cancer by 20%
  - cardiovascular disease by 35%
  - type-2 diabetes by 40%
  - colon cancer by 30%[11,12,13,14]

In fact, researchers believe that high cardiorespiratory fitness (i.e. healthy heart and lungs) can offset the risk of being at a higher weight.[15] As little as 2.5 hours of physical activity a week is enough to help those at a BMI above 40 to move from 'low' fitness to 'high' fitness category and reduce the risk of heart disease.[16] Compared to all the fear-mongering headlines and photographs of headless fatties in the news, imagine how empowering a public-health campaign built around moving your body for fun, pleasure, and excitement could be?

The last time I 'worked out' was PE at school!

Perhaps you're at the opposite end of the movement spectrum and you just can't get behind movement. Maybe the last time you did anything besides run for a bus was that super-traumatizing PE class where you slid down the hill in cross-country, violently winding yourself, catching your Adidas poppers on the way down, and revealing your pasty white fat legs to a bunch of fourteen-year-old meatheads in your class. Can't just be me.

I spoke to Anna Kessel to get some advice about how to rekindle the joy of movement if you hated PE at school.

'First of all, you're not alone. The majority of women and girls say they hated PE at school. And looking at the evidence – from the way women are taught to feel bad about their bodies, to the awful gym knickers that used to be PE kit, and the sexist approach of so many old-school teachers – it's little wonder that so many women and girls have a dysfunctional relationship to sport and moving our bodies.

'To move beyond the traumatic memories into a more positive space the first step is to give yourself permission to hate everything about sport and exercise. That way you can truly exorcize the ghosts. You are under no obligation to do anything at all, you certainly don't have to move to lose weight, or sculpt your bum or any of that crap. (Can I say crap? It's just that it really is crap.)

'Once you have established that moving your body is your own free choice, then you can begin to explore that a little more. Is there anything you like about moving your body? Do you like being outside in nature and having a walk? Or do you prefer to be indoors? Do you want music to accompany you? Do you like moving with friends, or would you rather have this as solitary time? Explore all these avenues and see where they take you. Maybe you love the feeling of being outside and discover that doing anything outdoors makes you feel good. Or maybe you love being in a team, or maybe it's all about the music and so dancing or zumba or soul cycle or basketball is what floats your boat. Try to observe what makes you feel good, both mentally and physically. It's important that you take both into account. Make sure that the environment you're in is right for you – that the teacher or coach or other participants make you feel good, and remember that you are under no requirement to keep the exercise or sport up. Keeping active is a lifelong journey, and it is not a linear thing. Activities will float in and out of our lives, what may be appealing at one time may fade at another, or life circumstances – such as having kids, starting a new job, moving house, falling ill – can also affect how active we are or which activities we are drawn to. So ignore all the "No Excuses" bullshit, and plot your own path.

'For me personally, moving my body brings each and every part of it alive. It is a helpful reminder that I am a person in my own right. That's essential to my well-being; without it my shoulders slump in front of my laptop and phone most days, my spine curves to one side as I constantly balance one of my children on my hip or carry shopping, and it can be easy to lose myself in the commitments of work, motherhood, and just keeping afloat. Movement grounds me – whether that's walking to the childminder and back, or a yoga session on a Sunday morning, running down the street laughing with my daughter as we try not to be late for school (again), a family walk in the park, or an adventure on the water with my friends. It's headspace, it's balance, it's thanking each and every part of me for holding me all together and functioning. The motions that our bodies perform every single day are incredible. In a world that obsesses over thigh gaps and pert buttocks we all too easily forget that.

'The mental and physical health benefits are huge. For this do not read "weight loss", and also no one should tell you that going for a run will solve your depression – let's not be simplistic. But the evidence out there around many female health problems – menstruation, fertility, osteoporosis, post-natal depression, menopause, libido – does suggest that with the right support being more physically active will bring benefits as part of a holistic approach to your health. There are also certain conditions – such as post-natal separation of the abdominals, affecting up to a third of women – that are directly remedied through gentle core work.

'Research also tells us that being sporty boosts your career chances – the likes of Hillary Clinton, Christine Lagarde, Emma Watson, Indra Nooyi, and Beyoncé all took part in sport in their formative years. An Ernst & Young study found that 94% of women in executive business roles played sport. Sport gave them confidence, the ability to work in a team, be disciplined, set goals, and – crucially – process criticism without being weighed down by it. Enjoy!'

CULTIVATING INTUITIVE MOVEMENT

Intuitive movement refers to your body's innate ability to communicate how, when, how much, and how often to move. It moves us away from looking at exercising and working out as a means to control our body and towards a way of grounding down into and being in our body.

1 **Reject expectations.** Only you know the type, intensity, frequency, and duration of exercise that's appropriate and feels good for your body. Not Instagram fitness models, not some fitness plan or activity tracker, not your mates or your partner.

2 **Pay attention to how, when, and for how long your body wants to move, rather than gadgets**. Activity trackers are distracting and inaccurate. They reduce movement down to calorie burning, and take you away from the experience of being in your body. Forget about the numbers.

3 **Reframe exercise as something that is enjoyable, that isn't punishing, and that's intuitive and feels good in your body.** Exercise that's tied to aesthetics will keep you tethered to the diet mentality and self-objectification, leading to unrealistic and unsustainable levels of activity.

FOCUS ON HOW IT FEELS

—

When you're considering the type of movement you want to do, consider how it *feels* in your body. For instance, do you:

- feel less stressed or anxious?
- have more energy?
- feel more alert?
- have better concentration?
- sleep better?
- improve your mood?
- feel better in your body?
- have fewer aches and pains?
- get your heart pounding (in a good way!)?
- feel stronger?
- improve flexibility?
- have more stamina?
- have fun?
- feel joy?

If you're used to defining the 'success' of your workout by numbers, it can be difficult to tune into intuitive movement, so sometimes it's helpful to work *backwards*. The most obvious example of this is when you *haven't* been able to move much. Maybe you do a lot of sitting for your job. You might get some tension through your shoulders and neck, and there's no better feeling than stretching it out or going for a gentle walk. Notice when you're in periods of relative inactivity and use that as your baseline; then compare that to how you feel when you do incorporate some movement into your day. You'll probably notice that it feels pretty good, so long as you're eating *enough* and not overdoing it and giving yourself plenty of rest.

Speaking of which, I've heard a lot of chat about 'active rest' from influencers and #fitspo folks; essentially what this means is that on days you aren't pushing past your 'threshold' you should still be pretty active (long brisk walks, yoga, etc). Just hold the phone a second. That sounds an awful lot like **1** a rule and **2** exercise addiction. So I want to make it abundantly clear that this type of mentality around rest is disordered. Rest isn't just important, it's essential. It allows your body to repair, it prevents overuse injury, amenorrhoea, infection, and everything else associated with overdoing it. How much rest is totally your call, but just know that rest is normal and healthy.

HOW DO WE KNOW IT'S TIME FOR A REST?

I spoke to personal trainer Hollie Grant (of Pilates PT) about how to know when it's time for a break.

- Feeling exhausted and totally wiped out (and exercise leaves you more drained as opposed to energized)
- It takes a long time for aches to go away between workouts (4–5 days as opposed to 2–3)
- Injuries that are taking a long time to heal
- If you are particularly stressed out, high-intensity activity may exacerbate it (consider a rest or some gentle activity)
- You get a lot of infections; too much activity weakens the immune system

Rest is important to allow us to assimilate the benefits of the activity we've done; changes and increases to our fitness levels occur *after* the exercise. It can also take up to forty-eight hours to restore glycogen levels in between tough workouts (like HIIT, for example). Glycogen is the body's storage form of carbohydrate in the form of small units of glucose joined together in long chains in the muscles and liver. Glycogen gets depleted through exercise (the more intense, the more rapidly it will get used up) and needs to be replenished by eating, you guessed it, carbs! Rest days are not 'an excuse' or laziness; they're important and healthy, and you categorically shouldn't feel bad about having a duvet day. Even if you're not doing formal exercise at a class, you're probably still doing some form of movement, whether that's cleaning the house, walking to the shops, or playing with kids; remember that still counts.

What's your motivation for moving?

Meredith Noble @madeonagenerousplan

In our diet-obsessed culture, we're taught that we need to exercise to make our bodies aesthetically appealing to others. We learn to choose the exercises we do based on how many calories they'll burn and how much muscle they'll help us build. We learn to feel guilty when we miss a workout, and often weaponize that guilt to force ourselves to keep going back to the gym.

The problem, as a lot of gym-goers know, is that motivating ourselves to move our bodies using guilt is not terribly sustainable long term. This is why most new year's resolutions to go to the gym don't lead to new, sustained movement practices!

Of course, we blame ourselves when this happens. But really, using guilt as a tool for motivation is usually doomed to fail in the long run.

Know what is a sustainable tool for motivation? Pleasure.

Yep, as humans, we're hard-wired to seek out things that bring us pleasure. And that's where the concept of intuitive movement (also known as 'joyful movement') comes in. It flips our typical diet-culture-informed relationship with movement on its head and says: we are much more likely to move our bodies regularly if we tap into what feels good.

Movement truly can feel awesome, when it's the right amount at the right time, but we're so busy chasing the ideal body that sometimes we don't slow down and let ourselves enjoy what it feels like to move our bodies. We also often force ourselves to move beyond what feels energizing and supportive to the point of exhaustion and/or pain. The truth is though, our bodies don't need to be pushed to extremes to benefit mightily from movement.

You can start practising intuitive movement by taking time to listen to your body on a daily basis. Just check in – how is your body feeling? Does it feel like it wants to stretch? Or burn off some energy? Or get its blood pumping to overcome a bit of fatigue? Ask yourself what type and amount of movement would feel good.

See if you can honour your body's requests without holding up one type of movement as 'better' than another. Although our society holds intense workouts in high regard, the truth is that movement doesn't have to be 'hardcore' to feel good or to benefit your body. Having an impromptu dance party in your living room is just as valid a choice as would be a Crossfit workout.

As you do a particular form of movement, see if you can practise staying connected to your body and listening to its response. Learning to have active conversations with your body is the best way to stay connected to pleasure and to your own intuition. Your body will react differently at different times, and the only way to truly honour its needs is to continue listening.

People often get stuck with intuitive movement when it comes to exercises that are used to support or prevent certain health conditions (e.g. physiotherapy). These exercises may feel non-negotiable, but one option is to try to bring more pleasure into them to make them more fun. Perhaps you blast your favourite music while you do them or call a friend to chat. Bottom line, any way you can bring more enjoyment into your movement practice, the more sustainable it will be.

DON'T HAVE TIME TO INCORPORATE MOVEMENT?

——

Are you looking for ways to incorporate movement but find you're struggling to fit it into an otherwise busy schedule? It might be a sign that you are chronically overscheduled. If so, does that mean you are struggling to look after yourself the way you would like to? How can you redress the balance? I've noticed a pattern that when clients aren't feeling good about their bodies and having bad body-image days/ weeks, it's usually a symptom that their lives are so full that they don't have time even for basic self-care. If this is you, think about ways you can prioritize things so that you get all your needs met. How can you prioritize movement? How can you get more sleep (if you need it!)? How can you find more time for yourself?

You might also consider how to make movement less of a burden and more part of your normal routine or day:

● Schedule it in like you would a meeting, it's not a commitment to go to the class or whatever, but at least you have the option

● Walking meeting – ask your colleague(s) if you can walk and talk. This is easiest if you're just discussing ideas and don't need a computer

● Take the stairs instead of the lift

● Find a personal trainer or instructor who can come to you at home – or ask your colleagues if they'd be interested in starting a lunchtime yoga/Pilates class at the office. You can find an instructor who will come to you as long as you have a minimum number of people committed per week.

● Have an active commute – walking or cycling to work (or you could be that person with a scooter)

● And remember, things you might not have considered as activity can all count: walking the dog, gardening, cleaning and hoovering, carrying heavy shopping home

THINGS TO CONSIDER WHEN BUILDING A MORE INTUITIVE RELATIONSHIP WITH MOVEMENT

———

I'm hoping by now that you're beginning to untangle yourself from diet culture, and the diet-mentality thoughts are fewer and further between. However, there are a few things related to exercise that are worth considering as you think about building a more intuitive relationship with your body and exercise.

Activity trackers: at the beginning of the book I pretty unequivocally told you to ditch any calorie or activity trackers. And while at this stage in the process, there's perhaps a little more room for nuance, I still, on the whole, am not a fan. Speaking from my own experience, and experience with clients, the temptation to track steps or calories burned can become not just a little obsessive, but it can switch on that disordered part of the brain, even for a fleeting second, especially on bad body-image days. So what I will say is, if you think there's even an outside chance of that being you, keep it in the box or the sock drawer or wherever. However, I realize that for people who are interested in endurance sports, they're kind of a necessary evil and you may need them for keeping pace during training. I don't think there's anything inherently wrong with that, but my advice is to turn off the calorie-tracking component where possible, and to limit wearing it when not exercising. Otherwise, trace your route on a map ahead of time, and use a good old-fashioned stopwatch or the function in your phone. There are also wearables that remind you to get up and have a stretch every hour or so if you're sitting at your desk, which isn't a bad idea. If you can isolate that function and turn off calorie or step options, then that probably won't trigger diet mentality. Otherwise, why not try setting a timer on your phone or a reminder in your Google calendar to have periodic stretches or take a little five-minute walk? Just remember that these trackers are rarely accurate and are rarely calibrated to the type of exercise you're doing; there will always be a temptation to reduce calorie intake to make up for deficit in activity – or to over exercise.

Gym culture looks suspiciously like diet culture: when thinking about developing a more intuitive relationship with movement, consider the environment you're working out in. Gyms can be a cesspool of diet-culture bullshit – messages to push yourself to the limit, questionable nutrition advice, people working out in short shorts, and the list goes on. I remember having a conversation once with a client who told me that when she went to the gym she'd compare herself with other people there who were working harder and longer than she was, and then got herself into a tailspin about being 'too fat' and needing to 'work out more'. She was already pretty active, so I had to give her a talking-to. We don't know shit about what's going on with other people we see in the gym. Are they professional athletes? Do they have an eating disorder or body dysmorphia? Are they training for a competition? Or do they have a really unhealthy relationship with food and their body? If you find yourself comparing yourself with other people at the gym, or feeling less than great about yourself when you go in or leave, then why not try taking a step back from the gym for a while (most places will let you put your membership on hold for a bit until you figure out what you want to do). A community centre or church hall, park, or yoga mat thrown down on your living-room floor are all as valid places to move as gyms, and are diet-culture-free spaces.

MOVEMENT IN A BIGGER BODY

There's an enormous fat-phobic double standard in society, where fat people are 'expected' to work out (because fat people should want to lose weight, duh), yet are often excluded from the conversation around activity and not given access to the same tools and resources as thin people. For example, not having sports bras or other active wear available in your size, or spaces that aren't adapted for bigger bodies. Gyms can be a hostile environment for anyone, but especially if you're at the higher end of the weight spectrum and have concerns about being judged or shamed while you're trying get your sweat on.

Ditto if you want to go for a swim but are afraid of being semi-undressed in public and people scrutinizing your body. Even for the most motivated of people this can create a barrier to actually engaging in movement. This is always a tricky thing to navigate with my fat clients and it usually involves a lot of experimenting and figuring out what works for them and their lifestyle. Some clients have zero fucks to give about doing their thing in a fat body, for others it's a source of anxiety, mostly because they're concerned about what other people think. If you fall into the latter group, it might be helpful to keep doing some work around internalized fat phobia (chapter 5). Here are some other tips that fat clients have found helpful; take what resonates with you, and leave the rest.

- **Find fat-positive classes:** They may be less common but more and more fat-friendly classes are popping up all over the place, especially thanks to the rise of the body-positive movement. 'Body positive', 'plus size', and 'curves', are all great search terms to help you find what you're looking for.
- **Build community:** Finding fat friends to make movement social, supportive, and fun can be key in building a sustainable practice.
- **Start your own group:** No fat-positive classes? No community? No problem! Become a goddamn hero in your community and start your own fat-positive group: use the power of social media to advertise or kick it old school and hand out flyers and stick up posters in the community centre. Chances are, you're not the only person in a bigger body who wants a fat-positive group or network to hang out and have fun with. It doesn't have to be a fat-only group (although that's cool too), so long as people of all shapes and sizes are respectful, friendly, and down for fun. You could rent a community hall and do a dance or yoga class, or just start a walking group.
- **Find a fat-positive PT:** Find a personal trainer who isn't going to push their bullshit weight-loss agenda on you. Look out for trainers who emphasize the physical and mental-health benefits of activity and movement, and who don't show shaming

before/after pictures on their site. The Health at Every Size® community has a register of different fat-positive professionals (including nutrition professionals/doctors and trainers). Go to: https://haescommunity.com/search/ – if you can't find someone in your area then don't be afraid to call around a few different people until you find someone you click with. You can explain that you are interested in increasing fitness/stamina/flexibility or just want to feel stronger in your body and you don't want to be weighed or have your body measurements taken (you can explain that you find this triggering for you). Most PTs will give you a free taster session to see if you vibe with them. And if you are a fat-positive PT yourself, make sure you add yourself to the list so people can find you.

● **YouTube:** There are so many great classes and trainers available for free online. These are great if you're short on time, don't want to fork out for a gym membership, or you feel uncomfortable getting your move on in public. Search 'plus size fitness'. I've noticed there are some videos trying to push weight loss so you might want to avoid these (they usually mention it in the title or description) – or if you feel like it won't trigger diet mentality and you want to give the video a go, then hit it. There are also videos for any fitness level; if you're a super-beginner, then you can start simple with chair yoga or walking workouts that are relatively gentle, and then kick up the intensity as and when you're ready.

● **Find active wear that works for you:** It's harder to come across cool, plus-size active wear, but it does exist. The fact that you might have to get it online isn't ideal, but it's encouraging to see that brands are beginning to take plus-size active wear more seriously and offering affordable options that perform the way you need them to. Nike have recently launched a cool range that goes up to a UK size 32. Having the right gear and feeling good in well-fitting, high-performing active wear can help give you a confidence boost for moving more in ways that feel good to you. Be comfortable, and wear supportive shoes.

- **Follow plus-size fitness accounts:** Get advice, ideas, tips, and motivation from other people in larger bodies (as opposed to #fitspo that might leave you feeling less than cute about yourself). Some of my favourites are listed in the resources section.

A NOTE ON BEING UNCOMFORTABLE IN YOUR BODY

Clients often tell me that they just want to lose weight because they don't feel good in their bodies and want to feel more comfortable. They may have joint pains or it might ache more after a workout than it used to. While a regular exercise routine might cause some weight loss, most studies show that exercise doesn't result in weight loss *per se*. However, regularly moving your body is likely to help increase fitness, stamina, strength, and flexibility, as well as make you feel more at home in your body, no matter what your size. If you are an exercise newbie or have taken a break from movement, don't go too hard too fast. This can cause injuries or excessive muscle soreness, to the point where you feel like you need to diet again or in a way that triggers diet mentality. It's helpful to put things into perspective. As we get older, our joints get achier. If we have been in a period of relative inactivity, we lose fitness and need to build it back up again. This doesn't just happen to people in bigger bodies, it happens to everyone, independent of weight, but it's all too easy to blame it on our bodies, especially on our weight. If you've put on weight, or feel like your body is holding you back from moving the way you want to, consider the following.

- Could I benefit from medication to help with joint or muscle pain? Talk to your doctor about painkillers or anti-inflammatories while you build your fitness level up. We have a culture of pill shaming in the UK, and the lifestyle medicine set are always pushing diet and exercise over medicine. And while we have to be mindful of over-prescribing, it might just be that medicine can reduce your pain to a point where it makes it easier and more enjoyable to engage in exercise to reach a stage where you can build up strength and stamina and then re-evaluate your meds.
- Could I get a referral to physiotherapy to work on joint mobility or injury rehabilitation?
- Was I going too hard and over exercising? Can I take a step back and gradually build up strength and stamina? I've definitely had more than one client tell me that they need to lose weight because it hurts when they exercise, when in reality, when we've looked at it more objectively, they've gone from 0 to 100 way too quick, pushing their body too hard and causing aches and pains. It's easy to blame this on your weight but, remember, this would also happen to a thin person who had low fitness who suddenly thought they were an Olympian. Instead, try taking a step back and build your strength and fitness up incrementally.
- Can I get help from a personal trainer who can work with me at my current fitness level? There are loads of trainers who offer affordable programmes online that are designed to move with you, based on your fitness level.
- Remember that weight loss isn't a time machine and thin people get aches and pains in their joints too.

CHALLENGE
Try something new or different

Over the next few weeks I want you to challenge yourself to try something new or different that you've always been intrigued about but never had the cajones to do. Pick something fun and joyful that will leave you invigorated and with a huge smile on your face. Not something that pushes you past your limit. Here are some ideas:

- find a fun new YouTube channel – try dance, Barre, walking workouts, yoga, etc
- try a new team sport
- adult ballet
- Beyoncé (or whoever) themed dance class
- restorative yoga
- trampoline fit class (or get your own little rebounder for the house, they are so fun!)
- take your bike out for a spin and feel the breeze in your hair

Whatever you pick, think joyful, intuitive movement – it's not about punishment. Maybe it's some 'you time' or maybe it's a social activity; no matter what, make it fun!

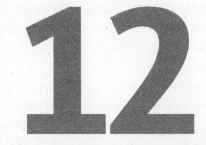

GENTLE NUTRITION

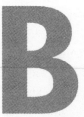efore we get started, I just want to make one thing clear. If you feel you might still be caught in the diet mentality or have any lingering thoughts about using IE for weight loss, stop right there. Go back and read through the areas you're still struggling with (use the quiz in the introduction to help you). If you think there's a risk of you turning nutritional concepts into a rule, then it might be best to back off for a bit, and return to this when you feel like you can be more relaxed. Often people seek out nutrition information to try and justify disordered eating patterns, so ask yourself, are you seeking out this information based on fear and restriction? Or is it coming from a place of curiosity and non-judgement? If it's the former then you may want to back off for a while.

How do you know if you're ready for a little gentle nutrition action? Well, you're probably ready for it when you're not that concerned about it, truthfully. From experience, if you're Captain Keen and desperately seeking out nutrition information, then it might be too soon. Here's a simple way to test it: think of a meal you ate recently, one you really enjoyed, maybe at a restaurant or something. Now list out what you ate in your journal. Next to the description I want you to write down all the words you associate with that meal. It might be positive words like tasty, delicious, satisfying; it might be more neutral, words like balanced, or something about the company you were with. Lastly you may have some negative words or judgements: high in carbs, used a lot of oils. Look at the balance of positive, neutral, or negative statements. How many of them pertain to nutrition? Even if they are positive statements (really high in veg!) about nutrition (as opposed to taste or satisfaction), then you might still be thinking of food in terms of good/bad. I'd hold off from moving forward until you've gone back to chapter 6 and worked on food neutrality some more.

If you feel like you're in a good place with food, your eating behaviours have stabilized (i.e. not bingeing, not restricting), then that's a sign you're probably in a good place and ready to take on nutrition information without internalizing it as a rule.

HOW FOOD MAKES YOU FEEL

If you've spent a long time stuck in your head when it comes to food and nutrition, it can be hard to approach food from a more relational perspective. In other words, instead of asking how much, you should have been asking what do I feel like having? How does food *make you feel?* What is your body telling you it wants to eat? Connecting with your body can seem like it's pretty tough, BUT you're probably more in touch than you think you are. For instance, I have one client who insisted that she couldn't tune in to what her body wanted. And session after session she demonstrated that she knew exactly what her body was after. The problem wasn't that her body didn't have the wisdom to figure this shit out; she just didn't have the confidence to let her body lead the way. Instead she was way too in her head. She'd tell me things like she felt she was coming down with a cold and was craving a hot, spicy curry. The chances are, you already know more than you think you know.

Let's do an experiment. Look at the diagram overleaf.

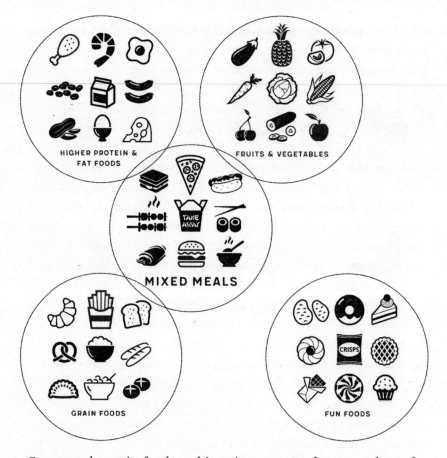

Cover up the grain foods and imagine your meals were only made up of fruits/veg or protein – like a chicken salad. Chances are it would feel like something was missing. It wouldn't be particularly satisfying or filling, you'd be low on energy and hungry again soon after. Now cover up the higher protein/fat group and imagine a meal with just grains and veg – like a salad sandwich. Again not super-satisfying or tasty. Now think about a chicken sandwich without salad. You probably wouldn't feel particularly energized or have a sense of well-being. Having a balanced meal just feels better in our bodies. Now cover up the main food groups, so you're left with the desserts. How does it feel to only eat these foods? Now cover up the desserts; how does it feel to *never* have those foods? Neither option feels great! Let's try a few more examples.

I want you to imagine a meal made up of foods from each of the three main groups. It could be a Thai green coconut chicken curry with aubergine and broccoli and rice:

vegetables   higher-protein/fat foods   grain

Or how about a snack like peanut butter and banana on toast?

 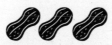

fruit   higher-protein/fat foods   grain

Or pick your own selection of foods based on something you like to eat. You can even write them out in a note on your phone using emojis.

FRUIT/VEGETABLE + HIGHER-PROTEIN/FAT FOOD + GRAIN

Now, use your hand or a piece of paper to cover the vegetable/fruit component. How does that change the way the meal makes you feel when you eat it? How do you feel after the meal compared to when the fruit/vegetable was there?

- more/less energized
- more/less bloated
- more/less satisfied
- more/less sustained
- more/less stamina
- more/less well
- more/less focused and able to concentrate
- more/less happy

Now, use your hand or a piece of paper to cover the higher-protein/fat component. How does that change the way the meal makes you feel when you eat it? How do you feel after the meal compared to when the higher-protein/fat food was there?

- more/less energized
- more/less bloated
- more/less satisfied
- more/less sustained
- more/less stamina
- more/less well
- more/less focused and able to concentrate
- more/less happy

Lastly, use your hand or a piece of paper to cover the grain. How does that change the way the meal makes you feel when you eat it? How do you feel after the meal compared to when the grain was there?

- more/less energized
- more/less bloated
- more/less satisfied
- more/less sustained
- more/less stamina
- more/less well
- more/less focused and able to concentrate
- more/less happy

You probably don't have to imagine too hard what the various permutations feel like. If you've ever been on the Paleo/low-carb diet then you'll know that by skipping the grains (bread, rice, pasta) you feel like shit or you're starving a few hours later. If you've ever tried a super-low-fat, low-calorie diet where you basically have to subsist on raw vegetables and rice cakes, you'll know how you can't focus, can't concentrate and are liable to snap at any second.

But what about when you put all three together? That's the sweet spot, right? You have energy, you feel satisfied, you feel content without being uncomfortable. You feel comfortably full for an appropriate amount of time before the gentle creep of hunger again. And the most important part is, in between meals and snacks you're not really thinking about food all that much. It doesn't demand all of your attention; you don't spend all of your time worrying about it.

This is the essence of gentle nutrition.

Of course, there's a bit more nuance to it than that. But ultimately, by paying attention to how different combinations of foods feel, you can't go too far wrong. If you think back to our thought experiment from chapter 8 you'll remember that if you eat ice cream day in, day out, after a while, you're not going to feel so hot. Likewise, if you have strict or rigid rules about takeaways and or only eat them accompanied by guilt and self-judgement, that doesn't feel good either. Given the freedom from food rules and restrictions, from food guilt and judgement, most people naturally gravitate towards a healthy balance of foods without over-thinking it. That's because it feels good to eat well most of the time. Remember though, this isn't a magic formula, it's not a hard and fast rule. Not every meal will be perfectly balanced, and it doesn't have to be.

THERE'S NO SUCH THING AS A PERFECT DIET

—

Diet culture, with its endless stream of food rules, good and bad foods, restrictions, exclusions, and fear-mongering can make it seem that if you just get the formula right, you can live for eternity without gaining weight or getting so much as a cold. But the reality is nutrition isn't a perfect science. Sure, we've figured out generally what you need to be healthy and well, but it's not a guarantee of immortality. You can't make yourself disease-proof, and worrying about the minutiae of detail of your diet and freaking out about every tiny nutrient is unlikely to actually make you any healthier because the hyper-focus on nutrition causes anxiety and food obsession. Food worry may even have negative physiological consequences, as we explored in chapter 7. Besides, if you're worried about food you can't actually enjoy it. To me, the best diet means having a healthy balance of foods *and* a healthy relationship to food. It's flexible; without rigid rules or restrictions.

PORTION CONTROL

A lot of nutrition advice is grounded in the idea that we constantly have to monitor and control our portions. Because serving sizes have increased over time, and because we have highly palatable foods available wherever we go, nutrition professionals often argue that we need to be vigilant about the portions we eat. But anyone who has ever counted or weighed their food, or even just compared what they eat to the size of their hand, will know that this is still an external regulation of food control, which draws us away from self-regulating our own intake based on hunger, fullness, and satisfaction.

I was taught to teach nutrition in terms of a palm-sized amount of this or a deck of cards-sized amount of that, but who wants to think of cubes of cheese relative to dice? The problem with this approach is that it undermines trust in our bodies to regulate our feeding. Who's to say that a thumb of peanut butter is the right amount for you? I don't know your life. I don't know how hungry you are, how satisfying you find particular foods, your activity level, how full a food leaves you feeling. Hopefully by now you realize that **a portion size depends on your hunger and fullness levels, and how satisfied a food leaves you**. Sure, there are suggested serving sizes on a package, but nine times out of ten they'll be too much, or too little, or they will make you fucking miserable trying to keep tabs on them. Trusting your body to self-regulate is where it's at when it comes to portion control. It may take a little while to really get to the point where you're not second-guessing and over-thinking this – that's totally normal – just give it some time, and you'll find that it becomes second nature and not something you have to consciously put a lot of effort into. I will add this little caveat though: if you are really, really struggling to know what an appropriate amount of food is for you, then you can use serving sizes on packaging as a guide. But remember that it's not a hard and fast rule; be curious and see if a serving is too much, too little, or not satisfying to you – remember to Goldilocks that shit!

DEALING WITH LEFTOVERS

———

Like I said, portion sizes being served in restaurants have increased over time, and even if they hadn't, it's unlikely that a standardized serving in a restaurant will be the exact right amount of food for everyone who orders a particular dish. At the risk of repeating myself, everyone's appetite is different from day to day and meal to meal, so it's impossible that your order will perfectly meet your exact requirements. Applying your mindful-eating skills will help you find the amount of food that's appropriate for you. Sometimes that means having leftovers. Clients seem to really struggle with this, especially because there's a big emphasis on reducing food waste. So here are some ideas for dealing with leftovers:

- Ask for any leftovers to be boxed up (take your own containers if you're super-organized)
  - eat them the next day
  - give them to your housemate, kid, or partner
  - offer them to a rough sleeper
- If you know a place has huge portions or you know you're not that hungry, consider sharing the dish (and maybe ordering a few sides to go along with it)

There are definitely times I've gone out to a restaurant for dinner and by the time dessert rolls around I know that I'll be uncomfortably full but I still want the dessert because this place is amazing and you never really get to go. You have two options here as I see it: **1** have the dessert and deal with the consequences without guilt (after all, full-ness will pass) or **2** get the dessert boxed up to take home and enjoy it later when you've made some space; no rules, so you get to decide.

THE FOUNDATION OF A HEALTHY DIET

—

I hope you're sitting down because I'm going to reveal to you the secrets of a healthy diet. Ready? Cos this might just blow your socks off!

Balance and variety.

I know, right? Mind-bending. OK, so maybe not the most revolutionary advice ever: certainly not as cool as drinking green juice or as fear-mongering as 'coffee will give you cancer, wait, no, coffee cures cancer' and the permanent state of confusion the media likes to keep you in. But, it's pretty fucking solid advice. And, chances are, you're already nailing it, and if you're not, you're doing better than you think.

Balance: For a lot of health bloggers, #balance looks like this: a massive plate of vegetables, little to no carbs, followed by a caption that says, 'had a tub of Ben & Jerry's and a bag of Reece's Pieces after #yolo'. Hate to be the one to say it (who am I kidding?), but that's not balance, that feels pretty disordered to me. In nutrition, when we talk about balance, we mean balance achieved over time. We don't mean every single meal has to be perfectly balanced, we don't even mean every single day; your body doesn't magically reset at midnight. Balance is achieved over days, weeks, and months; it's an average over time not a single meal or single day. You're not going to get a deficiency if you don't eat 5-a-day for one day!

Too often sensible dietary advice is taken to extremes. Public-health messages to be mindful of sugar intake have been warped and manipulated into 'sugar is a toxic poison and you must cut it out immediately'. But we know that restriction and deprivation can totally backfire and go too far the other way, causing us to overeat or binge on these forbidden foods. When we pay attention to how food makes us feel, and eat according to hunger, fullness, and satisfaction, moderation tends to take care of itself. We gravitate towards a balance of foods because that's what feels good, and we stop feeling compulsive around former shit list foods.

Variety: Restrictive diets tend to be, well, restrictive. That means we don't always get the most variety, preferring to stick to 'safe' foods. We end up eating the same foods over and over. When we eat more intuitively, and bring mindful awareness to what we're eating, we tend to get lots of variety because that's what's satisfying and tastes good, but this is also helpful from a nutrition perspective as it means we'll get a wider, broader range of foods and nutrients to help us cover all our nutritional bases too.

I want to add a fourth dimension to the foundation of a healthy diet: **taste**.

We've talked a lot about the pleasure principle in chapter 8, but I just want to drive home the point that eating nutritious foods shouldn't come at the expense of taste. If there's a food you really can't stand, even if it's high in nutrients, YOU DON'T HAVE TO EAT THAT SHIT. Gentle nutrition is not about deprivation or eating things you don't like. You don't have to eat spirulina-coated raw granola because it has fractionally more iron (or whatever, I'm making this up). If it tastes like crap, don't eat it. Think of new, creative ways to enjoy veggies or whole grains. Don't like quinoa, no problem, there are approximately infinity other combinations of foods that will help you get enough fibre and protein. Don't like kale? Don't mess with it! Nutrition shouldn't come at the expense of taste, and it doesn't have to! I mean, this might seem obvious, but it's something I really have to hammer into my clients who are low-key depriving themselves of delicious foods throughout the day and still bingeing at night. If you're stuck for inspiration, buy yourself a new cookbook (not a clean-eating one, but one by an actual professional cook or chef) or check out some blogs.

Here are some suggestions for making some nutrient-dense foods more fun.

Regular version	Fun version
raw carrot sticks	honey-roasted carrots
smoked salmon fillet	salmon fish cakes
literally anything	add garlic
boring veggies and grains	add a fun sauce – like cheese sauce to roasted cauliflower

NUTRITION 101

—

I find that, if anything, my clients have *too much* nutrition knowledge; things they've picked up from diets, social media, magazines, and the rest. But a lot of it is convoluted and bogged down in details that are irrelevant or cause them to be overly concerned. For example, I once had a client tell me that while almond butter was a 'superfood', peanut butter was unhealthy. When I probed a little, it was pretty clear this was just something she'd read on a blog and not something grounded in science. From a nutrition perspective, nuts are all fairly similar in terms of their nutrition composition and benefits. We really couldn't give two shits about which particular nut, so long as you enjoy it and aren't allergic to it. There's a ton of detail I could go into, ongoing debates in nutritional sciences, new advances and developments, groundbreaking research. But, in all honesty, these rarely change the advice on what we should actually be eating to support good health. So let's keep it simple.

First let's discuss some specific nutrients and their function.

The big leagues: macronutrients

Makro: somewhere you do your shopping in bulk – like a poor man's Costco.

Macro: a dietary component that contributes energy (calories).

In the simplest terms possible a macronutrient provides energy – aka calories. Carbs, protein, fats, and alcohol all provide energy when they're broken down, so they're macros. Fat has about double the energy density of protein and carbs; I don't say that to freak you out, but just to say that if you skip a source of fat at a meal, you may feel hangry sooner rather than later. So, all macronutrients give us energy. But that's not their only role. Each macronutrient has a specific job in the body.

Carbs are cool

Carbs are my FAVOURITE nutrient. Most people hate on carbs, and it makes me sad because carbs are so misunderstood; probably because people get confused between carbs and sugars and fibre and it gets a little tricky. In the most basic terms, carbs can be broken down into two groups: simple and complex.

Basically, all carbs are made up of simple sugars – sometimes they just have two sugars joined together like in table sugar, other times there are loads and loads strung together like a beaded necklace as is the case in fibre. Confused? You should be!

Let's break it down. What actually is a sugar?

Well, the fancy name for sugar is saccharide. Say it with me: 'SACK-A-RIDE'. Their main job is to provide us with energy. Saccharides are made up of three elements; just like water is made up of hydrogen and oxygen, saccharides are made up of hydrogen, oxygen, and, drumroll . . . carbon! Carbs. Carbon. Get it? In fact, carbon is the main element in carbohydrates. I know, surprising, right? So, there are three main saccharides that get joined up in different configurations to make up all carbohydrates – they're kinda like the building blocks. They are glucose, galactose, and fructose. You've probably even heard of them. Well, maybe not galactose because it's not really that important. But you've definitely heard of glucose and fructose.

Since each of these sugars is a single unit, or monomer, they're called monosaccharides (mono meaning one). Sugars made up of two monosaccharide units are called disaccharides. Between three and nine units and you've got an oligosaccharide. Above nine, all bets are off. Joke, they're called polysaccharides.

The table over the page summarizes the role of simple and complex carbs.[1]

SUGARS IN FOOD

—

Type of suger	Role	Food sources
Simple sugars		
Monosaccharides	**Fructose:** sugars are sweet, right? And fructose is the sweetest of the monosaccharides.	You find it in fruit (no shit!), root veg and honey.
	Glucose: this bad boy is also in fruits and veg, but it can come from the digestion (breakdown) of longer chains of carbohydrates – or polysaccharides too. When you hear of 'blood sugar levels', what people really mean is 'blood glucose concentration'. Loads of the cells in our body run on glucose – like our red blood cells, which carry oxygen through the body and the central nervous system, including the brain, where nerve impulses carry messages back and forth from our brains to our organs and muscles. Glucose is much less sweet than fructose.	Table sugar, fruits, vegetables

	Galactose: galactose is kinda the meh monosaccharide – like I said before, he's not up to much; the only thing he does really is join up with glucose to make lactose, that's a disaccharide sugar found in milk.	Cow and breast milk
Dissacharides These guys come about when two monosaccharides bond together.	**Sucrose:** aka table sugar. This is what you put on your Rice Krispies when you were a kid, and what you use to make cake. It's made up of a unit of glucose and a unit of fructose joined together.	It comes from sugar cane and sugar beet (natural AF). Other sweeteners like maple syrup and coconut sugar also contain loads of sucrose (~70%) and the rest is made up of free glucose and fructose.
	Lactose: made up from glucose and galactose. If you have a lactose intolerance, you'll know all about it.	It makes up about 40% of the dry weight of cow's milk, and about 60% of the dry weight of human breast milk. You with me so far? Time to kick it up a level.

Oligos Oligosaccharides are made of 3–9 monosaccharide units and can be split into two major groups: digestible and resistant.	**Digestible:** pretty self-explanatory – these types of sugars can easily be digested and absorbed in the small intestine. An example of these is maltodextrin: basically, a chain of glucose units that get digested into glucose in the small intestine.	They're usually added to foods to make them sweeter.
	Resistant: resistant oligosaccharides have this inspired name because they resist digestion in the upper gastrointestinal tract. That means they pass all the way through our gastrointestinal tracts to the large intestine, where they get fermented by the bacteria that live there. In other words they act as a prebiotic. The main resistant oligosaccharides are called inulin and fructo-oligosaccharides.	Artichoke, chicory root, wheat, rye, asparagus, onion, leeks, garlic, bananas

	Health benefits: Although human studies are quite limited, some animal studies suggest that resistant oligosaccharides can help reduce blood cholesterol and help maintain healthy blood glucose levels.	
Complex carbs		
Polysaccharides Polysaccharides are made of more than 9 monosaccharide units and primarily come from two groups: starches and non-starch polysaccharides.	**Starches:** Starches are the main source of carbohydrate that people eat; they're the main storage carbohydrate in most plants. These are made of long chains of glucose bound together.	Bread, pasta, beans, pulses, legumes, potatoes, wheat flour, cereals
	Fibres are neither digested nor absorbed by humans so they pass all the way through our digestive tracts to the large intestine, where they are fermented by the tens of trillions bacteria that live there – known as the microbiota. In other words, the fibre acts as food for the bacteria.	(See table overleaf) wheat, corn, rice, oats, barley, rye, beans, legumes

The bacteria chomp down on the fibre, which helps them multiply. Different fibre acts as food for different bacteria – food for bacteria is known as a prebiotic.

Prebiotics: prebiotics are defined as 'selectively fermented ingredients that result in specific changes, in the composition and/or activity of the gastrointestinal microbiota, thus conferring benefit(s) upon host health'.

High-fibre foods

In general, we aren't eating enough fibre, and adding some can have health benefits including a lower risk of heart disease, stroke, type-2 diabetes and bowel cancer.[2]

Group	Foods
Beans/lentils/pulses	Black beans, black-eyed peas, chickpeas, hummus, green and red lentils, split peas, baked beans
Whole grains	Oatmeal, wholegrain bread/pasta, baked potatoes (leave skin on for fibre hit), sweet potato, high-fibre breakfast cereal like Weetabix
Vegetables	Peas, sweetcorn, carrots, green beans, parsnips, beetroot
Fruits	Apples, bananas, raspberries, blackberries, strawberries, pears, citrus fruits, pineapple, mango, raisins, dates
Nuts	Peanuts, pistachios, cashews, almonds, walnuts, pine nuts, nut butters like almond or peanut
Seeds	Pumpkin seeds, sunflower seeds, flax seeds, chia seeds

Protein

Protein is made up of long chains of amino acids. There are relatively few amino acids but they constitute the building block of between 30,000 and 50,000 different proteins in our bodies. Protein is essential for growth and repair, building muscles and organs, hair, skin, nails, enzymes that carry out reactions in the body, hormones, blood cells and more. In fact, protein is the major structural component of all cells. Despite a large proportion of our body being made out of protein (yes, people, we are essentially just a slab of meat), relatively speaking, we require little protein in our day-to-day diets. In other words we don't have to eat our weight in protein every day for our bodies to work optimally. This is because protein gets 'recycled' (it's also called protein turnover, if you want to be fancy). This means that proteins are broken back down into their constituent amino acids and are repackaged as new proteins by the body. Some proteins, like enzymes, might be broken down relatively quickly, in a matter of minutes or hours; others may take days or weeks. When we don't get adequate carbohydrate in our diets, the body will use proteins and fats to generate energy – both from the food we eat and from those already in our body. In the UK, we tend to get about twice as much protein as we need, so in general it's not too much of a concern. Older adults may benefit from eating some extra protein as they're not as efficient at recycling it. But, for the most part, if you are eating a wide variety of different foods and meeting your energy needs, you should be getting enough protein.[3]

Sources of protein: beans, nuts, legumes, seeds, milk, cheese, eggs, meat, fish, grains

Fats – aka vitamin F

It's rumoured that when fat was first discovered it was called vitamin F – too bad we didn't stick with that nomenclature! Fat plays so many critical roles in the body – cholesterol (which is a type of fat) is converted into vitamin D, it helps us absorb fat-soluble vitamins (A,D,E,K), it helps keep us warm and protects our internal organs; it's also a large part of the membrane that encloses every single cell in our bodies. Our brains are around 60% fat and the myelin sheath that coats the cells in our nervous system is made of fat.[4] Lastly, and most importantly, fat is responsible for dissolving flavour compounds in things like garlic and herbs; if we didn't cook those things in some oil, the flavours wouldn't develop – fat is what helps our food taste good.

There are two main types of fat in the food we eat: saturated and unsaturated. Saturated fats are usually solid at room temperature:

think butter, lard, and coconut oil. Unsaturated fats are typically liquid at room temperature. This is to do with the structure of the fats; saturated fats can pack together tightly, whereas unsaturated fats are a bit floppier, meaning the molecules can move over each other more easily, which is why they tend to be liquid. Unsaturated fats can be broken down farther into mono, poly, and trans fats. Trans fats occur naturally in foods like meat and dairy in small amounts, but are more commonly found in manufactured food products, where they have undergone a process called hydrogenation. This effectively makes trans fats behave more like saturated fats than unsaturated fats. This means they can raise blood-cholesterol levels, increasing our risk of heart disease. However, most manufacturers in the UK have stopped using trans fat as an ingredient in foods, and the population gets about half of the recommended maximum, so it's nothing to stress about.[5]

Monounsaturated fats (MUFA): help protect our heart health by supporting levels of 'good' cholesterol or high-density lipo-protein (HDL), and lowering 'bad' cholesterol, or low-density lipoprotein (LDL).

Sources: olives, olive oil, rapeseed/canola oil (and spreads made from these oils), avocado and avocado oil, nuts like almonds, brazil nuts, and peanuts

Polyunsaturated fats (PUFA): these can help lower the level of LDL cholesterol and can be further split up into two main groups – omega-6 fatty acids and omega-3 fatty acids. We can make most types of fat we need from other fats and from raw materials; however, there are some types of omega-3s and omega-6s that we cannot make ourselves and we need to get these from food we eat – these are called essential fatty acids.

Omega-6 fatty acid – linoleic acid (LA): this is a relatively short fatty acid that gets converted to a longer-chain fatty acid in the body. In general, we get plenty of omega-6 and LA in our diet, but less so omega-3s.

Sources of LA: vegetable oils, some nuts, eggs, and whole grains

Omega-3 fatty acids: are less common in our diet, and we tend to need to eat more of these. **α-linolenic acid (ALA)** is a plant-based source of essential fatty acids, whereas **eicosapentanoic acid (EPA)** and **docosahexanoic acid (DHA)** typically come from marine sources such as fish oils and oily fish. Your body can convert ALA to EPA and DHA, although not very effectively. Therefore, while technically ALA is the only truly essential fatty acid, DHA and EPA become conditionally essential, meaning they are essential under some circumstances.

Sources of ALA: flax seeds, walnuts, soybeans, tofu, kale, eggs enriched with omega-3

Sources of DHA/EPA: mackerel, kippers, herring, trout, sardines, salmon

Saturated fats: whereas all foods contain a mixture of saturated and unsaturated fats, too much saturated fat in the food you eat can raise 'bad' LDL cholesterol in the blood, which can increase the risk of heart disease and stroke. That's not to say you can never enjoy foods with saturated fat, but be mindful of how often you're eating these foods, particularly if you have a family history of high cholesterol, stroke, or heart disease. Studies consistently show that replacing the amount of saturated fat in the food we eat with other macronutrients – such as PUFAs and wholegrain carbohydrates – is associated with a lower risk of coronary heart disease.[6] In fact, replacing saturated fats with PUFAs may help reduce risk of heart disease by around 17%, including in people who are otherwise considered healthy.[7]

Sources of saturated fats: fatty cuts of meat, sausages, pies, butter, ghee, cream, ice cream, biscuits, cakes, pastries, coconut oil

The little leagues: micronutrients

Micronutrients are nutrients that don't provide any energy, that we need in much smaller amounts than macronutrients and include vitamins, minerals, and phytonutrients.

These come from a wide variety of foods, primarily fruits and vegetables, but significant amounts also come from grains (especially whole grains), dairy foods and alternatives, beans, nuts, seeds, and fortified cereals. In the table below I've summarized the function and sources of the major micronutrients. You don't have to memorize this or micromanage every tiny nutrient: it's just to help you see that nutrients come from a wide variety of different foods. The way nutrition is talked about makes it seem as though you can only get one nutrient from one food, but remember, nutrition isn't all or nothing. If you skip fruit and veg one day, OK, no worries, you're probably still getting some fibre and micronutrients from whole grains or fortified flours, for instance; it's not going to kill you. But notice how it feels when you skip those things (with curiosity, not judgement!). It *probably* feels better when you get some of all of those foods.

Name of nutrient	Function	Food sources
Fat-soluble vitamins		
Vitamin A	Adaption of vision in the dark, normal growth and development, immune system response, antioxidant, maintaining healthy skin	Retinol (from animal sources) – oily fish, liver, eggs Beta-carotene (from plant sources) – yellow and green (leafy) vegetables, yellow fruit
Vitamin D	Helps with calcium absorption in the gut, may protect against some types of cancer, helps muscle strength, and protects against fractures from falls as it's important for keeping bones strong. Adequate levels also help reduce risk of infection (cold/flu) and SAD	Cod liver oil, oily fish, milk, margarine, fortified breakfast cereals, eggs – in the winter months in the UK, it's advised to take a 10µg supplement of vitamin D per day

Vitamin E	Helps maintain healthy skin and eyes, and strengthen the body's natural defence against illness and infection, antioxidant	Plant oils like soya, corn, sunflower, and olive oil; nuts and seeds, cereal products
Vitamin K	Blood coagulation, wound healing, keeping bones healthy	Green leafy vegetables – such as broccoli and spinach – vegetable oils, cereal grains. Small amounts in meat and dairy products
Water-soluble vitamins		
Vitamin B1 (thiamine)	Metabolism of fat, carbohydrate, and alcohol; keeping the nervous system healthy	Cereals, fortified flour, pulses, nuts
Vitamin B2 (riboflavin)	Helps normal growth, keeps skin, eyes, and the nervous system healthy, helps the body release energy from food	Eggs, milk, fortified cereals
Vitamin B3 (niacin)	Metabolism of fat and carbohydrate, keeps the nervous system and skin healthy	Meat, eggs, milk, wheat flour

Vitamin B5 (pantothenic acid)	Metabolism of fat and carbohydrate	Almost all meat and vegetables, but especially chicken, beef, potatoes, oats, tomatoes, eggs, broccoli, and whole grains
Vitamin B6 (pyridoxine)	Hormone metabolism, haemoglobin formation, allows the body to use and store energy from protein and carbohydrates in food	Meat, fish, whole grains, fortified cereals, pulses
Vitamin B7 (biotin)	Required by enzymes involved in fat synthesis and metabolism, glucose production and metabolism of some amino acids	At low levels in many foods, but especially liver, kidney, milk, eggs and dairy products
Vitamin B9 (folate/ folic acid)	Helps the body form red blood cells, reduces the risk of central neural tube defects in unborn babies, involved in synthesis of DNA	Broccoli, Brussels sprouts, leafy greens such as spinach and kale, chickpeas, fortified bread, and cereals

Vitamin B12 (cobalamin)	Brain development and keeping the nervous system healthy, production of red blood cells, releasing energy from food	Meat, fish, dairy, eggs, fortified cereals and other products
Vitamin C	Antioxidant, wound healing, maintaining healthy skin, blood vessels, bones and cartilage	A wide variety of fruit and vegetables: citrus fruits, red and green peppers, berries, broccoli, Brussels sprouts
Minerals		
Calcium	Essential for building strong teeth and bones, control of muscles and nerve signals, blood clotting	Milk, cheese, yoghurt, fortified cereals, white bread, beans, lentils and chickpeas, fish that you eat the bones, dark green leafy veg, tofu that has been set with calcium
Phosphorus	Another component of strong bones and teeth and helps release energy from food	Milk and dairy products (except butter), fish, red meat, poultry, nuts, fruits and vegetables, bread, oats

Iron	Part of red blood cells that carry oxygen around the body	Meat, beans, nuts, dried fruits like apricot, whole grains like brown rice, fish, eggs, fortified breakfast cereals, dark green leafy vegetables
Zinc	Breaking down alcohol, making new cells, wound healing, releasing energy from food	Whole grains, pork, dairy products, eggs, lamb, root vegetables, shellfish, beef
Copper	Helps produce red and white blood cells, important for the immune system	Nuts, shellfish, offal, cereals and cereal products
Iodine	Helps make thyroid hormones, which help keep cells and the metabolic rate – the speed at which chemical reactions take place in the body – healthy	Fish, shellfish, milk and dairy products, seaweed, iodized salt
Selenium	Helps keep the reproductive and immune systems healthy, antioxidant function	Brazil nuts, fish, meat, eggs

Magnesium	Helps release energy from food, ensures the parathyroid glands (which produce hormones important for bone health) work normally	Green vegetables, pulses, wholegrain cereals, meat, nuts, fish, meat, peanut butter, avocados
Manganese	Helps make and activate some of the enzymes in the body. Enzymes are proteins that help the body carry out chemical reactions, such as breaking down food	Tea, bread, nuts, cereal, green vegetables like peas and runner beans
Molybedenum	Helps make and activate some of the proteins involved in chemical reactions (enzymes) that help with repairing and making genetic material	Offal, nuts, bread, cereals like oats, peas
Chromium	Thought to influence how the hormone insulin behaves in the body. This means chromium may affect the amount of energy we get from food	Meat, whole grains, lentils, broccoli, potatoes, spices

THE DIETARY GUIDELINES

In 2016, Public Health England launched the latest set of dietary guidance for the UK – the guidelines, known as The Eatwell Plate, represent the best available evidence-based nutrition science, distilled down into recommendations for consumers to make sure they get a healthy balance of foods. Here I have highlighted the key messages from the guidelines to help you navigate the best ways to support your health. I have removed specific numbers or amounts because the guidelines are exactly that – a framework, not a rigid prescription, that allows for you to be flexible and adapt to your needs.

Eat a variety of fruit and vegetables: This is kind of a no-brainer. Check out the 'Eat the rainbow' and 'Eating more plants' sections below. We all know that fruit and veg are great for us. That doesn't mean you have to go vegan or plant-based, and you don't need to eat ten portions a day to get the benefits. Try and get a variety of fruit and veg each day (although if you go a day or two without it, which is actually pretty hard to do, it's not the end of the world). Fresh, frozen, canned and dried all count. Just be mindful of added sugars/syrups and salt in canned products. Also remember that fruit juices, while they totally count as a portion of fruit, have the fibre removed from them so won't contribute towards your fibre intake for the day (but are still delicious) and you can easily get around this by adding in higher-fibre foods, like having a bowl of oatmeal with a side of OJ in the morning.

Base meals on potatoes, bread, rice, pasta, or other starchy carbohydrates; choosing wholegrain versions where possible: Remember that whole grains tend to be more nutrient-dense, and include more fibre, helping support your gut health and reducing risk of disease. They also help keep your blood sugar levels, and therefore energy, more steady. Check out the high-fibre foods table above, and again, if you love white bread for toast, don't sweat it, think about other higher-fibre grains and foods.

Have some dairy or dairy alternatives (such as soya drinks): Dairy is a great source of calcium; if you are vegan/plant-based, make sure your plant-based milks, yoghurts, etc are fortified with calcium to help reduce the risk of osteoporosis.

Eat some beans, pulses, fish, eggs, meat, and other proteins: Proteins are generally satiating and therefore satisfying foods. If you eat fish, consider adding a portion of oily fish to your weekly shopping list. We know that 'superfood' is a made-up marketing term, but if there was such a thing, it would for sure be beans, pulses, and legumes; not only are they a great source of protein, starchy carbs, and fibre, they also count as a portion of veg. BOOM.

Choose unsaturated oils and spreads: Remember that fats help us absorb fat-soluble vitamins, and unsaturated fats especially can help reduce our risk of heart disease.

Drink 6–8 cups/glasses of fluid a day.

Be mindful of foods higher in salt or sugar: This doesn't mean you can't have them or that they're 'bad', but as with all foods, we want to be mindful of how they make us feel physically and mentally. Too little can feel restrictive and cause us to feel as though these foods are calling our name. Likewise, too much might not make us feel too hot either. Find a balance that feels right for you.

THE REAL FOOD GUIDE

The REAL food guide stands for the Recovery from Eating Disorders for Life and was developed to help guide nutrition and food decisions for people who have a troubled or broken relationship with food. I have adapted it slightly for use here as I think it's an enormously valuable tool to help visually represent the ideas of balance, moderation and variety that form the basis of a healthy diet, but also emphasize a healthy relationship with food. If it's helpful for you, use this as a guide to help reassure you that you're getting something from each of the food groups represented here most of the time. Remember it's not an all-or-nothing, hard and fast rule. One meal or day's worth of eating in a particular way won't make or break your health. No single food or meal can make us healthy, just as no single meal or food can make us unhealthy. The REAL food guide is designed to help you achieve balance and variety over time; don't sweat it if eating doesn't look like this every single day.[8]

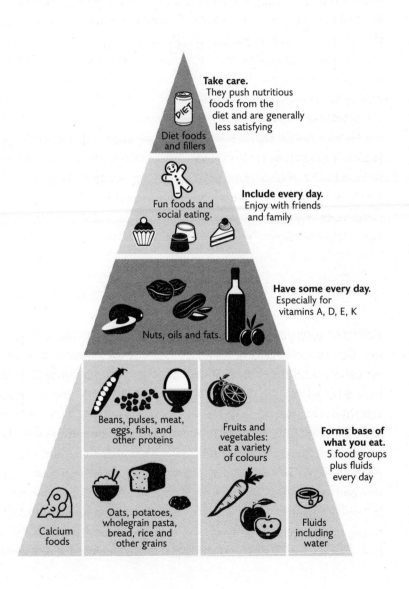

A caution on nutrition information: Keep in mind that if the nutrition information you're receiving strays too far from common sense, is promoting miracle cures, eliminating entire food groups, or vilifying certain foods or nutrients then it's probably not coming from the most reliable or evidence-based source. Check out the resources section for reliable sources of evidence-based nutrition, and if you're unsure, go back and look at Pixie's Bullshit Detector in chapter 7.

EAT THE RAINBOW
—

OK, so I'm not talking about Skittles here, although they are delicious and I really have a thing for the sour ones, but if you overdo it they kinda hurt your tongue. When we talk about eating the rainbow in terms of nutrition, we just mean get a load of different colours in there. It's not just so your plate is Instagrammable though! Fruits, vegetables, and grains have been shown to protect against chronic diseases like cardiovascular disease, some cancers, and type-2 diabetes, and this is down (at least in part) to the phytochemicals. Literally plant chemicals.

So what are these bad boys and what do they do? Well, these aren't like regular nutrients, these are cool nutrients. While the vitamins and minerals we talked about before remedy specific deficiencies, you're not going to get scurvy if you don't have enough phytochemicals in your meal, BUT having plenty of them in the diet may help lower your risk of chronic disease. They are non-nutritive compounds that are bioactive. Many phytochemicals are antioxidants, meaning they scavenge free radicals (like reactive oxygen and nitrogen species) in the body. Free radicals can cause damage to DNA in our cells, which can lead to cancer, age-related degeneration and Alzheimer's disease. SCARY-SOUNDING SHIT. It's important to note that our bodies produce free radicals all the time, it's not abnormal or unusual; they're not going to kill, so cool your jets. Our bodies produce free radicals in response to eating, breathing, exercise, stress, and just general life stuff. They also send important messages in our body and can help with wound healing and help fight infections. A certain amount of free radicals are actually helpful for keeping us healthy. But chronic oxidative stress from too many free radicals can lead to disease, and because our bodies are smart they also produce antioxidants to neutralize these free radicals. My favourite is called superoxide dismutase. If it sounds like a fucking superhero, it's because it is. SOD along with an army of other antioxidant enzymes helps keep us healthy.

Phytochemicals are like a back-up, second-line defence, just in case shit gets too real. Over 10,000 phytochemicals have been identified, but a large proportion are still unknown to scientists. The following table lists some of the more well-studied phytonutrients and their posited benefits.[9,10] It's important to note, though, that while some of these compounds have been very well studied in test tubes and animals, their effect is less well known in humans. That said, eating a wide variety of different foods helps ensure you get all the nutrients you need, and may have the added bonus of helping to prevent disease.

Group	Phyto-chemical	Colour	Food source	Disease it helps prevent
Carotenoids[11]	Lycopene	Red	Tomatoes, watermelon	Cardio-vascular disease, cancer, (diabetes)
	Lutein	Yellow	Kale, spinach, chard	Diabetes, cataracts, macular degeneration
	β-carotene	Orange	Carrots	Cancer
Organo-sulphur compound[12,13]	Allicin	White	Garlic, spring onions, chives	Reduces total and 'bad' (LDL) cholesterol, raises 'good' cholesterol, cancer
	Glucosinolates	White	Cruciferous vegetables (cauliflower, cabbage, Brussels sprouts)	Cancer
Flavonoids	Anthocyanins	Red/purple	Parsley, blueberries, black tea, citrus, red onion	Heart disease
	Flavanols	Colourless	Cocoa, wine	May help prevent dementia
	Flavonols	Yellow	Onions, broccoli, kale, apples, tea, buckwheat	Reduced blood pressure, diabetes, cancer

So, in general, antioxidants from food are helpful and beneficial and we should try to include a variety of fruits, vegetables, and whole grains to get the benefits.

BUT that's not a free pass to start hammering mega-doses of supplements containing these compounds; super-high doses of antioxidant supplements can actually *increase* disease risk. Magazines love to tell you to smash a ton of different supplements without acknowledging that *too much* of anything can cause more harm than good.

EAT MORE PLANTS

—

Plants are a great way to get more disease-fighting phytochemicals and fibre up in there. Here are some delicious ways to increase plant intake:

- add vegetables to your pizza or have a side salad
- chop a banana over your Weetabix in the morning
- add a tablespoon of ground flax seed into your porridge and/or top with fresh or frozen berries
- make a door-stop sandwich on sourdough with hummus, avocado, baby spinach leaves, sauerkraut, and sliced pickled beetroot
- swap white pasta for wholegrain (if you like it, no shame in white pasta though; wholegrain pasta in mac 'n'cheese? Over my dead body)
- make a black bean and lentil veggie chilli with chopped tomatoes, red peppers, and big spice
- a homemade smoothie (they aren't sieved like shop-bought ones, so more of the fibre remains intact)
- add some fruit and nutty, oaty granola to your yoghurt
- BBQ jackfruit tacos with guacamole and chopped tomato salsa
- veggie burgers with sweet-potato wedges
- channa masala curry with chickpeas and cauliflower in creamy coconut sauce
- vegetable lasagne
- veggie stir-fry with tofu

It sounds good in theory, right? You stop restricting yourself and eventually, once you've stopped losing your shit over pizza, you'll calm down and gravitate towards a healthy balance and variety of foods that are pretty much in line with your nutritional needs. I mean, that sounds almost too good, and when I explain it to people who are new to the concept of intuitive eating, they kind of give me the side-eye. And although more research needs to be done to elucidate this relationship, it appears that intuitive eaters may eat more nutritious foods overall, including eating more vegetables and fewer foods higher in sugar and fat, compared to people who intentionally restrict those foods.[14,15,16,17,18]

MEAL PLANNING AND INTUITIVE EATING

—

I often get asked if it's OK to meal plan when you're doing intuitive eating, and the simple answer is yes! Totally. Meal planning can be a really important part of self-care if you know that you will benefit in the future from having a batch of something ready to heat up when you get home after a long day. Where it becomes tricky is if you have been caught in the trap of rigid meal prepping that is very controlled and restrictive; going to meal planning from a place of self-care can trigger diet mentality. I encourage clients to plan meals that they know will be balanced and satisfying using recipes that they know they love and not from some prescriptive meal plan or clean-eating cookbook. Find recipes from actual chefs and cooks, make sure you're getting loads of variety and not just eating the same meal for five days in a row (if you can avoid it). But give yourself the freedom to be flexible if you decide what you really need is to order a pizza!

VEGETARIANISM AND VEGANISM

——

Another super-common question is where does vegetarianism or veganism fit within intuitive eating? Is it restricting yourself? This is a really important question because vegetarianism and veganism are often used to 'disguise' or legitimize disordered-eating behaviours. It's helpful to get very clear about your intentions behind choosing vegetarianism or veganism. Are you doing it to restrict the foods you eat or because you think it's the healthiest way to eat? Is it a decision based on fear? Or is it coming from a place of animal welfare or environmental concern? Be completely honest with yourself.

The way I interpret gentle nutrition is this: if eating a particular food doesn't make you feel good, then don't mess with it. Coffee gives me an upset stomach, so I don't drink it very often. If eating animal products doesn't feel good to you, then you don't have to. It is important to make sure that you are getting adequate nutrition and are eating a wide variety of foods within that though.

If being veggie or vegan is about ethics, then cool. But if it's about restriction, be very cautious. It's also worth considering if you really even have to slap a label on it? Sometimes holding off on labelling your diet can give you a little extra freedom to explore all different foods and see how they feel. For instance, maybe you want to eat mostly plant-based, but you know that you'll feel restricted without cheese. Ditching the 'vegan' label might help give you a little space to have cheese when you want it, while still honouring your commitment to animal and environmental ethics. It's also important to recognize that there are other ways besides your diet to support those causes, and if you have a history of disordered eating, it might be best to engage in activism outside of what's on your plate.

Tuning in to what I want to eat

When we're dieting, restricting, or otherwise in a funky relationship with food the effects of food on our bodies can be disguised by feelings of guilt or shame. Once we've ditched all the emotional baggage around food, we can gain a little perspective on how food makes us feel. We can use this information to guide our eating decisions. We can ask ourselves:

- What do I want to eat?
- What's going to taste good?
- How's this going to make me feel?
- What's going to feel good?
- How's this going to make my body feel?

Don't worry if you don't get it straight away, it can take time to figure out how different foods feel in your body (as opposed to how diet culture tells us it should feel!). Be patient, look for clues, and remember to Goldilocks the crap out of it! Eventually you won't have to think too hard about how food makes you feel and you will make food choices more intuitively or instinctively. If you find yourself second-guessing how food makes you feel and you are taking forever to deliberate, then you may be over-thinking it. If that's the case then you may just have to commit to something and *then* consider how it made you feel in retrospect: whether you want to feel that way again, whether you want to feel that way often or only some of the time. Ultimately, if healthy eating is pleasurable *and* feels good, that's going to be a lot more sustainable than the all-or-nothing scarcity mindset that's rooted in deprivation!

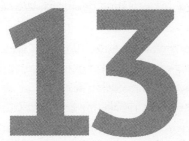

PUTTING IT ALL
TOGETHER

———

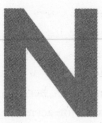 ow you're familiarized with the principles of IE I want to share some common 'road bumps' or sticking points that people have difficulty putting into place. I've asked some of my favourite non-diet friends to share pieces of inspiration and advice to really help you solidify the last little pieces of the IE process, and to refer back to if you need a little refresher without having to re-read the whole book.

How to move past the allure of weight loss
Fiona Sutherland, APD, @TheMindfulDietitian

Thanks to diet culture, there will always be an allure around weight loss. Just a temptation to try one more diet and then I can nail this intuitive eating business. You might not even be acting on it at all but the mentality, the diet mentality, just that little whisper is there. And that's pretty normal so give yourself a break. It's OK to grieve dieting, to let go of what you've put so much time, energy, money, and resources towards for so many years; letting go of that is pretty full on!

Give yourself some self-compassion; you're only human and when you've invested so much in this, it's like a stock market crash! All of a sudden, your stocks aren't coming to fruition – like you've invested in them, and what does that mean? That's actually a big step when people can kind of move past that, like that's when life opens really. But that's the one thing that people have is that grief process or the 'thin me' dream, or just the diet mentality hanging around, knocking.

If I'm not dieting then am I just letting myself go?
Julie Duffy Dillon, RD, @foodpeacedietitian

People often say to me, 'I know diets don't work for me, I've done them so many times, I just know they're not going to have a different outcome, but if I stop dieting, then I'm letting myself go.' And there's a cognitive distortion going on, an all-or-nothing mentality: 'If I'm not dieting then I'm just this gluttonous sloth sitting on the couch never doing anything again.' But this misses a lot of nuance and variation; choosing to not diet is a very active process because it's

Laoghaire Rathdown Libraries
nsgrsnge

tomer name: **Dobson, Margaret**
tomer ID: **********6208

s that you have borrowed

t eat it : how intuitive eating can help you
 your shit together around food
DLR27000043857
: **19 July 2022**
sages:

l items: 1
4/2022 16:18
ow 4
rdue: 0
l requests: 0
dy for collection: 0

s that you already have on loan

: Sisters
DLR20000224547
: **30 June 2022**
sages:

: First sight
300003100133444
: **19 July 2022**
sages:

: If you were me
DLR20000377990
: **19 July 2022**
sages:

nk you for using the SelfCheck System.
7

counter-cultural, and you could be thinking about it every day, multiple times a day. And it's important to remember it's a very health-promoting choice, it's just choosing to live in a way that's completely different. It sucks because diet culture teaches us 'if you don't choose me, then you're destined for failure', and again, because it's counter-cultural it just feels that way, but that's not accurate. Rejecting diet culture takes a lot of effort but the benefits can be enormous in terms of your mental and physical health, and your relationship to food.

I am fat, surely I should be on a diet?
Meredith Noble, Certified Body Trust®
Provider, @madeonagenerousplan

If you identify as plus-sized or fat, it can sometimes feel extra scary to give up pursuing weight loss through dieting. My clients routinely tell me their fears of never finding romantic partners, being ostracized socially, and not being able to participate in the same activities as thin people.

I never try to downplay the effects of fat oppression because they're unfortunately very real. At the same time, it can also be incredibly liberating to notice the pain we cause ourselves when we implicitly agree with what fat-phobic people say about us. When we agree with people that we're less worthy than them, the effects of fat oppression can be greatly amplified. When we rise up and gain confidence in ourselves no matter our size, we can adopt a much more resilient, strong posture in the face of negativity.

From that stance, we can also start to notice the places in our lives where we might be making incorrect assumptions about what we can and can't do as fat people. We can stop artificially limiting ourselves (from things like wearing certain clothes, seeking love, and taking other social risks) and truly start to thrive.

I keep freaking out about my body, what should I do?
Sumner Brooks @IntuitiveEatingRD

What a bad body-image day is really about:

Very often a difficult body-image day is like a little red flag going up that can tell you something more meaningful is going on for you. For the most part, we learn to associate stress in life with our body not being good enough. This can be true even if it is 'good' stress, like going on a date with someone you like. You may be excited about the date, and at the same time it may mean a lot to you for it to go well, so that stress manifests into thoughts about body image. For example, if someone didn't get a great review on an important assignment or in her job, then she might suddenly feel worse about her body, her weight, or her appearance. Or if someone is getting ready to deliver a speech in front of a large group of people and is having a very tough time getting dressed, she may be attributing the stress of wanting to do well at her speech with 'I have to look perfect' or 'I don't look good enough to do this'. This is very common, but all too often we get lost inside the body-image thoughts and we don't recognize it is simply a message that something important is going on.

What to do about it?

It can help greatly to pause and discover what in fact is truly bothering you. For the example about the stress of going on a date, the deeper issue could be: 'it's really important to me that I feel acceptable and treated well on this date' or 'clearly I care what this person thinks. That could be a good sign that I might really like him/her!' By recognizing the deeper message, it is so much easier to turn the negative into a neutral or even a positive mindset. If you're really struggling even after recognizing the message within your body-image discomfort, try and be very kind to yourself. Wear clothing that feels good on your body as this is critical for not carrying around a reminder all day that you're feeling uncomfortable in your body. Use things like your favourite-smelling lotion, listen to feel-good music, eat and/or drink comforting foods and beverages like hot tea or a homemade meal to satisfy yourself and demonstrate that even on a tough body-image day, you will not abandon self-kindness. You do not have to be perfect to be worthy, valuable, special, accepted, and respected. Anyone who can't respect you as you are today, doesn't deserve your time or energy. Lastly, try to look at yourself beyond your physical appearance. How we speak, listen, show up, relate, teach, care, and behave are great things to turn your attention to when you're feeling stuck in negative body image.

Help! I'm still eating past the point of comfortable fullness!
Paige Smathers, RD, @PaigeSmathersRD

Letting go of dieting and learning to tune in to and honour your body is a practice. If you're struggling to stop eating past the point of fullness, there are a few things to consider, experiment with, and practise. Ask yourself if you are eating small amounts or grazing throughout the day, causing primal, desperate hunger at night. Can you create a sense of curiosity around this, instead of judgement, experimenting with different things to see if they help you tune in to your cues? For some, answers about eating beyond fullness lie in simply eating intentional, satisfying meals throughout the day (rather than skipping meals or eating very small amounts) that help to lessen chaos with food later. Can you experiment with reminding yourself that food isn't scarce and you'll get what you need? Sometimes eating past fullness is a result of subconscious or conscious fears that food is scarce, leading you to feel compelled to eat beyond full right now. Can you give yourself that unconditional permission to eat and allow yourself to feel secure in food always being there? Experiment non-judgementally with these things in the spirit of curiosity, and you'll eventually uncover what works best for you. And remember, this is something we're practising each day, and with time you'll improve and learn more what is best for you.

Help! I'm still eating past the point of comfortable fullness! (Part 2): Laura

Following on from Paige (above), if you have established that you are giving yourself full unconditional permission and eating intentional and satisfying meals throughout the day, could it be that you are blaming your eating habits for your body not fitting into aesthetic ideals? In other words, do you perceive you are eating 'too much' simply because you're not happy with your body? Judging food choices may be a sign that you have some work to do on body image and internalized fat phobia. Remember that your body knows how to regulate itself without you having to micromanage it. Go back to chapter 5 on body image and revisit the exercises on body neutrality.

How to deal with fears around giving yourself unconditional permission
Haley Goodrich, RD, @hgoodrichrd

Giving yourself permission to give up dieting is a radical and counter-cultural act. Dieting gives you a false sense of control because you are told exactly what, how much, and when to eat. The problem is this is not sustainable and disconnects you from your body's needs. It is normal to fear that without these rules you will never stop eating; however, our bodies know how to give us the appropriate signals once we have made food available consistently. Hunger and fullness cues can be just as reliable as shivering when you are cold, sweating when you are hot, or feeling your bladder is full. Giving yourself permission to eat foods unconditionally and experience joy and pleasure isn't a sign of weakness. It doesn't mean that you are giving up or disregarding your health. Giving permission is a sign of strength and acceptance, and makes more room for you to take care of yourself. By giving yourself permission, you are gaining your inner voice of authority. You are the boss of your body and you know what is best for it.

Will I ever not crave highly palatable foods all the time? If I keep eating what I'm craving I feel like I'm going to eat brownies, ice cream, pizza, etc all the time?
Robyn Nohling, RD, FNP, @thereallife_rd

Giving yourself full permission to eat any and all foods at any and all times in any and all amounts is a foundational step in intuitive eating. Additionally, coming to a neutral place with all foods where you don't see any foods as 'good' or 'bad' is another foundational step. Moving through these two principles can take a while, so give yourself lots of patience. Any sort of physical, mental, or emotional restriction is going to trigger your biological drive to eat and interfere with your ability to make intuitive food choices. So if you are still having trouble giving yourself permission to eat brownies, it makes total sense that you'd crave them often because they are a forbidden food. Our brains crave what they can't have. Over time, you will come to a place where you can freely say, 'Sure, a cupcake sounds so good right now' and you can also freely say, 'I don't really feel like that cupcake, but thanks.' You'll still crave these foods occasionally, but they won't always be on your brain. Intuitive eating allows you to move away from chaotic or guilty experiences with food and teaches you how to feel competent around highly palatable foods. Remember food is supposed to be pleasurable and satisfying. Intuitive eating allows you to eat these pleasurable foods in a nourishing amount when you are craving them. Again, remember you won't always crave these foods for every meal/ snack but until you give yourself full permission to eat them without judgement you will crave them all the time. Be patient. Give yourself time. This is all part of the process.

How do I know if I'm still restricting/in diet mentality or if I REALLY want to eat the broccoli?
Christy Harrison, RD, @chr1styharrison

You're still in diet mentality if you're choosing foods you think are 'healthy' because you fear what will happen if you don't. If there's fear, there's probably some restrictive thinking at play. This is obviously distinct from the fear of, say, eating peanuts when you have a peanut allergy, which is an understandable and life-saving fear. But barring serious food allergies like that, you really don't feel afraid of eating (or not eating) anything when you're in the mindset of intuitive eating and gentle nutrition. Instead the operative emotions are desire and self-care – that is, you genuinely WANT the veggies (or whatever food) because they sound delicious/refreshing/crunchy/flavourful/etc, and you'd like to have some veggies that day because you know it helps your digestive system keep running smoothly. Note that it's possible to have the self-care impulse AND still be stuck in diet mentality, and the way you'll know is fear – fear of damaging your health by making the 'wrong' choice, and of course fear of gaining weight.

> **I know that diets don't work for me, but accepting I won't be thin/as thin as I imagined is really hard!**
> Meredith Noble, Certified Body Trust®
> Provider, @madeonagenerousplan

For a great many of us, embarking on a non-diet journey involves learning to accept that our bodies will never match the 'ideal' presented to us by society. It can also mean having to come to terms with the energy, time, and money we've wasted trying to reach that ideal.

It can be helpful to acknowledge the torrent of emotions this inner work can trigger. In fact, many practitioners have likened it to a grieving process, where we spend time bouncing between feelings of denial, anger, bargaining, depression, and acceptance.

It's important to know how completely normal it is to have strong emotions as you do this work. Giving up on the goal we once thought was the ticket to our happiness is not an easy task, but you can absolutely get to the other side. What will help most is giving yourself plenty of permission and time to process whatever emotions come up for you, whether that's through journalling, talking to friends, getting professional support, or something similar.

INTUITIVE EATING: FINDING *YOUR* NORMAL
—

Intuitive eating is a framework to help you get back to your version of normal – whatever that looks like for you. Intuitive eating is not prescriptive in terms of what, when, or how much you should eat. I don't want this to become yet another thing we have to do because it's cool or trendy. Intuitive eating is about you taking charge of your mental and physical health and rejecting dogmatic ideas about health being predicated on your weight or unrealistic beauty standards that were imposed on you before you were even conceived. It will look different on everyone, and that's OK! My favourite description of normal eating was written in 1983 by Ellyn Satter in her book *Secrets of Feeding a Healthy Family*[1], and she totally nails it:

> *Normal eating is going to the table hungry and eating until you are satisfied. It is being able to choose food you enjoy and eat it and truly get enough of it – not just stop eating because you think you should. Normal eating is being able to give some thought to your food selection so you get nutritious food, but not being so wary and restrictive that you miss out on enjoyable food. Normal eating is giving yourself permission to eat sometimes because you are happy, sad or bored, or just because it feels good. Normal eating is mostly three meals a day, or four or five, or it can be choosing to munch along the way. It is leaving some cookies on the plate because you know you can have some again tomorrow, or it is eating more now because they taste so wonderful. Normal eating is overeating at times, feeling stuffed and uncomfortable. And it can be undereating at times and wishing you had more.*
>
> *Normal eating is trusting your body to make up for your mistakes in eating. Normal eating takes up some of your time and attention, but keeps its place as only one important area of your life. In short, normal eating is flexible. It varies in response to your hunger, your schedule, your proximity to food, and your feelings.*

Normal eating is flexible, dynamic, and adapts to different situations and circumstances. Sometimes we are busy and stressed and need to make food choices that help support our immediate needs for energy and sustenance, with little regard for long-term health. Other times we have time, space, and energy to lovingly prepare home-cooked meals for our family for the whole week. Sometimes we order a pizza, sometimes we eat a salad, sometimes we eat both. Sometimes we eat a little too much birthday cake, other times we pass on the birthday cake. Sometimes we eat past the point of comfortable fullness, other times we don't eat enough and wake up with a rumbling tummy. All of this is intuitive eating, all of this is OK. You decide.

My wish for you is that by this point in the book you feel a million times better about food and body image. But also, if you're not there yet, seriously, don't sweat it. Intuitive eating is a practice; an iterative process that you can go back to as many times as you need to until you have taken what you need from it. The quiz on page 21 can help you identify the areas you might want to focus on (although you probably have a pretty good idea of this on your own). From experience, though, clients tend to think they're doing a lot worse than they really are (remember negativity bias). Remember we're not aiming for perfection here, but flexible, adaptive eating that makes you feel healthy and strong without feeling restricted or deprived.

NOW THE REAL WORK BEGINS

—

So where to now? Now that we're done with diets and body-checking, and restriction and deprivation, what comes next? Here's the part I come clean and level with you. My intention with this book was to help you get your shit together around food, but this was also a massive decoy, because getting your shit together around food is only the beginning of this story and the work that needs to be done. Make no mistake, food and body hang-ups are intentional and deliberate distractions engineered by a capitalist patriarchal society that thrives on insecurity, fabricated inadequacies, and keeping women from realizing their full power.

In this sense, getting your shit together around food is subversive; the patriarchy has weaponized food and our bodies against us under the guise of diet culture, 'wellness', and the beauty and fashion industries. Diet culture wants us to stay oppressed, fearful, consumed, and confused by navigating a system that intentionally shape-shifts and morphs to keep us just subdued and hungry enough not to realize what's going on.

But when we can shake off the ideals and the power that oppress us, only then can we push back against the tyranny, forging new paths, and making way for the real work to begin. The work of social justice and equality. Not just equal pay for white middle-class women, but equal pay for all women. Period. Pay is only one domain where we have work to do; there are countless others. The point here is this, and I'm going to be blunt so please forgive me, but there is way more important shit going on in the world that justifies and deserves our attention, resources, energy, and spirit than worrying about food, and when we look outside of ourselves at the pain and suffering of others around us it can help us gain clarity and perspective on our own hang-ups.

- In the UK one in ten girls have been unable to afford sanitary wear, and one in seven girls have struggled to afford sanitary wear.[2]
- The Trussell Trust, the largest food-bank network in the UK, handed out 1.2 million food packages in 2016/17 compared with around 41,000 food packages in 2009/10.[3]
- We are amidst the biggest refugee crisis since WWII, with over 65.6 million people displaced from their homes in 2016 due to war, violence, and persecution.[4]
- One in eight trans employees have been physically attacked by a colleague or customer in the last year and a quarter have experienced homelessness.[5]
- Socio-economic inequalities are the biggest driver of health disparities with people in the lowest socio-economic groups having a life expectancy seven years shorter than those in the highest socio-economic group. What's more, the richest people in society can enjoy seventeen more years disease/disability free compared to the poorest in society.[6] The World Health Organization has stated that social inequalities in health arise because of inequalities in the conditions of daily life and the fundamental drivers that give rise to them: inequities in power, money, and resources. If we are serious about improving health, we need to get serious about reducing inequality.[7]

Period poverty, homelessness, food inequality, LGBTQIA+ rights, and social inequalities present a fraction of the issues that plague society, and I'm certainly not suggesting that any one individual can take down all that stuff on their own. But imagine if the two-thirds of people on diets in the UK channelled all the energy, strength, grit, and determination usually reserved for dieting, and used it as a force for social change? Collectively, if each of us harnessed even a proportion of that energy into taking action, whether that's online activism, protesting, canvassing for a political party, volunteering with a charity, donating time or money, craftivism, starting a community group, or just helping your neighbour out with their shopping, imagine the ripple effect that would have?

Look, I'm not saying you need to become a martyr or a saint. I want you to live your dreams beyond dieting and exercise. Being free of diet culture means having the space and energy to create a fulfilling life (think about what you can do, what you can achieve, right now, in this body). What I'm saying though, is that if we pull together, we can make real and meaningful changes that not only enrich our lives, but help raise up those most vulnerable in our society, making it more fair and equitable for all of us. That is the real magic in unsubscribing from diet culture and it's time to take our power back.

RESOURCES

MORE ABOUT EATING DISORDERS

Eating disorders are serious mental-health conditions and need to be treated as soon as possible; the longer an ED persists, the longer the treatment time, and the higher the chance of relapse. I usually recommend that if you are concerned about whether you or someone you know has an ED, head to beateatingdisorders.org.uk – BEAT is the UK's leading eating-disorder charity and has lots of great information, resources, and support, as well as advice for how to seek treatment.

Do you have an eating disorder?

SCOFF is an eating-disorder screening tool geared towards screening for anorexia and bulima nervosa; it cannot diagnose an eating disorder, but it can help you identify whether you are at risk and help you decide if you need to get professional support.

Do you make yourself sick because you feel uncomfortably full?

Do you worry you have lost control over how much you eat?

Have you recently lost more than one stone in a three-month period?

Do you believe yourself to be fat when others say you are too thin?

Would you say that food dominates your life?

*One point for every 'yes'; a score of ≥2 indicates a likely case of anorexia nervosa or bulimia

Does someone you know have an eating disorder?

The ED charity, BEAT, has put together this helpful infographic opposite on helping spot EDs.

BEAT also has a great downloadable leaflet that you can bring along with you to your GP to help explain your experiences, and help make sure you get appropriate treatment. It covers common misconceptions GPs may have such as 'your weight isn't low enough' and how to respond and advocate for yourself. Just Google 'BEAT GP leaflet' and it should pop up.

EATING DISORDERS.
KNOW THE FIRST SIGNS?

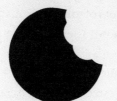

Lips
Are they obsessive
about food?

Flips
Is their behaviour
changing?

Hips
Do they have
distorted beliefs about
their body size?

Kips
Are they often tired
or struggling to
concentrate?

Nips
Do they disappear to the
toilet after meals?

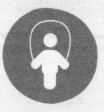

Skips
Have they started
exercising excessively?

If you're worried someone you care about is showing
any signs of an eating disorder – even if they're not on
our list – act quickly and get in touch. We can give you
the answers and support you need to help them on
the road to recovery as soon as possible.

Don't delay. Visitbeateatingdisorder.org.uk/tips

FURTHER READING

If you'd like to do a bit more reading around the topics of body image, non-diet nutrition, and mental health, then consider following some of these Instagram accounts, pick up these books or listen to these podcasts.

Fat and body-positive accounts to follow

These are just a few of the amazing accounts out there so make sure you have a look around and fill your feed up with supportive accounts that leave you feeling better than before you looked at their page!

@bodyposipanda
@iamdaniadriana
@nourishandeat
@scotteeisfat
@notoriouslydapper
@calliethorpe
@nerdabouttown
@glitterandlazers
@scarrednotscared
@bodypositivememes
@amandalacount
@themilitantbaker
@virgietovar
@sonyareneetaylor
@sonnyturner__
@theslumflower
@madeonagenerousplan
@hellostefanienicole
@gabifresh
@ceceolisa
@Mynameisjessamyn
@round_the_way_gal
@nolatrees
@diannebondyyoga
@lousiegreen_bigfitgirl
@gracevictory
@chairbreaker
@the_feeding_of_the_fox

@munroebergdorf
@antidietriotclub
@notplantbased
@kenziebrenna
@florencegiven
@makedaisychains
@rubyetc_
@watchshayslay
@meandmyed.art
@shooglet

INTUITIVE EATING AND WEIGHT-INCLUSIVE NUTRITIONISTS, DIETITIANS, AND THERAPISTS

@reallife_RD
@immaeatthat
@themindfuldietitan
@chrıstyharrison
@marcird
@paigesmathersrd
@alissarumseyrd
@foodpeacedietitian
@hgoodrichrd
@intuitiveeatingrd
@bodyimage_therapist

BOOKS ON BODY IMAGE / FAT ACCEPTANCE

Baker, Jess, *Landwhale: On Turning Insults Into Nicknames, Why Body Image Is Hard, and How Diets Can Kiss My Ass* (Seal Press, 2018)

Baker, Jess, *Things No One Will Tell Fat Girls* (Seal Press, 2015)

Cash, Thomas, *The Body image Workbook: An Eight-Step Program for Learning to Like Your Looks* (2nd Revised Edition: New Harbinger, 2008)

Cooper, Charlotte, *Fat Activism: A Radical Social Movement* (HammerOn Press, 2016)

Crabbe, Megan Jayne, *Body Positive Power: How to stop dieting, make peace with your body and live* (Vermilion, 2017)

Elman, Michelle, *Am I Ugly?* (Anima, 2018)

Harding, Kate and Marianne Kirby, *Lessons From the Fat-O-Sphere: Quit Dieting and Declare a Truce with Your Body* (Tarcherperigee, 2009)

MacLean, Roz, *The Body Book* (Promontory Press Inc., 2017)

Miller, Kelsey, *Big Girl: How I Gave Up Dieting and Got a Life* (Grand Central Publishing, 2016)

Sobczak, Connie, *Embody: Learning to Love Your Unique Body (and quiet that critical voice!)* (Gurze Books, 2014)

Taylor, Sonya Renee, *The Body is Not an Apology: The Power of Radical Self-Love* (Berrett-Koehler Publishers, 2018)

Tovar, Virgie, *You Have the Right to Remain Fat* (Melville House UK, 2018)

Wann, Marilyn, *Fat! So?: Because You Don't Have to Apologise for Your Size* (Ten Speed Press, 1998)

West, Lindsey, *Shrill: Notes from a Loud Woman* (Quercus, 2017)

Wolf, Naomi, *The Beauty Myth: How Images of Beauty Are Used Against Women* (Vintage: 1991)

BOOKS ON HEALTH / NON-DIET NUTRITION / MOVEMENT

Bacon, Linda, and Lucy Aphramor, *Body Respect: What Conventional Health Books Get Wrong, Leave Out, and Just Plain Fail to Understand about Weight* (BenBella Books, 2014)

Bacon, Linda, *Health At Every Size: The Surprising Truth About Your Weight* (BenBella Books, 2010)

Stanley, Jessamyn, *Every Body Yoga* (Workman Publishing, 2017)

Tandoh, Ruby, *Eat Up: Appetite and Eating What You Want* (Serpent's Tail, 2018)

Tribole, Evelyn, and Elyse Resch, *Intuitive Eating: A Revolutionary Program that Works* (Revised ed. Edition: Griffin, 2012)

Tribole, Evelyn, and Elyse Resch, *The Intuitive Eating Workbook: Ten Principles for Nourishing a Healthy Relationship with Food* (New Harbinger, 2017)

Turner, Pixie, *The Wellness Rebel* (Anima, 2018)

Warner, Anthony, *The Angry Chef: Bad Science and the Truth About Healthy Eating* (Oneworld Publications, 2018)

BOOKS ON MENTAL HEALTH

Brotheridge, Chloe, *The Anxiety Solution: A Quieter Mind, a Calmer You* (Michael Joseph, 2017)

Brown, Brené, *The Gifts of Imperfection: Let Go of Who You Think You're Supposed to Be and Embrace Who You Are* (Hazelden FIRM, 2010)

Devon, Natasha, *A Beginner's Guide to Being Mental: An A-Z* (Bluebird, 2018)

Gordon, Bryony, *Mad Girl* (Reprint edition: Headline, 2016)

Haig, Matt, *Reasons to Stay Alive* (Canongate Books Ltd., 2015)

Neff, Kristin, and Christopher Germer, *The Mindful Self-Compassion Workbook: A Proven Way to Accept Yourself, Build Inner Strength, and Thrive* (Guildford Press, 2018)

Van der Kolk, Bessel, *The Body Keeps the Score: Mind, Brain and Body in the Transformation of Trauma* (Penguin, 2015)

Watt, Tessa, *Mindfulness: Your step-by-step guide to a happier life* (Icon Books Ltd., 2015)

NON-DIET / INTUITIVE EATING-FOCUSED PODCASTS

Podcasts are an awesome way to feel supported on your intuitive eating journey – download liberally.

Don't Salt My Game – this is my podcast, come join us!

Body Kindness – Rebecca Scritchfield

Body Love Podcast – Jessi Haggerty

Food Psych – Christy Harrison

Love, Food – Julie Diffy Dillon

Made of Human – Sofie Hagen

Nutrition Matters – Paige Smathers

She's All Fat Pod – April Quioh and Sophia Carter Kahn

The Mindful Dietitian – Fiona Sutherland

REFERENCES

—

INTRODUCTION

1 Zang J, Shen M, Du S, Chen T, Zou S. 'The Association between Dairy Intake and Breast Cancer in Western and Asian Populations: A Systematic Review and Meta-Analysis'. J Breast Cancer [Internet]. Dec 2015 [cited 3 Mar 2018]; 18(4):313. Available from: http://www.ncbi.nlm.nih.gov/pubmed/26770237

2 Bağcı Bosi AT, Çamur D, Güler Ç. 'Prevalence of orthorexia nervosa in resident medical doctors in the faculty of medicine (Ankara, Turkey)'. Appetite [Internet]. Nov 2007 [cited 13 Jan 2018]; 49(3):661–6. Available from: http://www.ncbi.nlm.nih.gov/pubmed/17586085

3 Herranz Valera J, Acuña Ruiz P, Romero Valdespino B, Visioli F. 'Prevalence of orthorexia nervosa among ashtanga yoga practitioners: a pilot study'. Eat Weight Disord - Stud Anorexia, Bulim Obes [Internet]. 23 Dec 2014 [cited 13 Jan 2018]; 19(4):469–72. Available from: http://link.springer.com/10.1007/s40519-014-0131-6

4 Bo S, Zoccali R, Ponzo V, Soldati L, De Carli L, Benso A, et al. 'University courses, eating problems and muscle dysmorphia: are there any associations?' J Transl Med [Internet]. 7 Dec 2014 [cited 29 Jan 2018]; 12(1):221. Available from: http://translational-medicine.biomedcentral.com/articles/10.1186/s12967-014-0221-2

5 Satherley R, Howard R, Higgs S. 'Disordered eating practices in gastrointestinal disorders'. Appetite [Internet]. Jan 2015 [cited 13 Jan 2018]; 84:240–50. Available from: http://www.ncbi.nlm.nih.gov/pubmed/25312748

6 'Disordered Eating or Eating Disorder: What's the Difference?' Psychology Today [Internet]. [cited 13 Jan 2018]. Available from: https://www.psychologytoday.com/blog/contemporary-psychoanalysis-in-action/201402/disordered-eating-or-eating-disorder-what-s-the

7 Survey finds disordered eating behaviors among three out of four American women — UNC School of Medicine [Internet]. [cited 13 Jan 2018]. Available from: http://www.med.unc.edu/www/newsarchive/2008/april/survey-finds-disordered-eating-behaviors-among-three-out-of-four-american-women

8 Neumark-Sztainer D, Wall M, Larson NI, Eisenberg ME, Loth K. 'Dieting and disordered eating behaviors from adolescence to young adulthood: findings from a 10-year longitudinal study'. J Am Diet Assoc [Internet]. Jul 2011 [cited 10 Feb 2018]; 111(7):1004–11. Available from: http://www.ncbi.nlm.nih.gov/pubmed/21703378

9 Bould H, De Stavola B, Lewis G, Micali N. 'Do disordered eating behaviours in girls vary by school characteristics?' A UK cohort study. Eur Child Adolesc Psychiatry [Internet]. 15 Mar 2018 [cited 18 Apr 2018]; 1–9. Available from: http://link.springer.com/10.1007/s00787-018-1133-0

10 Shisslak CM, Crago M, Estes LS. 'The spectrum of eating disturbances'. Int J Eat Disord [Internet]. 1 Nov 1995 [cited 18 Apr 2018]; 18(3):209–19. Available from: http://doi.wiley.com/10.1002/1098-108X%281995%291%2918%3A3%3C209%3AAID-EAT2260180303%3E3.0.CO%3B2-E

11 Tylka TL, Kroon Van Diest AM. 'The Intuitive Eating Scale–2: Item refinement and psychometric evaluation with college women and men'. J Couns Psychol [Internet]. Jan 2013 [cited 5 Jan 2018];

60(1):137–53. Available from: http://www. ncbi.nlm.nih.gov/pubmed/23356469

12 Linardon J, Mitchell S. 'Rigid dietary control, flexible dietary control, and intuitive eating: Evidence for their differential relationship to disordered eating and body-image concerns'. Eat Behav [Internet]. Aug 2017 [cited 14 Sep 2017]; 26:16–22. Available from: http://linkinghub.elsevier.com/retrieve/pii/S147101531630201X

CHAPTER 1

1 'Orthorexia nervosa: Obsessive clean eating "imprisons" sufferers and endangers health, psychologist says'. The *Independent* [Internet]. [cited 15 Jun 2018]. Available from: https://www.independent.co.uk/life-style/health-and-families/orthorexia-nervosa-obsessive-clean-eating-disorder-endangers-health-sufferers-imprisoned-nhs-a7990616.html

2 'Beat Eating Disorders'. Orthorexia - What is Orthorexia [Internet]. 2017 [cited 7 Mar 2018]. Available from: https://www.beateatingdisorders.org.uk/types/orthorexia

3 British Dietetic Association. Top 5 worst celeb diets to avoid in 2017 [Internet]. 2016 [cited 7 Mar 2018]. Available from: https://www.bda.uk.com/news/view?id=153

4 Turner PG, Lefevre CE. 'Instagram use is linked to increased symptoms of orthorexia nervosa'. Eat Weight Disord - Stud Anorexia, Bulim Obes [Internet]. 1 Jun 2017 [cited 18 Jul 2017]; 22(2):277–84. Available from: http://www.ncbi.nlm.nih.gov/pubmed/28251592

5 Dunn TM, Bratman S. 'On orthorexia nervosa: A review of the literature and proposed diagnostic criteria'. Eat Behav [Internet]. Apr 2016 [cited 7 Mar 2018]; 21:11–17. Available from: http://linkinghub.elsevier.com/retrieve/pii/S1471015315300362

6 Stein K. 'Severely Restricted Diets in the Absence of Medical Necessity: The Unintended Consequences'. J Acad Nutr Diet [Internet]. Jul 2014 [cited 8 Mar 2018]; 114(7):986–94. Available from: http://www.ncbi.nlm.nih.gov/pubmed/24731508

7 Turner PG, Lefevre CE. Instagram use is linked to increased symptoms of orthorexia nervosa. Eat Weight Disord - Stud Anorexia, Bulim Obes [Internet]. 1 Jun 2017 [cited 18 Jul 2017]; 22(2):277–84. Available from: http://www.ncbi.nlm.nih.gov/pubmed/28251592

8 Neumark-Sztainer D, Wall M, Larson NI, Eisenberg ME, Loth K. 'Dieting and disordered eating behaviors from adolescence to young adulthood: findings from a 10-year longitudinal study'. J Am Diet Assoc [Internet]. Jul 2011 [cited 10 Feb 2018]; 111(7):1004–11. Available from: http://www.ncbi.nlm.nih.gov/pubmed/21703378

9 Crow S, Eisenberg ME, Story M, Neumark-Sztainer D. 'Psychosocial and behavioral correlates of dieting among overweight and non-overweight adolescents'. J Adolesc Health [Internet]. May 2006 [cited 13 Feb 2018]; 38(5):569–74. Available from: http://linkinghub.elsevier.com/retrieve/pii/S1054139X05002867

10 Shisslak CM, Crago M, Estes LS. 'The spectrum of eating disturbances'. Int J Eat Disord [Internet]. 1 Nov 1995 [cited 18 Apr 2018]; 18(3):209–19. Available from: http://doi.wiley.com/10.1002/1098-108X%281995I

1%2918%3A3%3C209%3A%3AAID-
EAT2260180303%3E3.0.CO%3B2-E

11 Marsh S. 'Eating disorders: NHS
reports surge in hospital admissions'
[Internet]. The *Guardian*. 2018 [cited 20
May 2018]. Available from: https://www.
theguardian.com/society/2018/feb/12/
eating-disorders-nhs-reports-surge-in-
hospital-admissions

12 Marsh S. 'Eating disorders in men rise
by 70% in NHS figures' [Internet]. The
Guardian. 2017 [cited 20 May 2018].
Available from: https://www.theguardian.
com/society/2017/jul/31/eating-disorders-
in-men-rise-by-70-in-nhs-figures

13 Boepple L, Thompson JK. 'A content
analysis of healthy living blogs: Evidence
of content thematically consistent with
dysfunctional eating attitudes and
behaviors'. Int J Eat Disord [Internet].
1 May 2014 [cited 9 Aug 2017]; 47(4):362–7.
Available from: http://doi.wiley.
com/10.1002/eat.22244

14 Turner PG, Lefevre CE. 'Instagram use
is linked to increased symptoms of
orthorexia nervosa'. Eat Weight Disord
- Stud Anorexia, Bulim Obes [Internet].
1 June 2017 [cited 2017 Jul 18]; 22(2):277–84.
Available from: http://www.ncbi.nlm.nih.
gov/pubmed/28251592

15 Mingoia J, Hutchinson AD, Wilson C,
Gleaves DH. 'The Relationship between
Social Networking Site Use and the
Internalization of a Thin Ideal in Females:
A Meta-Analytic Review'. Front Psychol
[Internet]. 2017 [cited 19 Jan 2018]; 8:1351.
Available from: http://www.ncbi.nlm.nih.
gov/pubmed/28824519

16 Fredrickson BL, Roberts TA, Noll SM,
Quinn DM, Twenge JM. 'That swimsuit
becomes you: sex differences in self-

objectification, restrained eating, and
math performance'. J Pers Soc Psychol
[Internet]. Jul 1998 [cited 9 Feb 2018];
75(1):269–84. Available from: http://www.
ncbi.nlm.nih.gov/pubmed/9686464

17 Cohen R, Newton-John T, Slater A.
'Selfie'-objectification: The role of selfies
in self-objectification and disordered
eating in young women'. Comput Human
Behav [Internet]. 1 Feb 2018 [cited 9 Feb
2018]; 79:68–74. Available from: https://
www.sciencedirect.com/science/article/
pii/S0747563217306003?via%3Dihub

18 Fox J, Rooney MC. 'The Dark Triad and
trait self-objectification as predictors of
men's use and self-presentation behaviors
on social networking sites'. Pers Individ
Dif [Internet]. Apr 2015 [cited 26 May
2018]; 76:161–5. Available from: http://
linkinghub.elsevier.com/retrieve/pii/
S0191886914007259

19 McLean SA, Paxton SJ, Wertheim EH,
Masters J. 'Photoshopping the selfie: Self
photo editing and photo investment are
associated with body dissatisfaction in
adolescent girls'. Int J Eat Disord
[Internet]. Dec 2015 [cited 10 Feb 2018];
48(8):1132–40. Available from: http://www.
ncbi.nlm.nih.gov/pubmed/26311205

20 Fredrickson BL, Roberts T-A.
'Objectification Theory: Toward
Understanding Women's Lived
Experiences and Mental Health Risks'.
Psychol Women Q [Internet]. 24 Jun 1997
[cited 9 Feb 2018]; 21(2):173–206. Available
from: http://journals.sagepub.com/
doi/10.1111/j.1471-6402.1997.tb00108.x

21 Fredrickson BL, Roberts TA, Noll SM,
Quinn DM, Twenge JM. 'That swimsuit
becomes you: sex differences in self-
objectification, restrained eating, and
math performance'. J Pers Soc Psychol

[Internet]. Jul 1998 [cited 9 Feb 2018]; 75(1):269–84. Available from: http://www. ncbi.nlm.nih.gov/pubmed/9686464

22 Hebl MR, King EB, Lin J. 'The Swimsuit Becomes Us All: Ethnicity, Gender, and Vulnerability to Self-Objectification'. Personal Soc Psychol Bull [Internet]. 2 Oct 2004 [cited 9 Feb 2018]; 30(10):1322–31. Available from: http:// journals.sagepub.com/ doi/10.1177/0146167204264052

23 Martins Y, Tiggemann M, Kirkbride A. 'Those Speedos Become Them'. Personal Soc Psychol Bull [Internet]. 17 May 2007 [cited 26 May 2018]; 33(5):634–47. Available from: http://journals.sagepub. com/doi/10.1177/0146167206297403

24 Hawkins N, Richards PS, Granley HM, Stein DM. 'The Impact of Exposure to the Thin-Ideal Media Image on Women'. Eat Disord [Internet]. Jan 2004 [cited 19 Jan 2018]; 12(1): 35–50. Available from: http:// www.tandfonline.com/doi/abs/10.1080/ 10640260490267751

25 Ibid

26 Rubinstein S, Caballero B. 'Is Miss America an undernourished role model?' JAMA [Internet]. [cited 20 May 2018]; 283(12):1569. Available from: http://www. ncbi.nlm.nih.gov/pubmed/10735392

27 Mingoia J, Hutchinson AD, Wilson C, Gleaves DH. 'The Relationship between Social Networking Site Use and the Internalization of a Thin Ideal in Females: A Meta-Analytic Review'. Front Psychol [Internet]. 2017 [cited 19 Jan 2018]; 8:1351. Available from: http://www.ncbi.nlm.nih. gov/pubmed/28824519

28 Robinson E, Aveyard P. 'Emaciated mannequins: a study of mannequin body

size in high street fashion stores'. J Eat Disord [Internet]. 2 Dec 2017 [cited 21 Apr 2018]; 5(1):13. Available from: http:// jeatdisord.biomedcentral.com/ articles/10.1186/s40337-017-0142-6

29 Boyce JA, Kuijer RG. 'Focusing on media body ideal images triggers food intake among restrained eaters: A test of restraint theory and the elaboration likelihood model'. Eat Behav [Internet]. 1 Apr 2014 [cited 20 May 2018]; 15(2):262–70. Available from: https://www. sciencedirect.com/science/article/pii/ S1471015314000294?via%3Dihub

30 Hawkins N, Richards PS, Granley HM, Stein DM. 'The Impact of Exposure to the Thin-Ideal Media Image on Women'. Eat Disord [Internet]. Jan 2004 [cited 19 Jan 2018]; 12(1): 35–50. Available from: http:// www.tandfonline.com/doi/abs/10.1080/ 10640260490267751

31 Ibid

32 Mingoia J, Hutchinson AD, Wilson C, Gleaves DH. 'The Relationship between Social Networking Site Use and the Internalization of a Thin Ideal in Females: A Meta-Analytic Review'. Front Psychol [Internet]. 2017 [cited 19 Jan 2018]; 8:1351. Available from: http://www.ncbi.nlm.nih. gov/pubmed/28824519

33 'Weight bias and obesity stigma: considerations for the WHO European Region' (2017) [Internet]. World Health Organization; Oct 2017 Oct [cited 25 Jan 2018]. Available from: http://www.euro. who.int/en/health-topics/ noncommunicable-diseases/obesity/ publications/2017/weight-bias-and-obesity-stigma-considerations-for-the-who-european-region-2017

34 Neumark-Sztainer D, Wall M, Larson NI, Eisenberg ME, Loth K. 'Dieting and disordered eating behaviors from adolescence to young adulthood: findings from a 10-year longitudinal study'. J Am Diet Assoc [Internet]. Jul 2011 [cited 10 Feb 2018]; 111(7):1004–11. Available from: http://www.ncbi.nlm.nih.gov/pubmed/21703378

35 'Weight bias and obesity stigma: considerations for the WHO European Region' (2017) [Internet]. World Health Organization; Oct 2017 Oct [cited 25 Jan 2018]. Available from: http://www.euro.who.int/en/health-topics/noncommunicable-diseases/obesity/publications/2017/weight-bias-and-obesity-stigma-considerations-for-the-who-european-region-2017

36 Hebl MR, King EB, Lin J. 'The Swimsuit Becomes Us All: Ethnicity, Gender, and Vulnerability to Self-Objectification'. Personal Soc Psychol Bull [Internet]. 2 Oct 2004 [cited 9 Feb 2018]; 30(10):1322–31. Available from: http://journals.sagepub.com/doi/10.1177/0146167204264052

37 Ibid

38 Sturgiss E, Jay M, Campbell-Scherer D, van Weel C. 'Challenging assumptions in obesity research'. BMJ [Internet]. 22 Nov 2017 [cited 25 Jan 2018]; 359:j5303. Available from: http://www.ncbi.nlm.nih.gov/pubmed/29167093

39 CSDH. 'Closing the gap in a generation'. [Internet]. 2008 [cited 17 Apr 2018]; 246. Available from: http://apps.who.int/iris/bitstream/handle/10665/43943/9789241563703_eng.pdf;jsessionid=FD7626BD75178D19E3DF93F998BE8848?sequence=1

40 Tarlov AR. 'Public policy frameworks for improving population health'. Ann N Y Acad Sci [Internet]. 1999 [cited 8 Aug 2017]; 896:281–93. Available from: http://www.ncbi.nlm.nih.gov/pubmed/10681904

41 Choi E, Sonin J. 'Determinants of Health' [Internet]. 2016 [cited 31 Jan 2018]. Available from: http://www.goinvo.com/features/determinants-of-health/

42 Crawford R. 'Healthism and the Medicalization of Everyday Life'. Int J Heal Serv [Internet]. Jul 1980 [cited 31 Jan 2018]; 10(3):365–88. Available from: http://journals.sagepub.com/doi/10.2190/3H2H-3XJN-3KAY-G9NY

43 Scrinis G. 'On the Ideology of Nutritionism'. Gastrinomica [Internet]. 2008 [cited 3 Mar 2018]; 8(1):39–48. Available from: http://gyorgyscrinis.com/wp-content/uploads/2013/05/GS-Ideology-of-Nutritionism-Gastronomica.pdf

44 Eckel RH. 'Eggs and beyond: is dietary cholesterol no longer important?' Am J Clin Nutr [Internet]. 1 Aug 2015 [cited 27 Feb 2018]; 102(2):235–6. Available from: https://academic.oup.com/ajcn/article/102/2/235/4614547

45 Jacobs DR, Gross MD, Tapsell LC. 'Food synergy: an operational concept for understanding nutrition'. Am J Clin Nutr [Internet]. 1 May 2009 [cited 3 Mar 2018]; 89(5):1543S–1548S. Available from: http://www.ncbi.nlm.nih.gov/pubmed/19279083

46 Bath S, British Dietetic Association D. Iodine Food Fact Sheet. [cited 27 Feb 2018]. Available from: https://www.bda.uk.com/foodfacts/Iodine.pdf

47 Mintel. 'Brits lose count of their calories: Over a third of Brits don't know

how many calories they consume on a typical day'. Mintel.com [Internet]. [cited 31 Jan 2018]. Available from: http://www. mintel.com/press-centre/food-and-drink/ brits-lose-count-of-their-calories-over-a-third-of-brits-dont-know-how-many-calories-they-consume-on-a-typical-day

48 Berge JM, Winkler MR, Larson N, Miller J, Haynos AF, Neumark-Sztainer D. 'Intergenerational Transmission of Parent Encouragement to Diet From Adolescence Into Adulthood'. Pediatrics [Internet]. 1 Apr 2018 [cited 9 Apr 2018]; 141(4):e20172955. Available from: http:// www.ncbi.nlm.nih.gov/pubmed/29511051

49 Rice K, Prichard I, Tiggemann M, Slater A. 'Exposure to Barbie: Effects on thin-ideal internalisation, body esteem, and body dissatisfaction among young girls'. Body Image [Internet]. 2016 [cited 20 May 2018]; 19:142–9. Available from: https://cfe.keltyeatingdisorders.ca/sites/ default/files/resource/1-s2.0-S1740144516300730-main.pdf

50 Tylka TL, Annunziato RA, Burgard D, Daníelsdóttir S, Shuman E, Davis C, et al. 'The weight-inclusive versus weight-normative approach to health: evaluating the evidence for prioritizing well-being over weight loss'. J Obes [Internet]. 2014 [cited 2017 Jul 18];2014:983495. Available from: http://www.ncbi.nlm.nih.gov/ pubmed/25147734

51 Tribole E, Resch E. Intuitive eating. 3rd ed. St. Martin's Griffin; 2012. 320 p.

52 Linardon J, Mitchell S. 'Rigid dietary control, flexible dietary control, and intuitive eating: Evidence for their differential relationship to disordered eating and body image concerns'. Eat Behav [Internet]. 2017 Aug [cited 2017 Sep 14];26:16–22. Available from: http:// linkinghub.elsevier.com/retrieve/pii/ S147101531630201X

53 Tylka TL, Calogero RM, Daníelsdóttir S. 'Is intuitive eating the same as flexible dietary control? Their links to each other and well-being could provide an answer'. Appetite [Internet]. 2015 Dec [cited 2018 Feb 1];95:166–75. Available from: http:// www.ncbi.nlm.nih.gov/pubmed/26162949

54 Linardon J, Mitchell S. 'Rigid dietary control, flexible dietary control, and intuitive eating: Evidence for their differential relationship to disordered eating and body-image concerns'. Eat Behav [Internet]. Aug 2017 [cited 14 Sep 2017]; 26:16–22. Available from: http:// linkinghub.elsevier.com/retrieve/pii/ S147101531630201X

55 Duarte C, Ferreira C, Pinto-Gouveia J, Trindade IA, Martinho A. 'What makes dietary restraint problematic? Development and validation of the Inflexible Eating Questionnaire'. Appetite [Internet]. 1 Jul 2017 [cited 18 Jul 2017]; 114:146–54. Available from: http://www. ncbi.nlm.nih.gov/pubmed/28347777

56 Schaefer JT, Magnuson AB. 'A Review of Interventions that Promote Eating by Internal Cues'. J Acad Nutr Diet [Internet]. May 2014 [cited 7 Aug 2017]; 114(5):734–60. Available from: http://www. ncbi.nlm.nih.gov/pubmed/24631111

57 Clifford D, Ozier A, Bundros J, Moore J, Kreiser A, Morris MN. 'Impact of Non-Diet Approaches on Attitudes, Behaviors, and Health Outcomes: A Systematic Review'. J Nutr Educ Behav [Internet]. Mar 2015 [cited 20 Nov 2017]; 47(2):143–155.e1. Available from: http:// www.ncbi.nlm.nih.gov/pubmed/25754299

58 Ibid

59 Tribole E, MS R. 'Intuitive Eating: Research Update'. SCAN'S Pulse [Internet]. 2017; 36(3):1–5. Available from: file:///Users/laurathomas/Downloads/Tribole.IntuitiveEatingResearchUpdate. SCAN.2017.pdf

60 Tylka TL, Annunziato RA, Burgard D, Daníelsdóttir S, Shuman E, Davis C, et al. 'The weight-inclusive versus weight-normative approach to health: evaluating the evidence for prioritizing well-being over weight loss'. J Obes [Internet]. 2014 [cited 18 Jul 2017]; 2014:983495. Available from: http://www.ncbi.nlm.nih.gov/pubmed/25147734

61 Dyke N Van, Drinkwater EJ. 'Relationships between intuitive eating and health indicators: literature review'. Public Health Nutr [Internet]. [cited 17 Apr 2018]; 17(8):1757–66. Available from: https://www.cambridge.org/core/services/aop-cambridge-core/content/view/CBC03E81A54FBAAC49B2A8B2EC49631C/S1368980013002139a.pdf/review_article_relationships_between_intuitive_eating_and_health_indicators_literature_review.pdf

62 Tribole E, MS R. 'Intuitive Eating: Research Update' [Internet]. 2017 [cited 25 Sep 2017]. Available from: file:///Users/laurathomas/Downloads/Tribole.IntuitiveEatingResearchUpdate. SCAN.2017.pdf

63 Tribole E, Resch E. *The Intuitive eating workbook: ten principles for nourishing a healthy relationship with food.* New Harbinger; 2017. 244 p.

64 Garfinkel SN, Seth AK, Barrett AB, Suzuki K, Critchley HD. 'Knowing your own heart: Distinguishing interoceptive accuracy from interoceptive awareness'. Biol Psychol [Internet]. 1 Jan 2015 [cited 16 Feb 2018]; 104:65–74. Available from: https://www.sciencedirect.com/science/article/pii/S0301051114002294

65 Haycraft E, Blissett J. 'Predictors of Paternal and Maternal Controlling Feeding Practices with 2- to 5-year-old Children'. J Nutr Educ Behav [Internet]. Sep 2012 [cited 30 Jan 2018]; 44(5):390–7. Available from: http://www.ncbi.nlm.nih.gov/pubmed/21371945

66 Holley CE, Haycraft E, Farrow C. 'Why don't you try it again?' A comparison of parent led, home based interventions aimed at increasing children's consumption of a disliked vegetable. Appetite [Internet]. Apr 2015 [cited 30 Jan]; 87:215–22. Available from: http://www.ncbi.nlm.nih.gov/pubmed/25555540

67 Farrow CV, Haycraft E, Blissett JM. 'Teaching our children when to eat: how parental feeding practices inform the development of emotional eating – a longitudinal experimental design'. Am J Clin Nutr [Internet]. 1 May 2015 [cited 30 Jan 2018]; 101(5):908–13. Available from: http://www.ncbi.nlm.nih.gov/pubmed/25787999

CHAPTER 2

1 '$245 Billion Weight Loss and Weight Management Market, 2017-2022 by Equipment, Surgical Equipment, Diet, and Weight Loss Services'. Markets Insider [Internet]. [cited 12 Feb 2018]. Available from: http://markets.businessinsider.com/news/stocks/245-Billion-Weight-Loss-and-Weight-Management-Market-2017-2022-by-Equipment-Surgical-Equipment-Diet-and-Weight-Loss-Services-1005830884

2 Anderson JW, Konz EC, Frederich RC, Wood CL. 'Long-term weight-loss maintenance: a meta-analysis of US studies'. Am J Clin Nutr [Internet]. Nov 2001 [cited 20 Nov 2017]; 74(5):579–84. Available from: http://www.ncbi.nlm.nih.gov/pubmed/11684524

3 McEvedy SM, Sullivan-Mort G, McLean SA, Pascoe MC, Paxton SJ. 'Ineffectiveness of commercial weight-loss programs for achieving modest but meaningful weight loss: Systematic review and meta-analysis'. J Health Psychol [Internet]. 10 Oct 2017 [cited 1 Feb 2018]; 22(12):1614–27. Available from: http://www.ncbi.nlm.nih.gov/pubmed/28810454

4 Verstuyf J, Patrick H, Vansteenkiste M, Teixeira PJ. 'Motivational dynamics of eating regulation: a self-determination theory perspective'. [cited 13 Dec 2017]. Available from: https://ijbnpa.biomedcentral.com/track/pdf/10.1186/1479-5868-9-21?site=ijbnpa.biomedcentral.com

5 Tylka TL, Annunziato RA, Burgard D, Daníelsdóttir S, Shuman E, Davis C, et al. 'The weight-inclusive versus weight-normative approach to health: evaluating the evidence for prioritizing well-being over weight loss'. J Obes [Internet]. 2014 [cited 18 Jul 2017]; 2014:983495. Available from: http://www.ncbi.nlm.nih.gov/pubmed/25147734

6 Bacon L, Aphramor L, Kuller L, Savage M, Hirsch I, Siegler I, et al. 'Weight Science: Evaluating the Evidence for a Paradigm Shift'. Nutr J [Internet]. 24 Dec 2011 [cited 18 Jul 2017]; 10(1):9. Available from: http://nutritionj.biomedcentral.com/articles/10.1186/1475-2891-10-9

7 Sumithran P, Proietto J. 'The defence of body weight: a physiological basis for weight regain after weight loss'. Clin Sci [Internet]. 1 Feb 2013 [cited 22 Dec 2017]; 124(4):231–41. Available from: http://clinsci.org/lookup/doi/10.1042/CS20120223

8 Johannsen DL, Knuth ND, Huizenga R, Rood JC, Ravussin E, Hall KD. 'Metabolic Slowing with Massive Weight Loss despite Preservation of Fat-Free Mass'. J Clin Endocrinol Metab [Internet]. Jul 2012 [cited 1 Feb 2018]; 97(7):2489–96. Available from: http://www.ncbi.nlm.nih.gov/pubmed/22535969

9 Fothergill E, Guo J, Howard L, Kerns JC, Knuth ND, Brychta R, et al. 'Persistent metabolic adaptation 6 years after The Biggest Loser competition'. Obesity [Internet]. Aug 2016 [cited 5 Sep 2017]; 24(8):1612–9. Available from: http://doi.wiley.com/10.1002/oby.21538

10 Rosenbaum M, Kissileff HR, Mayer LES, Hirsch J, Leibel RL. 'Energy intake in weight-reduced humans'. Brain Res [Internet]. 2 Sep 2010 [cited 8 Feb 2018]; 1350:95–102. Available from: http://www.ncbi.nlm.nih.gov/pubmed/20595050

11 Tomiyama AJ, Mann T, Vinas D, Hunger JM, Dejager J, Taylor SE. 'Low calorie dieting increases cortisol'. Psychosom Med [Internet]. May 2010 [cited 1 Feb 2018]; 72(4):357–64. Available from: http://www.ncbi.nlm.nih.gov/pubmed/20368473

12 Nakamura Y, Walker BR, Ikuta T. 'Systematic review and meta-analysis reveals acutely elevated plasma cortisol following fasting but not less severe calorie restriction'. Stress [Internet]. 3 Mar 2016 [cited 1 Feb 2018]; 19(2):151–7. Available from: http://www.tandfonline.com/doi/full/10.3109/10253890.2015.1121984

13 Sumithran P, Proietto J. 'The defence of body weight: a physiological basis for weight regain after weight loss'. Clin Sci [Internet]. 1 Feb 2013 [cited 22 Dec 2017]; 124(4):231–41. Available from: http://clinsci.org/lookup/doi/10.1042/CS20120223

14 Johannsen DL, Knuth ND, Huizenga R, Rood JC, Ravussin E, Hall KD. 'Metabolic Slowing with Massive Weight Loss despite Preservation of Fat-Free Mass'. J Clin Endocrinol Metab [Internet]. Jul 2012 [cited 1 Feb 2018]; 97(7):2489–96. Available from: http://www.ncbi.nlm.nih.gov/pubmed/22535969

15 Dulloo AG, Montani J-P. 'Pathways from dieting to weight regain, to obesity and to the metabolic syndrome: an overview'. Obes Rev [Internet]. 1 Feb 2015 [cited 19 Sep 2017]; 16(S1):1–6. Available from: http://doi.wiley.com/10.1111/obr.12250

16 Tylka TL, Annunziato RA, Burgard D, Daníelsdóttir S, Shuman E, Davis C, et al. 'The weight-inclusive versus weight-normative approach to health: evaluating the evidence for prioritizing well-being over weight loss'. J Obes [Internet]. 2014 [cited 18 Jul 2017]; 2014:983495. Available from: http://www.ncbi.nlm.nih.gov/pubmed/25147734

17 Cereda E, Malavazos AE, Caccialanza R, Rondanelli M, Fatati G, Barichella M. 'Weight cycling is associated with body weight excess and abdominal fat accumulation: A cross-sectional study'. Clin Nutr [Internet]. Dec 2011 [cited 13 Jun 2018]; 30(6):718–23. Available from: http://www.ncbi.nlm.nih.gov/pubmed/21764186

18 Aphramor, L. A. 'Stages of Change Perpective to Diet, Non-Diet and Health Gain Approaches for Weight Concerns' Netw. Health Digest (2017 May); 124:20–26)

19 Seimon RV, Roekenes JA, Zibellini J, Zhu B, Gibson AA, Hills AP, et al. 'Do intermittent diets provide physiological benefits over continuous diets for weight loss? A systematic review of clinical trials'. Mol Cell Endocrinol [Internet]. Dec 2015 [cited 25 Apr 2018]; 418:153–72. Available from: http://linkinghub.elsevier.com/retrieve/pii/S0303720715300800

20 Zdrojewicz Z, Popowicz E, Szyca M, Michalik T, Śmieszniak B. 'TOFI phenotype – its effect on the occurrence of diabetes'. Pediatr Endocrinol Diabetes Metab [Internet]. 2017 [cited 13 Jun 2018]; 23(2):96–100. Available from: http://www.ncbi.nlm.nih.gov/pubmed/29073292

21 Anderson JW, Konz EC, Frederich RC, Wood CL. 'Long-term weight-loss maintenance: a meta-analysis of US studies'. Am J Clin Nutr [Internet]. Nov 2001 [cited 20 Nov 2017]; 74(5):579–84. Available from: http://www.ncbi.nlm.nih.gov/pubmed/11684524

22 Ibid

23 McEvedy SM, Sullivan-Mort G, McLean SA, Pascoe MC, Paxton SJ. 'Ineffectiveness of commercial weight-loss programs for achieving modest but meaningful weight loss: Systematic review and meta-analysis'. J Health Psychol [Internet]. 10 Oct 2017 [cited 1 Feb 2018]; 22(12):1614–27. Available from: http://www.ncbi.nlm.nih.gov/pubmed/28810454

24 Ibid

25 Fothergill E, Guo J, Howard L, Kerns JC, Knuth ND, Brychta R, et al. 'Persistent metabolic adaptation 6 years after The

Biggest Loser competition'. Obesity [Internet]. Aug 2016 [cited 5 Sep 2017]; 24(8):1612–19. Available from: http://doi.wiley.com/10.1002/oby.21538

26 '6 Years after The Biggest Loser, Metabolism Is Slower and Weight Is Back Up'. Scientific American [Internet]. [cited 12 Feb 2018]. Available from: https://www.scientificamerican.com/article/6-years-after-the-biggest-loser-metabolism-is-slower-and-weight-is-back-up/

27 Rosenbaum M, Kissileff HR, Mayer LES, Hirsch J, Leibel RL. 'Energy intake in weight-reduced humans'. Brain Res [Internet]. 2 Sep 2010 [cited 8 Feb 2018]; 1350:95–102. Available from: http://www.ncbi.nlm.nih.gov/pubmed/20595050

28 Kalm LM, Semba RD. 'They starved so that others be better fed: remembering Ancel Keys and the Minnesota experiment'. J Nutr [Internet]. Jun 2005 [cited 5 Sep 2017]; 135(6):1347–52. Available from: http://www.ncbi.nlm.nih.gov/pubmed/15930436

29 Johannsen DL, Knuth ND, Huizenga R, Rood JC, Ravussin E, Hall KD. 'Metabolic Slowing with Massive Weight Loss despite Preservation of Fat-Free Mass'. J Clin Endocrinol Metab [Internet]. Jul 2012 [cited 1 Feb 2018]; 97(7):2489–96. Available from: http://www.ncbi.nlm.nih.gov/pubmed/22535969

30 Fothergill E, Guo J, Howard L, Kerns JC, Knuth ND, Brychta R, et al. 'Persistent metabolic adaptation 6 years after 'The Biggest Loser' competition'. Obesity [Internet]. Aug 2016 [cited 5 Sep 2017]; 24(8):1612–19. Available from: http://doi.wiley.com/10.1002/oby.21538

31 Rosenbaum M, Kissileff HR, Mayer LES, Hirsch J, Leibel RL. 'Energy intake in

weight-reduced humans'. Brain Res [Internet]. 2 Sep 2010 [cited 8 Feb 2018]; 1350:95–102. Available from: http://www.ncbi.nlm.nih.gov/pubmed/20595050

32 Perello M, Sakata I, Birnbaum S, Chuang J-C, Osborne-Lawrence S, Rovinsky SA, et al. 'Ghrelin increases the rewarding value of high-fat diet in an orexin-dependent manner'. Biol Psychiatry [Internet]. 1 May 2010 [cited 22 Dec 2017]; 67(9):880–6. Available from: http://www.ncbi.nlm.nih.gov/pubmed/20034618

33 Challet E, Piggins HD, Yan L, Blasiak A, Gundlach AL, Hess G, et al. 'Interactions of Circadian Rhythmicity, Stress and Orexigenic Neuropeptide Systems: Implications for Food Intake Control'. Front Neurosci Artic Front Neurosci [Internet]. 2017 [cited 13 Sep 2017]; 11(11). Available from: https://www.ncbi.nlm.nih.gov/pmc/articles/PMC5357634/pdf/fnins-11-00127.pdf

34 Sohn J-W. 'Network of hypothalamic neurons that control appetite'. BMB Rep [Internet]. Apr 2015 [cited 4 Jan 2018]; 48(4):229–33. Available from: http://www.ncbi.nlm.nih.gov/pubmed/25560696

35 Sobrino Crespo C, Perianes Cachero A, Puebla Jiménez L, Barrios V, Arilla Ferreiro E. 'Peptides and Food Intake'. Front Endocrinol (Lausanne) [Internet]. 24 Apr 2014 [cited 4 Jan 2018]; 5:58. Available from: http://journal.frontiersin.org/article/10.3389/fendo.2014.00058/abstract

36 Beck B. Neuropeptide Y in normal eating and in genetic and dietary-induced obesity. Philos Trans R Soc Lond B Biol Sci [Internet]. 29 July 2006 [cited 13 Aug 2017]; 361(1471):1159–85. Available from:

http://www.ncbi.nlm.nih.gov/
pubmed/16874931

37 Smith KJ, Deschênes SS, Schmitz N.
'Investigating the longitudinal association
between diabetes and anxiety: a
systematic review and meta-analysis'.
Diabet Med [Internet]. 25 Mar 2018 [cited
13 Apr 2018]; Available from: http://doi.
wiley.com/10.1111/dme.13606

CHAPTER 3

1 Neff K, Germer C. 'Oxford Handbook of
Compassion Science' [Internet]. Doty J,
editor. Oxford University Press; 2017
[cited 13 Feb 2018]. Available from: http://
self-compassion.org/wp-content/
uploads/2017/09/Neff.Germer.2017.pdf

2 Braun TD, Park CL, Gorin A. 'Self-
compassion, body image, and disordered
eating: A review of the literature'. Body
Image [Internet]. 2016 [cited 12 Feb 2018];
17:117–31. Available from: http://self-
compassion.org/wp-content/
uploads/2016/06/Braun_2016.pdf

3 Slater A, Varsani N, Diedrichs PC.
'#fitspo or #loveyourself? The impact of
fitspiration and self-compassion
Instagram images on women's body
image, self-compassion, and mood'. Body
Image [Internet]. Sep 2017 [cited 27 Aug
2017]; 22:87–96. Available from: http://
www.ncbi.nlm.nih.gov/pubmed/28689104

4 Braun TD, Park CL, Gorin A. 'Self-
compassion, body image, and disordered
eating: A review of the literature'. Body
Image [Internet]. 2016 [cited 12 Feb 2018];
17:117–31. Available from: http://self-
compassion.org/wp-content/
uploads/2016/06/Braun_2016.pdf

5 Slater A, Varsani N, Diedrichs PC.
'#fitspo or #loveyourself? The impact of

fitspiration and self-compassion
Instagram images on women's body
image, self-compassion, and mood'. Body
Image [Internet]. Sep 2017 [cited 27 Aug
2017]; 22:87–96. Available from: http://
www.ncbi.nlm.nih.gov/pubmed/28689104

6 Albertson ER, Neff KD, Dill-
Shackleford KE. 'Self-Compassion and
Body Dissatisfaction in Women: A
Randomized Controlled Trial of a Brief
Meditation Intervention'. [cited 13 Feb
2018]. Available from: http://self-
compassion.org/wp-content/uploads/
publications/AlbertsonBodyImage.pdf

7 Fothergill E, Guo J, Howard L, Kerns JC,
Knuth ND, Brychta R, et al. 'Persistent
metabolic adaptation 6 years after The
Biggest Loser competition'. Obesity
[Internet]. Aug 2016 [cited 5 Sep 2017];
24(8):1612–19. Available from: http://doi.
wiley.com/10.1002/oby.21538

8 Adams CE, Leary MR. 'Promoting Self–
Compassionate Attitudes Toward Eating
Among Restrictive and Guilty Eaters'. J
Soc Clin Psychol [Internet]. Dec 2007
[cited 14 Feb 2018]; 26(10):1120–44.
Available from: http://guilfordjournals.
com/doi/10.1521/jscp.2007.26.10.1120

9 Rodriguez MA, Xu W, Wang X, Liu X.
'Self-Acceptance Mediates the
Relationship between Mindfulness and
Perceived Stress'. Psychol Rep [Internet].
Apr 2015 [cited 13 Feb 2018]; 116(2):513–22.
Available from: http://journals.sagepub.
com/doi/10.2466/07.PR0.116k19w4

10 'Issues – Oxford Mindfulness Centre'
[Internet]. [cited 15 Feb 2018]. Available
from: http://oxfordmindfulness.org/
for-you/issues-landing-page/

11 Beck D. *My feet aren't ugly: a girl's guide to loving herself from the inside out*; Beaufort Books; 2007.

CHAPTER 4

1 Zhang Q, Wang Y. 'Socioeconomic inequality of obesity in the United States: do gender, age, and ethnicity matter?' Soc Sci Med [Internet]. Mar 2004 [cited 9 Aug 2017]; 58(6):1171–80. Available from: http://www.ncbi.nlm.nih.gov/pubmed/14723911

2 Maclean PS, Bergouignan A, Cornier M-A, Jackman MR. 'Biology's response to dieting: the impetus for weight regain'. Am J Physiol Regul Integr Comp Physiol [Internet]. 2011 Sep [cited 2018 Jul 7];301(3):R581-600. Available from: http://www.physiology.org/doi/10.1152/ajpregu.00755.2010

3 Perello M, Sakata I, Birnbaum S, Chuang J-C, Osborne-Lawrence S, Rovinsky SA, et al. 'Ghrelin increases the rewarding value of high-fat diet in an orexin-dependent manner'. Biol Psychiatry [Internet]. 1 May 2010 [cited 22 Dec 2017]; 67(9):880–6. Available from: http://www.ncbi.nlm.nih.gov/pubmed/20034618

4 Sobrino Crespo C, Perianes Cachero A, Puebla Jiménez L, Barrios V, Arilla Ferreiro E. 'Peptides and Food Intake. Front Endocrinol' (Lausanne) [Internet]. 24 Apr 2014 [cited 4 Jan 2018]; 5:58. Available from: http://journal.frontiersin.org/article/10.3389/fendo.2014.00058/abstract

5 Jakubowicz D, Froy O, Wainstein J, Boaz M. 'Meal timing and composition influence ghrelin levels, appetite scores and weight loss maintenance in overweight and obese adults'. Steroids [Internet]. Mar 2012 [cited 12 Aug 2017];

77(4):323–31. Available from: http://linkinghub.elsevier.com/retrieve/pii/S0039128X11003515

6 Cummings DE, Weigle DS, Frayo RS, Breen PA, Ma MK, Dellinger EP, et al. 'Plasma Ghrelin Levels after Diet-Induced Weight Loss or Gastric Bypass Surgery'. N Engl J Med [Internet]. 2002 May 23 [cited 2018 Jun 15];346(21):1623–30. Available from: http://www.nejm.org/doi/abs/10.1056/NEJMoa012908

7 Ibid

8 Coutinho SR, Rehfeld JF, Holst JJ, Kulseng B, Martins C. 'Impact of weight loss achieved through a multidisciplinary intervention on appetite in patients with severe obesity'. Am J Physiol Metab [Internet]. 23 Jan 2018 [cited 28 May 2018]; ajpendo.00322.2017. Available from: http://www.ncbi.nlm.nih.gov/pubmed/29360396

9 Challet E, Piggins HD, Yan L, Blasiak A, Gundlach AL, Hess G, et al. 'Interactions of Circadian Rhythmicity, Stress and Orexigenic Neuropeptide Systems: Implications for Food Intake Control'. Front Neurosci Artic Front Neurosci [Internet]. 2017 [cited 13 Sep 2017]; 11(11). Available from: https://www.ncbi.nlm.nih.gov/pmc/articles/PMC5357634/pdf/fnins-11-00127.pdf

10 Wang J, Akabayashi A, Dourmashkin J, Yu HJ, Alexander JT, Chae HJ, et al. 'Neuropeptide Y in relation to carbohydrate intake, corticosterone and dietary obesity'. Brain Res [Internet]. 17 Aug 1998 [cited 27 Feb 2018]; 802(1–2):75–88. Available from: http://www.ncbi.nlm.nih.gov/pubmed/9748512

11 Sohn J-W. Network of hypothalamic neurons that control appetite. BMB Rep

[Internet]. Apr 2015 [cited 4 Jan 2018];
48(4):229–33. Available from: http://www.
ncbi.nlm.nih.gov/pubmed/25560696

12 Sobrino Crespo C, Perianes Cachero A,
Puebla Jiménez L, Barrios V, Arilla
Ferreiro E. 'Peptides and Food Intake'.
Front Endocrinol (Lausanne) [Internet].
24 Apr 2014 [cited 4 Jan 2018]; 5:58.
Available from: http://journal.frontiersin.
org/article/10.3389/fendo.2014.00058/
abstract

13 Beck B. 'Neuropeptide Y in normal
eating and in genetic and dietary-induced
obesity'. Philos Trans R Soc Lond B Biol
Sci [Internet]. 29 Jul 2006 [cited 13 Aug
2017]; 361(1471):1159–85. Available from:
http://www.ncbi.nlm.nih.gov/
pubmed/16874931

14 Fulton S, Woodside B, Shizgal P.
'Does neuropeptide Y contribute to the
modulation of brain stimulation reward
by chronic food restriction?' Behav Brain
Res [Internet]. Aug 2002 [cited 22 Dec
2017]; 134(1–2):157–64. Available from:
http://linkinghub.elsevier.com/retrieve/
pii/S0166432801004697

15 Ciampolini M, Lovell-Smith D,
Bianchi R, de Pont B, Sifone M, van
Weeren M, et al. 'Sustained Self-
Regulation of Energy Intake: Initial
Hunger Improves Insulin Sensitivity'.
J Nutr Metab [Internet]. 2010
[cited 27 Aug 2017]; 2010:1–7. Available
from: http://www.ncbi.nlm.nih.gov/
pubmed/20721291

16 Schaefer JT, Magnuson AB. 'A Review
of Interventions that Promote Eating by
Internal Cues'. J Acad Nutr Diet
[Internet]. May 2014 [cited 7 Aug 2017];
114(5):734–60. Available from: http://www.
ncbi.nlm.nih.gov/pubmed/24631111

17 Miller CK, Kristeller JL, Headings A,
Nagaraja H. 'Comparison of a mindful
eating intervention to a diabetes
self-management intervention among
adults with type 2 diabetes: a randomized
controlled trial'. Health Educ Behav
[Internet]. Apr 2014 [cited 25 Jul 2017];
41(2):145–54. Available from: http://www.
ncbi.nlm.nih.gov/pubmed/23855018

18 El Madden C, Leong SL, Gray A,
Horwath CC. 'Eating in response to
hunger and satiety signals is related to
BMI in a nationwide sample of 1601
mid-age New Zealand women'. Public
Health Nutr [Internet]. [cited 20 Jul 2017];
15(12):2272–9. Available from: https://pdfs.
semanticscholar.org/d7e0/851335
f147a33445143d1caeb07970f4e13f.pdf

19 Ciampolini M, Lovell-Smith D,
Bianchi R, de Pont B, Sifone M, van
Weeren M, et al. 'Sustained self-regulation
of energy intake: initial hunger improves
insulin sensitivity'. J Nutr Metab
[Internet]. 22 Jun 2010 [cited 13 Aug 2017].
Available from: http://www.ncbi.nlm.nih.
gov/pubmed/20721291

20 Garfinkel SN, Seth AK, Barrett AB,
Suzuki K, Critchley HD. Knowing your
own heart: Distinguishing interoceptive
accuracy from interoceptive awareness.
Biol Psychol [Internet]. 2015 Jan 1 [cited
2018 Feb 16]; 104:65–74. Available from:
https://www.sciencedirect.com/science/
article/pii/S0301051114002294

21 Tylka TL, Kroon Van Diest AM. 'The
Intuitive Eating Scale–2: Item refinement
and psychometric evaluation with college
women and men'. J Couns Psychol
[Internet]. Jan 2013 [cited 5 Jan 2018];
60(1):137–53. Available from: http://www.
ncbi.nlm.nih.gov/pubmed/23356469

22 Holt SH, Miller JC, Petocz P, Farmakalidis E. 'A satiety index of common foods'. Eur J Clin Nutr [Internet]. Sep 1995 [cited 19 Feb 2018]; 49(9):675–90. Available from: http://www.ncbi.nlm.nih.gov/pubmed/7498104

23 Pross N, Demazières A, Girard N, Barnouin R, Santoro F, Chevillotte E, et al. 'Influence of progressive fluid restriction on mood and physiological markers of dehydration in women'. Br J Nutr [Internet]. 28 Jan 2013 [cited 5 Jul 2017]; 109(2):313–21. Available from: http://www.ncbi.nlm.nih.gov/pubmed/22716932

CHAPTER 5

1 Stunkard AJ, Harris JR, Pedersen NL, McClearn GE. 'The Body-Mass Index of Twins Who Have Been Reared Apart'. N Engl J Med [Internet]. 24 May 1990 [cited 29 Jan 2018]; 322(21):1483–7. Available from: http://www.nejm.org/doi/abs/10.1056/NEJM199005243222102

2 Speakman JR, Levitsky DA, Allison DB, Bray MS, de Castro JM, Clegg DJ, et al. 'Set points, settling points and some alternative models: theoretical options to understand how genes and environments combine to regulate body adiposity'. Dis Model Mech [Internet]. Nov 2011 [cited 10 Feb 2018]; 4(6):733–45. Available from: http://www.ncbi.nlm.nih.gov/pubmed/22065844

3 Müller M, Bosy-Westphal A, Heymsfield SB. 'Is there evidence for a set point that regulates human body weight?' F1000 Med Rep [Internet]. 9 Aug 2010 [cited 10 Feb 2018]; 2:59. Available from: http://www.ncbi.nlm.nih.gov/pubmed/21173874

4 Yu Y-H, Vasselli JR, Zhang Y, Mechanick JI, Korner J, Peterli R.

'Metabolic vs. hedonic obesity: a conceptual distinction and its clinical implications'. Obes Rev [Internet]. Mar 2015 [cited 10 Feb 2018]; 16(3):234–47. Available from: http://www.ncbi.nlm.nih.gov/pubmed/25588316

5 Sandra Aamodt: Why dieting doesn't usually work. TED Talk. TED.com [Internet] [cited 8 Feb 2018]. Available from: https://www.ted.com/talks/sandra_aamodt_why_dieting_doesn_t_usually_work

6 Rosenbaum M, Kissileff HR, Mayer LES, Hirsch J, Leibel RL. 'Energy intake in weight-reduced humans'. Brain Res [Internet]. 2 Sep 2010 [cited 8 Feb 2018]; 1350:95–102. Available from: http://www.ncbi.nlm.nih.gov/pubmed/20595050

7 Chhabra KH, Adams JM, Jones GL, Yamashita M, Schlapschy M, Skerra A, et al. 'Reprogramming the body weight set point by a reciprocal interaction of hypothalamic leptin sensitivity and Pomc gene expression reverts extreme obesity'. Mol Metab [Internet]. 2016 Oct 1 [cited 2018 Jul 9];5(10):869–81. Available from: https://www.sciencedirect.com/science/article/pii/S2212877816301144?via%3Dihub#bib12

8 Ravussin Y, Gutman R, Diano S, Shanabrough M, Borok E, Sarman B, et al. 'Effects of chronic weight perturbation on energy homeostasis and brain structure in mice'. Am J Physiol Integr Comp Physiol [Internet]. 2011 Jun [cited 2018 Jul 9]; 300(6):R1352–62. Available from: http://www.physiology.org/doi/10.1152/ajpregu.00429.2010

9 Rosenbaum M, Leibel RL. '20 years of leptin: role of leptin in energy homeostasis in humans'. J Endocrinol [Internet]. 2014 Oct 1 [cited 2018 Jul

9];223(1):T83-96. Available from: http://www.ncbi.nlm.nih.gov/pubmed/25063755

10 Strohacker K, Carpenter KC, McFarlin BK. 'Consequences of Weight Cycling: An Increase in Disease Risk?' Int J Exerc Sci [Internet]. 2009 [cited 2018 Jul 9]; 2(3):191–201. Available from: http://www.ncbi.nlm.nih.gov/pubmed/25429313

11 Mehta T, Smith DL, Muhammad J, Casazza K, Casazza K. 'Impact of weight cycling on risk of morbidity and mortality'. Obes Rev [Internet]. 2014 Nov [cited 2018 Jul 9]; 15(11):870–81. Available from: http://www.ncbi.nlm.nih.gov/pubmed/25263568

12 Montani J-P, Viecelli AK, Prévot A, Dulloo AG. 'Weight cycling during growth and beyond as a risk factor for later cardiovascular diseases: the 'repeated overshoot' theory'. Int J Obes [Internet]. 2006 Dec 28 [cited 2018 Jul 9]; 30(S4):S58–66. Available from: http://www.nature.com/articles/0803520

13 Tribole E, Resch E. Intuitive Eating. 3rd ed. St. Martin's Griffin; 2012. 320 p.

14 Myers A, Rosen JC. 'Obesity stigmatization and coping: relation to mental health symptoms, body image, and self-esteem'. Int J Obes Relat Metab Disord [Internet]. Mar 1999 [cited 27 Feb 2018]; 23(3):221–30. Available from: http://www.ncbi.nlm.nih.gov/pubmed/10193866

15 'Spurious Correlations' [Internet]. [cited 28 May 2018]. Available from: http://www.tylervigen.com/spurious-correlations

16 O'Hara L, Taylor J. 'What's Wrong With the 'War on Obesity?' A Narrative Review of the Weight-Centered Health Paradigm and Development of the 3C Framework to Build Critical Competency for a Paradigm Shift'. SAGE Open [Internet]. 16 Apr 2018 [cited 28 May 2018]; 8(2):2158244018772288. Available from: http://journals.sagepub.com/doi/10.1177/2158244018772888

17 'Weight bias and obesity stigma: considerations for the WHO European Region' (2017) [Internet]. World Health Organization; Oct 2017 [cited 25 Jan 2018]. Available from: http://www.euro.who.int/en/health-topics/noncommunicable-diseases/obesity/publications/2017/weight-bias-and-obesity-stigma-considerations-for-the-who-european-region-2017

18 Swift JA, Hanlon S, El-Redy L, Puhl RM, Glazebrook C. 'Weight bias among UK trainee dietitians, doctors, nurses and nutritionists'. J Hum Nutr Diet [Internet]. Aug 2013 [cited 18 Jul 2017]; 26(4):395–402. Available from: http://www.ncbi.nlm.nih.gov/pubmed/23171227

19 Tylka TL, Annunziato RA, Burgard D, Daníelsdóttir S, Shuman E, Davis C, et al. 'The weight-inclusive versus weight-normative approach to health: evaluating the evidence for prioritizing well-being over weight loss'. J Obes [Internet]. 2014 [cited 18 Jul 2017]; 2014:983495. Available from: http://www.ncbi.nlm.nih.gov/pubmed/25147734

20 Schwartz MB, Chambliss HO, Brownell KD, Blair SN, Billington C. 'Weight Bias among Health Professionals Specializing in Obesity'. Obes Res [Internet]. Sep 2003 [cited 25 Jan 2018];11(9):1033–9. Available from: http://www.ncbi.nlm.nih.gov/pubmed/12972672

21 Lozano-Sufrategui L, Sparkes AC, McKenna J. Weighty: NICE's Not-So-Nice Words. Front Psychol [Internet]. 2016 [cited 18 Jul 2017]; 7:1919. Available from:

http://www.ncbi.nlm.nih.gov/
pubmed/27999560

22 Ramos Salas X. 'The ineffectiveness
and unintended consequences of the
public health war on obesity'. Can J Public
Health [Internet]. 3 Feb 2015 [cited 20
Nov 2017]; 106(2):e79-81. Available from:
http://www.ncbi.nlm.nih.gov/
pubmed/25955676

23 Major B, Hunger JM, Bunyan DP,
Miller CT. 'The ironic effects of weight
stigma'. J Exp Soc Psychol [Internet]. Mar
2014 [cited 18 Jul 2017]; 51:74–80. Available
from: http://linkinghub.elsevier.com/
retrieve/pii/S0022103113002047

24 Brewis, A. A. (2014) 'Stigma and the
perpetuation of obesity', Social Science &
Medicine, 118, pp. 152–158. doi: 10.1016/j.
socscimed.2014.08.003.

25 Levy BR, Pilver CE. 'Residual stigma:
psychological distress among the formerly
overweight'. Soc Sci Med [Internet]. Jul
2012 [cited 18 Jul 2017]; 75(2):297-9.
Available from: http://www.ncbi.nlm.nih.
gov/pubmed/22560867

26 Vadiveloo M, Mattei J. 'Perceived
Weight Discrimination and 10-Year Risk
of Allostatic Load Among US Adults'. Ann
Behav Med [Internet]. 23 Feb 2017 [cited
18 Jul 2017]; 51(1):94–104. Available from:
http://www.ncbi.nlm.nih.gov/
pubmed/27553775

27 Andreyeva T, Puhl RM, Brownell KD.
'Changes in Perceived Weight
Discrimination Among Americans,
1995–1996 Through 2004–2006'. Obesity
[Internet]. 28 May 2008 [cited 25 Jan
2018]; 16(5):1129–34. Available from: http://
www.ncbi.nlm.nih.gov/pubmed/18356847

28 'Weight bias and obesity stigma:
considerations for the WHO European
Region' (2017) [Internet]. World Health
Organization; Oct 2017 [cited 25 Jan 2018].
Available from: http://www.euro.who.int/
en/health-topics/noncommunicable-
diseases/obesity/publications/2017/
weight-bias-and-obesity-stigma-
considerations-for-the-who-european-
region-2017

29 Pearl RL, Wadden TA, Hopkins CM,
Shaw JA, Hayes MR, Bakizada ZM, et al.
'Association between weight bias
internalization and metabolic syndrome
among treatment-seeking individuals
with obesity. Obesity' [Internet]. Feb 2017
[cited 25 Jan 2018]; 25(2):317–22. Available
from: http://doi.wiley.com/10.1002/
oby.21716

30 Vadiveloo M, Mattei J. 'Perceived
Weight Discrimination and 10-Year Risk
of Allostatic Load Among US Adults'. Ann
Behav Med [Internet]. 23 Feb 2017 [cited
18 Jul 2017]; 51(1):94–104. Available from:
http://www.ncbi.nlm.nih.gov/
pubmed/27553775

31 'Weight bias and obesity stigma:
considerations for the WHO European
Region' (2017) [Internet]. World Health
Organization; Oct 2017 [cited 25 Jan 2018].
Available from: http://www.euro.who.int/
en/health-topics/noncommunicable-
diseases/obesity/publications/2017/
weight-bias-and-obesity-stigma-
considerations-for-the-who-european-
region-2017

32 Sturgiss E, Jay M, Campbell-Scherer D,
van Weel C. 'Challenging assumptions in
obesity research'. BMJ [Internet]. 22 Nov
2017 [cited 25 Jan 2018]; 359:j5303.
Available from: http://www.ncbi.nlm.nih.
gov/pubmed/29167093

33 Ikeda J, Amy NK, Ernsberger P, Gaesser GA, Berg FM, Clark CA, et al. 'The National Weight Control Registry: a critique'. J Nutr Educ Behav [Internet]. [cited 8 Aug 2017]; 37(4):203–5. Available from: http://www.ncbi.nlm.nih.gov/pubmed/16029691

34 Anderson JW, Konz EC, Frederich RC, Wood CL. 'Long-term weight-loss maintenance: a meta-analysis of US studies'. Am J Clin Nutr [Internet]. Nov 2001 [cited 20 Nov 2017]; 74(5):579–84. Available from: http://www.ncbi.nlm.nih.gov/pubmed/11684524

35 McEvedy SM, Sullivan-Mort G, McLean SA, Pascoe MC, Paxton SJ. 'Ineffectiveness of commercial weight-loss programs for achieving modest but meaningful weight loss: Systematic review and meta-analysis'. J Health Psychol [Internet]. 10 Oct 2017 [cited 1 Feb 2018]; 22(12):1614–27. Available from: http://www.ncbi.nlm.nih.gov/pubmed/28810454

36 Johannsen DL, Knuth ND, Huizenga R, Rood JC, Ravussin E, Hall KD. 'Metabolic Slowing with Massive Weight Loss despite Preservation of Fat-Free Mass'. J Clin Endocrinol Metab [Internet]. Jul 2012 [cited 1 Feb 2018]; 97(7):2489–96. Available from: http://www.ncbi.nlm.nih.gov/pubmed/22535969

37 Grodstein F, Levine R, Troy L, Spencer T, Colditz GA, Stampfer MJ. 'Three-year follow-up of participants in a commercial weight loss program. Can you keep it off?' Arch Intern Med [Internet]. 24 Jun 1996 [cited 8 Aug 2017]; 156(12):1302–6. Available from: http://www.ncbi.nlm.nih.gov/pubmed/8651838

38 Mehta T, Smith DL, Muhammad J, Casazza K, Casazza K. 'Impact of weight cycling on risk of morbidity and mortality'. Obes Rev [Internet]. Nov 2014 [cited 19 Sep 2017]; 15(11):870–81. Available from: http://www.ncbi.nlm.nih.gov/pubmed/25263568

39 Montani J-P, Schutz Y, Dulloo AG. 'Dieting and weight cycling as risk factors for cardiometabolic diseases: who is really at risk?' Obes Rev [Internet]. Feb 2015 [cited 8 Aug 2017]; 16:7–18. Available from: http://doi.wiley.com/10.1111/obr.12251

40 Beavers KM, Neiberg RH, Houston DK, Bray GA, Hill JO, Jakicic JM, et al. 'Body Weight Dynamics Following Intentional Weight Loss and Physical Performance: The Look AHEAD Movement and Memory Study'. Obes Sci Pract [Internet]. Oct 2015 [cited 19 Sep 2017]; 1(1):12–22. Available from: http://www.ncbi.nlm.nih.gov/pubmed/27453790

41 Madigan CD, Pavey T, Daley AJ, Jolly K, Brown WJ. 'Is weight cycling associated with adverse health outcomes? A cohort study'. Prev Med (Baltim) [Internet]. Mar 2018 [cited 8 Mar 2018]; 108:47–52. Available from: http://linkinghub.elsevier.com/retrieve/pii/S0091743517304966

42 Brownell KD, Greenwood MRC, Stellar E, Shrager EE. 'The effects of repeated cycles of weight loss and regain in rats'. Physiol Behav [Internet]. 1 Oct 1986 [cited 8 Mar 2018]; 38(4):459–64. Available from: https://www.sciencedirect.com/science/article/abs/pii/0031938486904117

43 Tylka TL, Annunziato RA, Burgard D, Daníelsdóttir S, Shuman E, Davis C, et al. 'The weight-inclusive versus weight-normative approach to health: evaluating the evidence for prioritizing well-being over weight loss'. J Obes [Internet]. 2014 [cited 18 Jul 2017]; 2014:983495. Available from: http://www.ncbi.nlm.nih.gov/pubmed/25147734

44 Flegal KM, Kit BK, Orpana H, Graubard BI. 'Association of all-cause mortality with overweight and obesity using standard body mass index categories: a systematic review and meta-analysis'. JAMA [Internet]. 2 Jan 2013 [cited 29 Jan 2018]; 309(1):71–82. Available from: http://jama.jamanetwork.com/article.aspx?doi=10.1001/jama.2012.113905

45 Benatti F, Solis M, Artioli G, Montag E, Painelli V, Saito F, et al. 'Liposuction Induces a Compensatory Increase of Visceral Fat Which Is Effectively Counteracted by Physical Activity: A Randomized Trial'. J Clin Endocrinol Metab [Internet]. Jul 2012 [cited 8 Feb 2018]; 97(7):2388–95. Available from: http://www.ncbi.nlm.nih.gov/pubmed/22539589

46 Klein S, Fontana L, Young VL, Coggan AR, Kilo C, Patterson BW, et al. 'Absence of an Effect of Liposuction on Insulin Action and Risk Factors for Coronary Heart Disease'. N Engl J Med [Internet]. 17 Jun 2004 [cited 8 Feb 2018]; 350(25):2549–57. Available from: http://www.ncbi.nlm.nih.gov/pubmed/15201411

47 Matheson EM, King DE, Everett CJ. 'Healthy Lifestyle Habits and Mortality in Overweight and Obese Individuals'. J Am Board Fam Med [Internet]. 1 Jan 2012 [cited 8 Feb 2018]; 25(1):9–15. Available from: http://www.ncbi.nlm.nih.gov/pubmed/22218619

48 Gaesser GA, Angadi SS, Sawyer BJ. 'Exercise and Diet, Independent of Weight Loss, Improve Cardiometabolic Risk Profile in Overweight and Obese Individuals'. Phys Sportsmed [Internet]. 13 May 2011 [cited 4 Mar 2018]; 39(2):87–97. Available from: http://www.ncbi.nlm.nih.gov/pubmed/21673488

49 Fogelholm M. 'Physical activity, fitness and fatness: relations to mortality, morbidity and disease risk factors'. A systematic review. Obes Rev [Internet]. Mar 2010 [cited 14 Jun 2018]; 11(3):202–21. Available from: http://www.ncbi.nlm.nih.gov/pubmed/19744231

50 Messier V, Malita FM, Rabasa-Lhoret R, Brochu M, Karelis AD. 'Association of cardiorespiratory fitness with insulin sensitivity in overweight and obese postmenopausal women: a Montreal Ottawa New Emerging Team study'. Metabolism [Internet]. Sep 2008 [cited 4 Mar 2018]; 57(9):1293–8. Available from: http://www.ncbi.nlm.nih.gov/pubmed/18702957

51 Velho S, Paccaud F, Waeber G, Vollenweider P, Marques-Vidal P. 'Metabolically healthy obesity: different prevalences using different criteria'. Eur J Clin Nutr [Internet]. 14 Oct 2010 [cited 4 Mar 2018]; 64(10):1043–51. Available from: http://www.ncbi.nlm.nih.gov/pubmed/20628408

52 Abd El-Kader SM. 'Aerobic versus resistance exercise training in modulation of insulin resistance, adipocytokines and inflammatory cytokine levels in obese type 2 diabetic patients'. J Adv Res [Internet]. 1 Apr 2011 [cited 14 Jun 2018]; 2(2):179–83. Available from: https://www.sciencedirect.com/science/article/pii/S2090123210001104

53 Olver I. 'It's all relative: how to understand cancer risk' [Internet]. The Conversation. 2016 [cited 2018 Jul 7]. Available from: https://theconversation.com/its-all-relative-how-to-understand-cancer-risk-55494

54 Lozano-Sufrategui L, Sparkes AC, McKenna J. 'Weighty: NICE's Not-So-Nice

Words. Front Psychol' [Internet]. 2016 [cited 18 Jul 2017]; 7:1919. Available from: http://www.ncbi.nlm.nih.gov/pubmed/27999560

55 Ramos Salas X. 'The ineffectiveness and unintended consequences of the public health war on obesity'. Can J Public Health [Internet]. 3 Feb 2015 [cited 20 Nov 2017]; 106(2):e79-81. Available from: http://www.ncbi.nlm.nih.gov/pubmed/25955676

56 Carbonneau E, Bégin C, Lemieux S, Mongeau L, Paquette M-C, Turcotte M, et al. 'A Health at Every Size® intervention improves intuitive eating and diet quality in Canadian women'. Clin Nutr [Internet]. Jun 2017 [cited 4 Mar 2018]; 36(3):747-54. Available from: http://www.ncbi.nlm.nih.gov/pubmed/27378611

57 Provencher V, Bégin C, Tremblay A, Mongeau L, Corneau L, Dodin S, et al. 'Health-At-Every-Size and Eating Behaviors: 1-Year Follow-Up Results of a Size Acceptance Intervention'. J Am Diet Assoc [Internet]. Nov 2009 [cited 18 Jul 2017]; 109(11):1854-61. Available from: http://www.ncbi.nlm.nih.gov/pubmed/19857626

58 Bacon L, Stern JS, Van Loan MD, Keim NL. 'Size Acceptance and Intuitive Eating Improve Health for Obese, Female Chronic Dieters'. J Am Diet Assoc [Internet]. Jun 2005 [cited 25 Jul 2017]; 105(6):929-36. Available from: http://www.ncbi.nlm.nih.gov/pubmed/15942543

59 Bacon L, Keim NL, Van Loan MD, Derricote M, Gale B, Kazaks A, et al. 'True'. Int J Obes [Internet]. 30 May 2002 [cited 8 Aug 2017]; 26(6):854-65. Available from: http://www.ncbi.nlm.nih.gov/pubmed/12037657

60 Carroll S, Borkoles E, Polman R. 'Short-term effects of a non-dieting lifestyle intervention program on weight management, fitness, metabolic risk, and psychological well-being in obese premenopausal females with the metabolic syndrome'. Appl Physiol Nutr Metab [Internet]. Feb 2007 [cited 4 Mar 2018]; 32(1):125-42. Available from: http://www.ncbi.nlm.nih.gov/pubmed/17332789

61 Ibid

62 Ibid

63 Gaesser GA, Angadi SS, Sawyer BJ. 'Exercise and Diet, Independent of Weight Loss, Improve Cardiometabolic Risk Profile in Overweight and Obese Individuals'. Phys Sportsmed [Internet]. 13 May 2011 [cited 4 Mar 2018]; 39(2):87-97. Available from: http://www.ncbi.nlm.nih.gov/pubmed/21673488

64 Messier V, Malita FM, Rabasa-Lhoret R, Brochu M, Karelis AD. 'Association of cardiorespiratory fitness with insulin sensitivity in overweight and obese postmenopausal women: a Montreal Ottawa New Emerging Team study'. Metabolism [Internet]. Sep 2008 [cited 4 Mar 2018]; 57(9):1293-8. Available from: http://www.ncbi.nlm.nih.gov/pubmed/18702957

65 Velho S, Paccaud F, Waeber G, Vollenweider P, Marques-Vidal P. 'Metabolically healthy obesity: different prevalences using different criteria'. Eur J Clin Nutr [Internet]. 14 Oct 2010 [cited 4 Mar 2018]; 64(10):1043-51. Available from: http://www.ncbi.nlm.nih.gov/pubmed/20628408

66 Association for Size Diversity and Health. 'HAES® Principles' [Internet]. [cited 4 Mar 2018]. Available from: https://

www.sizediversityandhealth.org/content.
asp?id=76

CHAPTER 6

1 Verstuyf J, Patrick H, Vansteenkiste M,
Teixeira PJ. 'Motivational dynamics of
eating regulation: a self-determination
theory perspective'. [cited 13 Dec 2017].
Available from: https://ijbnpa.
biomedcentral.com/track/
pdf/10.1186/1479-5868-9-21?site=ijbnpa.
biomedcentral.com

2 Ibid

3 Shah AK, Shafir E, Mullainathan S.
'Scarcity Frames Value'. Psychol Sci
[Internet]. 12 Apr 2015 [cited 10 Apr 2018];
26(4):402–12. Available from: http://www.
ncbi.nlm.nih.gov/pubmed/25676256

4 Shah AK, Mullainathan S, Shafir E.
'Some Consequences of Having Too Little'.
Science (80-) [Internet]. 2 Nov 2012 [cited
10 Apr 2018]; 338(6107):682–5. Available
from: http://www.sciencemag.org/cgi/
doi/10.1126/science.1222426

5 Polivy J, Herman CP. 'Distress and
eating: why do dieters overeat?' Int J Eat
Disord [Internet]. Sep 1999 [cited 5 Jan
2018]; 26(2):153–64. Available from: http://
www.ncbi.nlm.nih.gov/pubmed/10422604

6 Verstuyf J, Patrick H, Vansteenkiste M,
Teixeira PJ. 'Motivational dynamics of
eating regulation: a self-determination
theory perspective'. [cited 13 Dec 2017].
Available from: https://ijbnpa.
biomedcentral.com/track/
pdf/10.1186/1479-5868-9-21?site=ijbnpa.
biomedcentral.com

7 Tylka TL, Kroon Van Diest AM. 'The
Intuitive Eating Scale–2: Item refinement
and psychometric evaluation with college

women and men'. J Couns Psychol
[Internet]. Jan 2013 [cited 5 Jan 2018];
60(1):137–53. Available from: http://www.
ncbi.nlm.nih.gov/pubmed/23356469

8 Polivy J, Herman CP. 'Distress and
eating: why do dieters overeat?' Int J Eat
Disord [Internet]. Sep 1999 [cited 5 Jan
2018]; 26(2):153–64. Available from: http://
www.ncbi.nlm.nih.gov/pubmed/10422604

9 Tarlov AR. 'Public policy frameworks
for improving population health'. Ann N
Y Acad Sci [Internet]. 1999 [cited 8 Aug
2017]; 896:281–93. Available from: http://
www.ncbi.nlm.nih.gov/pubmed/
10681904

10 Kristeller JL, Wolever RQ.
'Mindfulness-Based Eating Awareness
Training for Treating Binge Eating
Disorder: The Conceptual Foundation'. Eat
Disord [Internet]. 28 Dec 2010 [cited 13
Jun 2018]; 19(1):49–61. Available from:
http://www.ncbi.nlm.nih.gov/
pubmed/21181579

11 Epstein LH, Carr KA, Cavanaugh MD,
Paluch RA, Bouton ME. 'Long-term
habituation to food in obese and
nonobese women'. Am J Clin Nutr
[Internet]. 1 Aug 2011 [cited 7 Feb 2018];
94(2):371–6. Available from: http://www.
ncbi.nlm.nih.gov/pubmed/21593492

12 Ibid

13 Turner PG, Lefevre CE. 'Instagram use
is linked to increased symptoms of
orthorexia nervosa'. Eat Weight Disord
– Stud Anorexia, Bulim Obes [Internet]. 1
Jun 2017 [cited 18 Jul 2017]; 22(2):277–84.
Available from: http://www.ncbi.nlm.nih.
gov/pubmed/28251592

14 Dunn TM, Bratman S. 'On orthorexia
nervosa: A review of the literature and

proposed diagnostic criteria'. Eat Behav [Internet]. Apr 2016 [cited 7 Mar 2018]; 21:11–17. Available from: http://linkinghub. elsevier.com/retrieve/pii/ S1471015315300362

15 Tremelling K, Sandon L, Vega GL, McAdams CJ. 'Orthorexia Nervosa and Eating Disorder Symptoms in Registered Dietitian Nutritionists in the United States'. J Acad Nutr Diet [Internet]. 1 Oct 2017 [cited 13 Jan 2018]; 117(10):1612–17. Available from: http://www.ncbi.nlm.nih. gov/pubmed/28624376

CHAPTER 7

1 Westwater ML, Fletcher PC, Ziauddeen H. 'Sugar addiction: the state of the science'. Eur J Nutr [Internet]. Nov 2016 [cited 14 Jun 2018]; 55(Suppl 2):55–69. Available from: http://www.ncbi.nlm.nih. gov/pubmed/27372453

2 Gearhardt AN, White MA, Potenza MN. 'Binge eating disorder and food addiction'. Curr Drug Abuse Rev [Internet]. Sep 2011 [cited 13 Dec 2017]; 4(3):201–7. Available from: http://www.ncbi.nlm.nih.gov/ pubmed/21999695

3 Lebwohl B, Cao Y, Zong G, Hu FB, Green PHR, Neugut AI, et al. 'Long term gluten consumption in adults without celiac disease and risk of coronary heart disease: prospective cohort study'. BMJ [Internet]. 2 May 2017 [cited 14 Jun 2018]; j1892. Available from: http://www.bmj. com/lookup/doi/10.1136/bmj.j1892

4 Sanz Y. 'Effects of a gluten-free diet on gut microbiota and immune function in healthy adult humans'. Gut Microbes [Internet]. 27 May 2010 [cited 14 Jun 2018]; 1(3):135–7. Available from: http:// www.ncbi.nlm.nih.gov/pubmed/21327021

5 De Palma G, Nadal I, Collado MC, Sanz Y. 'Effects of a gluten-free diet on gut microbiota and immune function in healthy adult human subjects'. Br J Nutr [Internet]. 18 Oct 2009 [cited 14 Jun 2018]; 102(08):1154. Available from: http:// www.ncbi.nlm.nih.gov/pubmed/19445821

6 European Commission – PRESS RELEASES – Press release – 'Questions and Answers on Food Additives' [Internet]. [cited 13 Jun 2018]. Available from: http://europa.eu/rapid/press-release_MEMO-11-783_en.htm

7 Ibid

8 Larsson MO, Sloth Nielsen V, Bjerre N, Laporte F, Cedergreen N. 'Refined assessment and perspectives on the cumulative risk resulting from the dietary exposure to pesticide residues in the Danish population'. Food Chem Toxicol [Internet]. Jan 2018 [cited 13 Apr 2018]; 111:207–67. Available from: http://www. ncbi.nlm.nih.gov/pubmed/29155356

9 Barański M, Rempelos L, Iversen PO, Leifert C. 'Effects of organic food consumption on human health; the jury is still out!' Food Nutr Res [Internet]. 6 Jan 2017 [cited 7 May 2018]; 61(1):1287333. Available from: http:// foodandnutritionresearch.net/index.php/ fnr/article/view/1154

10 Zipfel S, Sammet I, Rapps N, Herzog W, Herpertz S, Martens U. 'Gastrointestinal disturbances in eating disorders: clinical and neurobiological aspects'. Auton Neurosci [Internet]. 2006 Oct 30 [cited 2018 Oct 2];129(1–2):99–106. Available from: http://www.ncbi.nlm.nih.gov/ pubmed/16962383

11 De Palma G, Nadal I, Collado MC, Sanz Y. 'Effects of a gluten-free diet on gut microbiota and immune function in healthy adult human subjects'. Br J Nutr [Internet]. 2009 Oct 18 [cited 2018 Jun 14];102(08):1154. Available from: http://www.ncbi.nlm.nih.gov/pubmed/19445821

12 Levinovitz A. *The gluten lie: and other myths about what you eat.* Regan Arts; 2015. 272 p.

13 Ibid

14 Vernia P, Di Camillo M, Foglietta T, Avallone VE, De Carolis A. 'Diagnosis of lactose intolerance and the "nocebo" effect: The role of negative expectations'. Dig Liver Dis [Internet]. Sep 2010 [cited 6 Mar 2018]; 42(9):616–19. Available from: http://www.ncbi.nlm.nih.gov/pubmed/20227928

15 Levinovitz A. *The gluten lie: and other myths about what you eat.* Regan Arts; 2015. 272 p.

16 Mönnikes H, Tebbe JJ, Hildebrandt M, Arck P, Osmanoglou E, Rose M, et al. 'Role of Stress in Functional Gastrointestinal Disorders'. Dig Dis [Internet]. 2001 [cited 26 Feb 2018]; 19(3):201–11. Available from: http://www.ncbi.nlm.nih.gov/pubmed/11752838

17 Zernicke KA, Campbell TS, Blustein PK, Fung TS, Johnson JA, Bacon SL, et al. 'Mindfulness-Based Stress Reduction for the Treatment of Irritable Bowel Syndrome Symptoms: A Randomized Wait-list Controlled Trial'. Int J Behav Med [Internet]. 23 Sep 2013 [cited 7 May 2018]; 20(3):385–96. Available from: http://www.ncbi.nlm.nih.gov/pubmed/22618308

18 Peters SL, Yao CK, Philpott H, Yelland GW, Muir JG, Gibson PR. 'Randomised clinical trial: the efficacy of gut-directed hypnotherapy is similar to that of the low FODMAP diet for the treatment of irritable bowel syndrome'. Aliment Pharmacol Ther [Internet]. 1 Sep 2016 [cited 15 Jan 2018]; 44(5):447–59. Available from: http://doi.wiley.com/10.1111/apt.13706

19 Kavuri V, Raghuram N, Malamud A, Selvan SR. 'Irritable Bowel Syndrome: Yoga as Remedial Therapy'. Evidence-Based Complement Altern Med [Internet]. 2015 [cited 26 Feb 2018]; 2015:1–10. Available from: http://www.ncbi.nlm.nih.gov/pubmed/26064164

20 Moayyedi P, Ford AC, Talley NJ, Cremonini F, Foxx-Orenstein AE, Brandt LJ, et al. 'The efficacy of probiotics in the treatment of irritable bowel syndrome: a systematic review'. Gut [Internet]. 1 Mar 2010 [cited 18 Jun 2018]; 59(3):325–32. Available from: http://www.ncbi.nlm.nih.gov/pubmed/19091823

21 Irritable bowel syndrome in adults: diagnosis and management | Guidance and guidelines | NICE. [cited 2018 Oct 2]; Available from: https://www.nice.org.uk/guidance/cg61/chapter/1-Recommendations#dietary-and-lifestyle-advice

22 Howard S, Adams J, White M. 'Nutritional content of supermarket ready meals and recipes by television chefs in the United Kingdom: cross sectional study'. BMJ [Internet]. 14 Dec 2012 [cited 8 May 2018]; 345:e7607. Available from: http://www.ncbi.nlm.nih.gov/pubmed/23247976

23 Fiolet T, Srour B, Sellem L, Kesse-Guyot E, Allès B, Méjean C, et al. 'Consumption of ultra-processed foods and cancer risk: results from NutriNet-Santé prospective cohort'. BMJ [Internet]. 14 Feb 2018 [cited 7 May 2018]; 360:k322.

Available from: http://www.ncbi.nlm.nih.
gov/pubmed/29444771

24 BBC News. 'Ultra-processed foods
"linked to cancer"' [Internet]. [cited 7 May
2018]. Available from: http://www.bbc.
co.uk/news/health-43064290

CHAPTER 8

1 Williams M, Teasdale J, Segal Z,
Kabat-Zinn J. 'The Mindful Way through
Depression: Freeing Yourself from
Chronic Unhappiness' [Internet]. New
York: Guildford Press; 2007 [cited 18 Jun
2018]. Available from: http://
innovationecosystem.com/wp-content/
uploads/2017/02/Eating-One-Raisin2.pdf

CHAPTER 9

1 Crujeiras AB, Goyenechea E, Abete I,
Lage M, Carreira MC, Martínez JA, et al.
'Weight Regain after a Diet-Induced
Loss Is Predicted by Higher Baseline
Leptin and Lower Ghrelin Plasma Levels'.
J Clin Endocrinol Metab [Internet].
Nov 2010 Nov [cited 15 Jun 2018];
95(11):5037–44. Available from: http://
www.ncbi.nlm.nih.gov/pubmed/
20719836

2 Cella F, Adami G, Giordano G, Cordera
R. 'Effects of dietary restriction on serum
leptin concentration in obese women'. Int
J Obes [Internet]. 26 May 1999 [cited 15
Jun 2018]; 23(5):494–7. Available from:
http://www.nature.com/articles/0800847

CHAPTER 10

1 Espeset EMS, Gulliksen KS, Nordbø
RHS, Skårderud F, Holte A. 'The Link
Between Negative Emotions and Eating
Disorder Behaviour in Patients with
Anorexia Nervosa'. Eur Eat Disord Rev
[Internet]. Nov 2012 [cited 13 Jun 2018];

20(6):451–60. Available from: http://doi.
wiley.com/10.1002/erv.2183

2 Lavis A. 'Careful Starving: Reflections
on (Not) Eating, Caring and Anorexia'. In:
Abbots E-J, Lavis A, Attala L, editors.
Careful Eating: Bodies, Food and Care
[Internet]. 2015 [cited 13 Jun 2018].
p. 91–108. Available from: http://pure-oai.
bham.ac.uk/ws/files/22017582/Careful_
Starving_Final_Pre_pub.pdf

3 Chart adapted from: Cook-Cottone CP,
Guyker WM. 'The Development and
Validation of the Mindful Self-Care Scale
(MSCS): an Assessment of Practices that
Support Positive Embodiment'.
Mindfulness (N Y) [Internet]. 3 Feb 2018
[cited 20 Feb 2018]; 9(1):161–75. Available
from: http://link.springer.com/10.1007/
s12671-017-0759-1

4 Ibid

5 Irish LA, Kline CE, Gunn HE, Buysse
DJ, Hall MH. 'The role of sleep hygiene
in promoting public health: A review of
empirical evidence'. Sleep Med Rev
[Internet]. Aug 2015 [cited 20 Feb 2018];
22:23–36. Available from: http://
linkinghub.elsevier.com/retrieve/pii/
S1087079214001002

6 Sleep Statistics – Latest Research &
Data | American Sleep Assoc [Internet].
[cited 28 May 2018]. Available from:
https://www.sleepassociation.org/
about-sleep/sleep-statistics/

7 Irish LA, Kline CE, Gunn HE, Buysse
DJ, Hall MH. 'The role of sleep hygiene
in promoting public health: A review of
empirical evidence'. Sleep Med Rev
[Internet]. Aug 2015 [cited 21 Feb
2018];22:23–36. Available from: http://
www.ncbi.nlm.nih.gov/pubmed/25454674

8 Emotions Word Wheel reproduced with kind permission from Geoffrey Roberts.

9 Tribole E, Resch E. *The Intuitive eating workbook: ten principles for nourishing a healthy relationship with food.* New Harbinger; 2017. 244 p.

10 Garfinkel SN, Seth AK, Barrett AB, Suzuki K, Critchley HD. 'Knowing your own heart: Distinguishing interoceptive accuracy from interoceptive awareness'. Biol Psychol [Internet]. 1 Jan 2015 [cited 16 Feb 2018]; 104:65–74. Available from: https://www.sciencedirect.com/science/article/pii/S0301051114002294

CHAPTER 11

1 Hausenblas HA, Schreiber K, Smoliga JM. 'Addiction to exercise'. BMJ [Internet]. 26 Apr 2017 [cited 22 Feb 2018]; 357:j1745. Available from: http://www.ncbi.nlm.nih.gov/pubmed/28446435

2 Griffiths MD, Szabo A, Terry A. 'The exercise addiction inventory: a quick and easy screening tool for health practitioners'. Br J Sport Med [Internet]. 2005 [cited 24 Feb 2018]; 39. Available from: http://www.bjsportmed.com/cgi/content/full/39/6/e30

3 Hausenblas HA, Schreiber K, Smoliga JM. 'Addiction to exercise'. BMJ [Internet]. 26 Apr 2017 [cited 22 Feb 2018]; 357:j1745. Available from: http://www.ncbi.nlm.nih.gov/pubmed/28446435

4 Segar M, Spruijt-Metz D, Nolen-Hoeksema S. 'Go Figure? Body-Shape Motives are Associated with Decreased Physical Activity Participation Among Midlife Women'. Sex Roles [Internet]. Feb 2006 [cited 22 Feb 2018]; 54(3–4):175–87. Available from: http://link.springer.com/10.1007/s11199-006-9336-5

5 Segar ML, Eccles JS, Richardson CR. 'Type of Physical Activity Goal Influences Participation in Healthy Midlife Women'. Women's Health Issues [Internet]. Jul 2008 [cited 5 Mar 2018]; 18(4):281–91. Available from: http://www.ncbi.nlm.nih.gov/pubmed/18468920

6 Public Health England. 'Health matters: getting every adult active every day – GOV.UK' [Internet]. GOV.UK. [cited 14 Apr 2018]. Available from: https://www.gov.uk/government/publications/health-matters-getting-every-adult-active-every-day/health-matters-getting-every-adult-active-every-day

7 Jeukendrup A. 'LCHF diets and performance in elite athletes' [Internet]. [cited 28 May 2018]. Available from: http://www.mysportscience.com/single-post/2016/12/26/LCHF-diets-and-performance-in-elite-athletes

8 Burke LM, Ross ML, Garvican-Lewis LA, Welvaert M, Heikura IA, Forbes SG, et al. 'Low carbohydrate, high fat diet impairs exercise economy and negates the performance benefit from intensified training in elite race walkers'. J Physiol [Internet]. 1 May 2017 [cited 15 Jun 2018]; 595(9):2785–807. Available from: http://www.ncbi.nlm.nih.gov/pubmed/28012184

9 Burke LM, Hawley JA, Wong SHS, Jeukendrup AE. 'Carbohydrates for training and competition'. J Sports Sci [Internet]. 9 Jan 2011 [cited 14 Apr 2018]; 29(sup1):S17–27. Available from: https://www.tandfonline.com/doi/full/10.1080/02640414.2011.585473

10 Gaesser GA, Angadi SS, Sawyer BJ. 'Exercise and Diet, Independent of Weight Loss, Improve Cardiometabolic Risk Profile in Overweight and Obese Individuals'. Phys Sportsmed [Internet].

13 May 2011 [cited 22 Mar 2018]; 39(2):87–97. Available from: http://www.tandfonline.com/doi/full/10.3810/psm.2011.05.1898

11 Public Health England. 'Health matters: getting every adult active every day – GOV.UK' [Internet]. GOV.UK. [cited 14 Apr 2018]. Available from: https://www.gov.uk/government/publications/health-matters-getting-every-adult-active-every-day/health-matters-getting-every-adult-active-every-day

12 Gaesser GA, Angadi SS, Sawyer BJ. 'Exercise and Diet, Independent of Weight Loss, Improve Cardiometabolic Risk Profile in Overweight and Obese Individuals'. Phys Sportsmed [Internet]. 13 May 2011 [cited 22 Mar 2018]; 39(2):87–97. Available from: http://www.tandfonline.com/doi/full/10.3810/psm.2011.05.1898

13 Charansonney OL, Després J-P. 'Disease prevention – should we target obesity or sedentary lifestyle?' Nat Rev Cardiol [Internet]. 25 Aug 2010 [cited 22 Mar 2018]; 7(8):468–72. Available from: http://www.nature.com/articles/nrcardio.2010.68

14 Hajizadeh Maleki B, Tartibian B, Mooren FC, FitzGerald LZ, Krüger K, Chehrazi M, et al. 'Low-to-moderate intensity aerobic exercise training modulates irritable bowel syndrome through antioxidative and inflammatory mechanisms in women: Results of a randomized controlled trial'. Cytokine [Internet]. 1 Feb 2018 [cited 14 Apr 2018]; 102:18–25. Available from: https://www.sciencedirect.com/science/article/abs/pii/S1043466617303873

15 Charansonney OL, Després J-P. 'Disease prevention – should we target obesity or sedentary lifestyle?' Nat Rev Cardiol [Internet]. 25 Aug 2010 [cited 22 Mar 2018]; 7(8):468–72. Available from: http://www.nature.com/articles/nrcardio.2010.68

16 Do K, Brown RE, Wharton S, Ardern CI, Kuk JL. 'Association between cardiorespiratory fitness and metabolic risk factors in a population with mild to severe obesity'. BMC Obes [Internet]. 31 Dec 2018 [cited 14 Feb 2018]; 5(1):5. Available from: https://bmcobes.biomedcentral.com/articles/10.1186/s40608-018-0183-7

CHAPTER 12

1 Geissler C and Powers H. (eds) Human Nutrition: Twelfth Edition 2011, Churchill Livingston (pub).

2 SACN. 'Carbohydrates and Health'. 2015 [cited 14 May 2018]; Available from: https://assets.publishing.service.gov.uk/government/uploads/system/uploads/attachment_data/file/445503/SACN_Carbohydrates_and_Health.pdf

3 Geissler C and Powers H. (eds) Human Nutrition: Twelfth Edition 2011, Churchill Livingston (pub).

4 Ibid

5 Ibid

6 Zong G, Li Y, Wanders AJ, Alssema M, Zock PL, Willett WC, et al. 'Intake of individual saturated fatty acids and risk of coronary heart disease in US men and women: two prospective longitudinal cohort studies'. BMJ [Internet]. 23 Nov 2016 [cited 17 Apr 2018]; 355:i5796. Available from: http://www.ncbi.nlm.nih.gov/pubmed/27881409

7 Hooper L, Martin N, Abdelhamid A, Davey Smith G. 'Reduction in saturated fat intake for cardiovascular disease'. Cochrane Database Syst Rev [Internet]. 10 Jun 2015 [cited 17 Apr 2018]; Available from: http://doi.wiley. com/10.1002/14651858.CD011737

8 Chart reproduced with permission of the authors. Full reference: Hart, S. et al. (2018) 'Development of the "Recovery from Eating Disorders for Life" Food Guide (REAL Food Guide) – a food pyramid for adults with an eating disorder.' Journal of Eating Disorders. BioMed Central, 6, p. 6. doi: 10.1186/s40337-018-0192-4.

9 Zhang Y-J, Gan R-Y, Li S, Zhou Y, Li A-N, Xu D-P, et al. 'Antioxidant Phytochemicals for the Prevention and Treatment of Chronic Diseases'. Molecules [Internet]. 27 Nov 2015 [cited 28 Jan 2018]; 20(12):21138–56. Available from: http://www.mdpi.com/1420-3049/20/12/19753

10 Dias JS. 'Nutritional Quality and Health Benefits of Vegetables: A Review'. Food Nutr Sci [Internet]. 2012 [cited 29 Jan 2018]; 3:1354–74. Available from: http://dx.doi.org/10.4236/fns.2012.310179

11 Leoncini E, Nedovic D, Panic N, Pastorino R, Edefonti V, Boccia S. 'Carotenoid Intake from Natural Sources and Head and Neck Cancer: A Systematic Review and Meta-analysis of Epidemiological Studies'. Cancer Epidemiol Biomarkers Prev [Internet]. 1 Jul 2015 [cited 15 Jun 2018]; 24(7):1003–11. Available from: http://www.ncbi.nlm.nih.gov/pubmed/25873578

12 Nicastro HL, Ross SA, Milner, JA. 'Garlic and onions: their cancer prevention properties'. Cancer Prev Res (Phila) [Internet]. 1 Mar 2015 [cited 15 Jun 2018]; 8(3):181–9. Available from: http://www.ncbi.nlm.nih.gov/pubmed/25586902

13 Glade MJ. 'Food, nutrition, and the prevention of cancer: a global perspective'. American Institute for Cancer Research/World Cancer Research Fund, American Institute for Cancer Research, 1997. Nutrition [Internet]. 1 Jun 1999 [cited 15 Jun 2018]; 15(6):523–6. Available from: http://www.ncbi.nlm.nih.gov/pubmed/10378216

14 Schaefer JT, Magnuson AB. 'A Review of Interventions that Promote Eating by Internal Cues'. J Acad Nutr Diet [Internet]. May 2014 [cited 7 Aug 2017]; 114(5):734–60. Available from: http://www.ncbi.nlm.nih.gov/pubmed/24631111

15 El Madden C, Leong SL, Gray A, Horwath CC. 'Eating in response to hunger and satiety signals is related to BMI in a nationwide sample of 1601 mid-age New Zealand women'. Public Health Nutr [Internet]. [cited 20 Jul 2017]; 15(12):2272–9. Available from: https://pdfs.semanticscholar.org/d7e0/851335f147a33445143d1caeb07970f4e13f.pdf

16 Carbonneau E, Bégin C, Lemieux S, Mongeau L, Paquette M-C, Turcotte M, et al. 'A Health at Every Size® intervention improves intuitive eating and diet quality in Canadian women'. Clin Nutr [Internet]. Jun 2017 [cited 4 Mar 2018]; 36(3):747–54. Available from: http://www.ncbi.nlm.nih.gov/pubmed/27378611

17 Smith T, Steven R. 'Intuitive Eating, Diet Composition, and the Meaning of Food in Healthy Weight Promotion'. Hawks Am J Heal Educ — May [Internet]. 2006 [cited 17 Apr 2018]; 37(3). Available from: https://files.eric.ed.gov/fulltext/EJ795904.pdf

18 Camilleri GM, Méjean C, Bellisle F, Andreeva VA, Kesse-Guyot E, Hercberg S, et al. 'Intuitive Eating Dimensions Were Differently Associated with Food Intake in the General Population-Based NutriNet-Santé Study'. J Nutr [Internet]. Jan 2017 [cited 17 Apr 2018]; 147(1):61–9. Available from: http://www.ncbi.nlm.nih.gov/pubmed/27798333

CHAPTER 13

1 Ellyn Satter. Reproduced with permission from *Secrets of Feeding a Healthy Family: How to Eat, How to Raise Good Eaters, How to Cook*. For more information, go to www.EllynSatterInstitute.org.

2 Plan International. '#FreePeriods – research on period poverty and stigma'. Plan International UK [Internet]. [cited 17 Apr 2018]. Available from: https://plan-uk.org/media-centre/freeperiods-research-on-period-poverty-and-stigma

3 How many people use food banks? – Full Fact [Internet]. [cited 17 Apr 2018]. Available from: https://fullfact.org/economy/how-many-people-use-food-banks/

4 United Nations High Commissioner for Refugees (UNHCR). 'Forced displacement worldwide at its highest in decades' [Internet]. [cited 17 Apr 2018]. Available from: http://www.unhcr.org/afr/news/stories/2017/6/5941561f4/forced-displacement-worldwide-its-highest-decades.html

5 Stonewall. 'LGBT in Britain – Trans Report' (2017) [Internet]. [cited 17 Apr 2018]. Available from: https://www.stonewall.org.uk/lgbt-britain-trans-report

6 Strategic Review of Health Inequalities in England post 2010. 'Fair Society, Healthy Lives' [Internet]. [cited 17 Apr 2018]. Available from: http://www.instituteofhealthequity.org/resources-reports/fair-society-healthy-lives-the-marmot-review/fair-society- healthy-lives-full-report-pdf.pdf

7 CSDH. 'Closing the gap in a generation'. [Internet]. 2008 [cited 17 Apr 2018]; 246. Available from: http://apps.who.int/iris/bitstream/handle/10665/43943/978924156 3703_eng.pdf;jsessionid= FD7626BD75178D19E3DF93F998 BE8848?sequence=1

ACKNOWLEDGEMENTS

There are so many people that helped make this book a reality.

I'd first of all like to thank the amazing team at Bluebird. Their enthusiasm and genuine excitement for the book helped me keep pushing through when it felt like there was no end in sight. I'd especially like to thank my editors Carole and Martha for their guidance in shaping the book. Thanks too to Jess and Jodie for bigging me up and generally being super-cool.

A huge thank you to my literary agent Richard Pike at Conville and Walsh for seeing something in my work and for taking a risk. Your impeccably high standards have helped ensure this book found the best possible home.

Thank you to all the wonderful people who have contributed to this book or helped me with my research; I'm so grateful to you for allowing me to share your wisdom in these pages. Fiona Sutherland, Michelle Elman, Pixie Turner, The Rooted Project, Kimberley Wilson, Julie Duffy Dillon, Anna Kessel, Meredith Noble, Sumner Brooks, Paige Smathers, Haley Goodrich, Robyn Nohling, Christy Harrison, Jenni, Jim Stewart, Nichola Ludlam-Raine, Amy Slater, Deb Burgard.

Shout to Pixie Turner, Megan Rossi, Nic Ludlam-Raine, Rosie Saunt, Rosie Spinks, Anthony Warner and Izy Hossack for always having my back, professionally and personally.

I'm truly indebted to Captain Science for fact-checking the manuscript and making sure the science was as robust as it could be. Thank you for being sceptical, challenging me, and ultimately for being open-minded enough to shift your perspective when the science challenged everything you have believed up until this point. I'm so proud I can call you my friend.

An enormous thanks to my work wife, Helen West (and to Rosie for sharing her with me) for reassuring me when I (regularly) lost confidence in myself throughout the research and writing process. Thank you for each and every pep talk.

Special thank you to Claire Stewart, Maritza Martinez, Rhiannon McDonald, and Ashley Shepherd for not giving two shits about nutrition and reminding me about life outside of writing a book; you're always there for me whenever I need you the most. Let's hang out soon.

Major props to Sazzy and Fran Café for the constant supply of caffeine and peanut butter on toast; couldn't have done it without you guys.

So many thanks to anyone and everyone who has followed, shared, or otherwise supported my work through Don't Salt My Game, social media, and now through this book. I wish I could hug every single last one of you, but in lieu of that, please accept a gargantuan thank-you from the bottom of my heart. You guys are the best.

A massive thanks to my family for their unconditional love and support.

And finally, thank you to my husband, Dave. You are my everything and I couldn't have written this book without you holding me together (sometimes literally) through the anxiety, sleepless nights, and frequent meltdowns. Thank you for your unwavering conviction in me, even when others have lost faith; you give me strength every day. Everything I do is so that we can build a better life together. You're my favourite.